ATLAS OF CLINICAL
ENDOCRINOLOGY

ATLAS OF CLINICAL ENDOCRINOLOGY

Series Editor
Stanley G. Korenman, MD

Professor and Associate Dean
Department of Medicine
UCLA School of Medicine
UCLA Medical Center
Los Angeles, California

Volume II
DIABETES

Volume Editor
C. Ronald Kahn, MD

Mary K. Iacocca Professor of Medicine
Harvard Medical School;
Director and Executive Vice President
Joslin Diabetes Center
Boston, Massachusetts

With 19 contributors

b

**Blackwell
Science**

Developed by Current Medicine, Inc., Philadelphia

Current Medicine

CM — CURRENT MEDICINE

400 Market Street
Suite 700
Philadelphia, PA 19106

Developmental Editor:	*Marian A. Bellus*
Editorial Assistant:	*Forrest Perry*
Design and Layout:	*Christopher Allan*
Illustrators:	*Nicole Mock, Paul Schiffmacher, Larry Ward, Debra Wertz, Arlene Ligori*
Director of Product Development:	*Mary Kinsella*
Associate Art Director:	*Jerilyn Kauffman*
Art Department Manager:	*Debra Wertz*
Production:	*Lori Holland, Amy Giuffi*
Indexing:	*Alexandra Nickerson*

Diabetes / [edited by] C. Ronald Kahn
     p. cm.—(Atlas of clinical endocrinology; 2)
   Includes bibliographical references and index.
   ISBN 0-632-04399-7
   1. Diabetes Atlases.   I. Kahn, C. Ronald.   II. Series
  II. Series.
    [DNLM: 1. Diabetes Mellitus atlases. WK 17 A8806 1999 v. 2]
  RC649.A846 1999 vol. 2
  [RC660]
  616.4'0022'2 s—dc21
  [616.4'62—dc21]
  DNLM/DLC
  for Library of Congress   99—27959
                                           CIP

Printed in Hong Kong by Paramount Printing Group Limited

10 9 8 7 6 5 4 3 2 1

DISTRIBUTED WORLDWIDE BY BLACKWELL, SCIENCE, INC.

Series Preface

The human body depends on information even more than energy. The means of information transfer are chemical, whether at synapses or through the mediation of hormones at a distance (endocrine), between adjacent cells (paracrine), or within a single cell (autocrine). The body seems to be able to utilize any available molecule for signaling, including gases like nitric oxide and nutrients such as calcium and glucose. In endocrinology, the physician deals with signaling and its disorders, and in nutrition and metabolism, both signaling and energetics.

Endocrinology has been at the forefront of scientific medicine because the molecules involved are so potent that they produce measurable responses at low concentration, and the syndromes produced by an absence or an excess of hormones can be characterized. Furthermore, researchers purified hormones and elucidated their properties very early in the development of scientific medicine, which led to their introduction as pharmaceuticals for both diagnostic and therapeutic purposes. As new hormones and signaling and molecular response processes are elucidated, endocrinology continues to expand and become more sophisticated. Because the available knowledge is so extensive, it is relatively simple to place new information in context. Providing information to clinicians in an atlas format is particularly suitable for the field of endocrinology because the syndromes are often dramatic, molecular and metabolic pathways are well described, and algorithms for diagnosis and therapy can be developed. In fact, the reader will be struck by the remarkable thoroughness achievable in depicting this field in an atlas, namely, the *Atlas of Clinical Endocrinology*.

The Atlas of Clinical Endocrinology series includes five volumes: Thyroid Diseases, Diabetes, Osteoporosis, Neuroendocrinology and Pituitary Diseases, and Human Nutrition and Obesity. In each field, outstanding experts have contributed not only "state of the art" information but also their expert perspectives on the problems they cover. Throughout the field of endocrinology, major advances have strengthened the scientific base, the diagnostic armamentarium, and the therapeutic options.

In the Thyroid Diseases volume, the recent advances in our understanding of the thyroid hormone economy shed light on the alterations that occur with chronic illness, drugs, and aging. The contributors thoroughly illustrate the dilemmas associated with the management of thyroid nodules and thyroid cancer as well as thyroid disease in pregnancy and the complications of Graves' disease.

Advances in diabetes research and treatment have been dramatic. The volume on Diabetes illustrates the great advances in our understanding of the regulation of insulin secretion and the multiple mechanisms of its action. These advances, as well as the epidemiologic and genetic research that is covered, provide a strong foundation for understanding and managing the consequences of long-term hyperglycemia on the eye, kidney, nerves, and lipids, and on the cardiovascular system. Algorithms are provided for clinical treatment of deficient insulin action with newer agents as well as insulin in both types of diabetes.

Therapy to prevent osteoporotic fractures has become a mainstay in the health care of older women and now older men as well. The Osteoporosis volume describes the bone economy and illustrates the various syndromes leading to loss of bone mineral and the consequences of osteoporotic fracture. The authors describe and justify approaches to preventive and postfracture therapy, using both medications and nonpharmaceutical means.

In the Neuroendocrinology and Pituitary Diseases volume, major advances in understanding of the interrelationships between the central nervous system and control of pituitary and hypothalamic function are illustrated. Individuals with disorders of growth are characterized. The role of medical treatment in the management of acromegaly and prolactinomas and the approach toward the diagnosis of Cushing's syndrome are elucidated.

Disorders of nutrition, particularly obesity, are the most common disorders in advanced societies. In the Human Nutrition and Obesity volume, the regulation of appetite and eating is addressed; the nutritional requirements for growth and development are characterized; and the impact of diet on clinical conditions such as diabetes, hypertension, cardiovascular disease, cancer, aging and digestive diseases is discussed. The growing use of nutritional supplements is addressed and an integrated program for the management of obesity given.

We are grateful to Current Medicine and especially to Abe Krieger who saw the *Atlas of Clinical Endocrinology* as a dramatic and efficient medium for providing information about endocrinology and metabolism.

Stanley G. Korenman, MD

v

Preface

Diabetes mellitus is among the most common endocrine disorders affecting about 7% of the U.S. population. As a result, this disorder is seen frequently not only by the endocrinologist but also by internists and primary care physicians.

Diabetes mellitus is, in reality, a group of disorders that have in common hyperglycemia and a risk for long-term complications. Type 1 diabetes (formerly called insulin-dependent diabetes) is an autoimmune disease in which the beta cells of the pancreas are destroyed. This is classically a disease of children and young adults, but recent studies indicate that type 1 diabetes can occur at any age. Type 2 diabetes (formerly called non–insulin-dependent diabetes) classically occurs in adults, especially the elderly, but recently it is being diagnosed with increasing frequency in children. Several rare forms of diabetes mellitus include maturity onset diabetes of the young (MODY) and diabetes secondary to other disorders. Significant recent progress has been made in defining the genes and the immune mechanisms involved in type 1 diabetes. Type 2 diabetes also has strong genetic influences that lead to insulin resistance and relative beta-cell failure.

The long-term complications of diabetes are divided into the microvascular complications, affecting the eye, kidney and nerve, and the macrovascular complications with accelerated atherosclerosis and increased risk of amputation, myocardial infarction, and stroke. The basic mechanisms of each of these complications is a combination of the adverse effects of hyperglycemia on tissues, stimulation of various growth factors, and the secondary effects of conditions frequently associated with diabetes such as hypertension and hyperlipidemia.

Major clinical trials (the DCCT and the UKPDS) have indicated the importance of intensive treatment of both type 1 and type 2 diabetes. In the case of type1 diabetes, intensive therapy can reduce the incidence of complications by up to 60%. For type 2 diabetes, in general, therapy is less effective in normalizing glucose, and the reduction in complications is more modest. Aggressive treatment of associated disorders is also important, including management of hypertension and the abnormal lipid profile, which predispose to the microvascular and macrovascular complications.

The expanding knowledge with regard to the basic mechanisms of disease in both forms of diabetes is opening new avenues for therapy. Immunomodulation may delay or perhaps eventually prevent the onset of type 1 diabetes. Transplantation of whole pancreas is increasingly successful, and more clinical trials are now being performed on islet cell transplantation. New agents to increase insulin sensitivity, such as the thiazolidinediones, and insulin secretion are also improving the management of type 2 diabetes. However, even now, many patients do not receive optimal therapy, which requires both a concerted team effort on the part of the physician and medical personnel and a strongly motivated patient who participates actively in adjusting his or her therapy. Current research into agents that block the adverse effects of hyperglycemia on tissues may ultimately make management of the diabetic patient and prevention of complications a more easily achieved goal.

C. Ronald Kahn, MD

Contributors

DOMENICO ACCILI, MD
Chief of the Unit on Genetics and Hormone Action
National Institutes of Health
Bethesda, Maryland

LLOYD PAUL AIELLO, MD, PHD
Assistant Professor
Department of Ophthalmology
Harvard Medical School;
Investigator
Joslin Diabetes Center
Boston, Massachusetts

MARK A. ATKINSON, PHD
Professor
Department of Pathology
University of Florida School of Medicine
Gainesville, Florida

SUSAN BONNER-WEIR, PHD
Associate Professor
Department of Medicine
Harvard Medical School;
Senior Investigator
Joslin Diabetes Center
Boston, Massachusetts

MICHAEL BROWNLEE, MD
Professor
Department of Medicine
Albert Einstein College of Medicine
New York, New York

VERONICA M. CATANESE, MD
Assistant Professor
Department of Medicine and Cell Biology
New York University School of Medicine;
Associate Dean
New York University School of Medicine
New York, New York

ELE FERRANNINI, MD
Professor of Internal Medicine
University of Pisa School of Medicine;
Head, Metabolism Unit
CNR Institute of Clinical Physiology
Pisa, Italy

ROBERT R. HENRY, MD
Professor
Department of Medicine
University of California, San Diego;
Chief, Section of Endocrinology and Metabolism
VA Medical Center
San Diego, CA

C. RONALD KAHN, MD
Mary K. Iacocca Professor of Medicine
Department of Medicine
Harvard Medical School;
Director and Executive Vice President
Joslin Diabetes Center
Boston, Massachusetts

HIROKO KANNO, MD
Visiting Fellow
Unit on Genetics and Hormone Action
National Institutes of Health
Bethesda, Maryland

ABBAS E. KITABCHI, MD, PHD
Professor
Department of Medicine
University of Tennessee
Memphis, Tennessee

ELEFTHERIA MARATOS-FLIER, MD
Assistant Professor
Harvard Medical School;
Investigator
Joslin Diabetes Center
Boston, Massachusetts

Contributors, *continued*

SUNDER MUDALIAR, MD, MRCP

Assistant Clinical Professor
Department of Medicine/Endocrinology
University of California, San Diego;
Staff Physician
VA San Diego Health Care System
San Diego, California

DAVID M. NATHAN, MD

Associate Professor
Department of Medicine
Harvard Medical School;
Director, Diabetes Center
Massachusetts General Hospital
Boston, Massachusetts

F. JOHN SERVICE, MD, PHD

Professor
Department of Medicine
Consultant, Division of Endocrinology
Mayo Clinic
Rochester, Minnesota

ARUN J. SHARMA, PHD

Instructor
Department of Medicine
Harvard Medical School;
Assistant Investigator
Joslin Diabetes Center
Boston, Massachusetts

ROBERT C. STANTON, MD

Assistant Professor of Medicine
Department of Medicine0
Harvard Medical School;
Chief, Renal Division
Joslin Diabetes Center
Boston, Massachusetts

AARON I. VINIK, MD, PHD, FCP, FACP

Director of the Research Institutes: Pathology, Anatomy, Neurobiology
Professor of Medicine, Anatomy, and Neurobiology
Eastern Virginia Medical School;
Adjunct Professor
Old Dominion University;
Norfolk, Virginia

GORDON C. WEIR, MD

Professor
Department of Medicine
Harvard Medical School;
Senior Investigator
Joslin Diabetes Center
Boston, Massachusetts

Contents

Contents, *continued*

Contents, *continued*

Color Plates

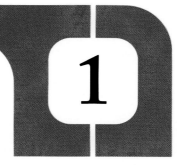

REGULATION OF INSULIN SECRETION AND ISLET CELL FUNCTION

Gordon C. Weir, Susan Bonner-Weir, and Arun Sharma

The β cells of the islets of Langerhans are the only cells in the body that make a meaningful quantity of insulin, a hormone that has evolved to be essential for life, exerting critical control over carbohydrate, fat, and protein metabolism. Islets are scattered throughout the pancreas; they vary in size but typically contain about 1000 cells of which about 80% are β cells located in a central core surrounded by a mantle of non–β cells A human pancreas contains about one million islets, which comprise only about 1% of the mass of the pancreas. Insulin is released into the portal vein, which means the liver is exposed to particularly high concentrations of insulin.

Insulin secretion from β cells responds very precisely to small changes in glucose concentration in the physiologic range, thereby keeping glucose levels within the range of 70–150 mg/dL in normal individuals. β-cells have a unique differentiation that permits linkage of physiologic levels of glucose to the metabolic signals that control the release of insulin. Thus, there is a close correlation between the rate of glucose metabolism and insulin secretion. This is dependent upon the oxidation of glucose-derived acetyl-CoA and also NADH generated by glycolysis, which is shuttled to mitochondria to contribute to ATP production. Insulin secretion is also regulated by various other physiologic signals. During eating insulin secretion is enhanced by not only glucose, but amino acids and the gut hormones GLP-1 and gastric inhibitory peptide (GIP). Free fatty acids (FFAs) can also modulate insulin secretion, particularly to help maintain insulin secretion during prolonged fasting. The parasympathetic nervous system has a stimulatory effect exerted by acetylcholine and probably the peptidergic mediator VIP, which may also contribute to enhanced insulin secretion during eating. The sympathetic nervous system with epinephrine from the adrenal medulla and norepinephrine from nerve terminals acts upon alpha adrenergic receptors to inhibit insulin secretion. This suppression of insulin is particularly useful during exercise. Important drugs include sulfonylureas, which have a stimulatory influence useful for the treatment of diabetes, and diazoxide with an inhibitory effect used for treatment of hypoglycemia caused by insulin-producing tumors.

Type 1 diabetes is caused by reduced β-cell mass resulting from autoimmune destruction of β cells, which leads to profound insulin deficiency that can progress to fatal hyperglycemia and ketoacidosis. The non–β-cells of the islet are spared, with glucagon secretion actually being excessive, which accounts for some of the hyperglycemia of the diabetic state. The situation is more complicated in type 2 diabetes, which has a strong genetic basis predisposing individuals to obesity and insulin resistance, a problem greatly magnified by our Western life style with its plentiful food and lack of physical activity. Diabetes, however, only develops when β cells are no longer able to compensate for this insulin resistance. Indeed, most people with insulin resistance never develop diabetes, but as our population ages, more β cell decompensation occurs and the prevalence of diabetes rises. Pathology studies indicate that β cell mass in type 2 diabetes is about 50% of normal and that islets often are infiltrated with amyloid deposits that may have a toxic effect upon β cells.

In all forms of diabetes, whether type 2 diabetes , early type 1 diabetes or failing pancreas or islet transplants, insulin secretory abnormalities are found that seem largely secondary to exposure of β cells to the diabetic milieu and that are reversible if normoglycemia can be restored. The most prominent abnormality is an impairment of glucose-induced insulin secretion, which is more severe for early release (first phase) than the longer second phase of secretion. In contrast, β cells responses to such non-glucose secretagogues as arginine, GLP-1, isoproterenol or sulfonylureas are more intact. The etiology of these β cell secretory abnormalities is not fully understood, but β cells exposed to abnormally high glucose concentrations lose the differentiation that normally equips them with the unique metabolic machinery needed for glucose-induced insulin secretion. Marked abnormalities are found at the level of gene expression that appear to have a crippling effect upon the metabolic integrity of the β cell. Abnormalities of glucagon secretion are also found in both forms of diabetes, with secretion not being appropriately suppressed by hyperglycemia or stimulated by hypoglycemia, which is problematic because glucagon is an important counterregulatory hormone for protection against hypoglycemia. This failure of glucagon to respond makes people with type 1 diabetes more vulnerable to the dangers of insulin-induced hypoglycemia.

Anatomy, Embryology, and Physiology

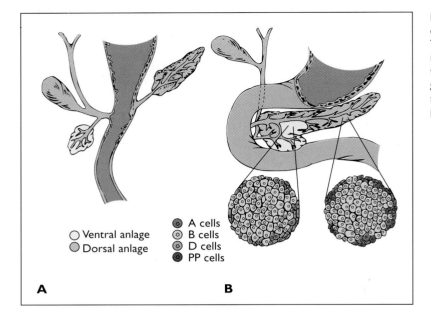

FIGURE 1-1. Embryologic origin of pancreas and islets. A dorsal anlage and one or two ventral anlagen form from the primitive gut (**A**) and later fuse (**B**) [1]. The ventral anlage forms the head of the pancreas and has pancreatic polypeptide rich islets with few if any A cells. The dorsal anlage forms the major portion of the pancreas, that being the tail, body and part of the head; here the islets are glucagon-rich and pancreatic polypeptide poor. Roughly the A and PP cells substitute for each other in number (15-25% of the islet cells) while the percentages of β cells (70-80%) and D cells (5%) remain the same.

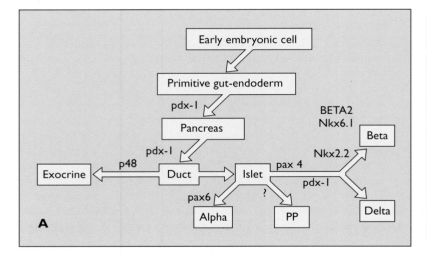

B. UNIQUE β-CELL DIFFERENTIATION

Increased expression	Decreased expression
GLUT2	Glucose-6-phosphatase
Glucokinase	Hexokinase
mGPDH	Lactate dehydrogenase
Pyruvate carboxylase	PEPCK
Insulin	c-myc
IAPP	
PDX-1	
Nkx 6.1	

FIGURE 1-2. Pancreatic and islet differentiation. The complex control of differentiation of the pancreas and its three major components, exocrine acinar cells, ducts, and islets of Langerhans are being elucidated by genetic analysis (**A** and **B**) [1–3]. At present only some of the transcription factors involved in the transition from endoderm to pancreas and then to the final mature pancreatic cell types are known; several of them (beta 2, Nkx 2..2, Nkx 6.1) are also involved in the development of the nervous system. One that is clearly necessary, but not sufficient, is pdx-1(ipf-1/stf-1/idx-1); without it no pancreas is formed and later it seems to be needed for β-cell differentiation. Both exocrine and islet cells differentiate from the pancreatic ductal epithelium, but whether they arise from the same precursor pool or even whether all the islet cells share a cell lineage remains unanswered. PP—pancreataic polypeptide. *Adapted from* Edlund [1].

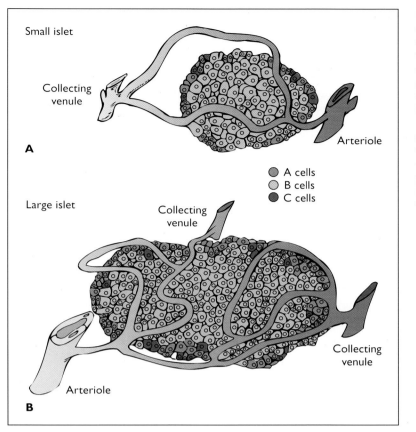

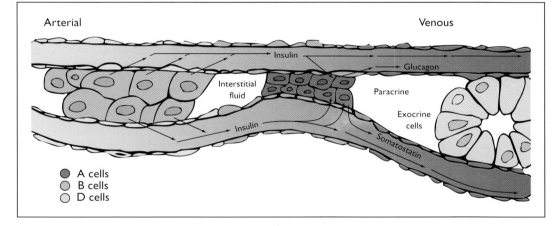

FIGURE 1-3. Islet vasculature and core/mantle relations. A diagrammatic summary of combined data from corrosion casts and the serial reconstructions of rat islets [2]. In both small and large islets, β cells make up the central core while the non–β cells (A, PP and D cells) form the surrounding mantle. The A cells which contain glucagon are found mainly in islets of the dorsal lobe of the pancreas, PP cells which contain pancreatic polypeptide and are found mainly in ventral lobe islets, and D cells containing somatostatin are found in islets of both lobes of the pancreas.

Short arterioles enter an islet at discontinuities of the non–β cell mantle and branch into capillaries that form a glomerular-like structure. After traversing the β cell mass, capillaries penetrate the mantle of non-(cells as the blood leaves the islet. In small islets (less than 160 um in diameter) (**A**), efferent capillaries pass through exocrine tissue before coalescing into collecting venules. In large islets (greater than 260 um diameter) (**B**), capillaries coalesce at the edge of the islet and run along the mantle as collecting venules.

FIGURE 1-4. The relationship between islet core and mantle, indicating potential intraislet portal-flow and paracrine interactions. This formulation is based about the known vascular anatomy and studies with passive immunization [4,5]. These relationships suggest that β cells being upstream are unlikely to be very much influenced by the glucagon and somatostatin produced by the A cells and D cells of the islet mantle, respectively. The downstream A cells, however, may be strongly influenced by insulin from the upstream β cells, which has a suppressive influence upon glucagon secretion. This helps explain why glucagon secretion can not be suppressed by the hyperglycemia of diabetes, which means that glucagon is secreted in excessive amounts, thus contributing further to the hyperglycemia of diabetes. This vascular pattern is know as the islet-acinar portal circulation, which means that islet hormones are released downstream directly onto exocrine cells; insulin in particular is thought to have a trophic effect upon the exocrine pancreas.

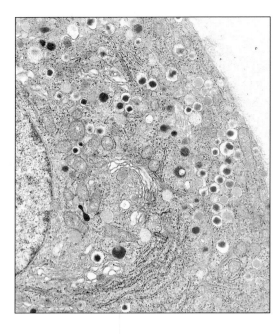

FIGURE 1-5. Electron micrograph of a β cell. There are four major endocrine cell types in mammalian islets: the insulin-producing β cell, the glucagon-producing A cell, the somatostatin-producing D cell and the pancreatic polypeptide-producing PP-cell. Ultrastructural and immunocytochemical techniques are used to distinguish these cell types. β cells are polyhedral, being truncated pyramids about 10 x 10 x 8 um, and are usually well granulated with about 10,000 secretory granules. There are two forms of insulin granules (250–350 nm in diameter): mature ones with an electron dense core that is visibly crystalline in some species and a loosely fitting granule-limiting membrane giving the appearance of a spacious halo, and immature granules with little or no halo and moderately electron dense contents. Immature granules have been shown to be the major, if not the only, site of proinsulin to insulin conversion [6]. In each granule, besides insulin, there are at least 100 other peptides, including IAPP/amylin [7].

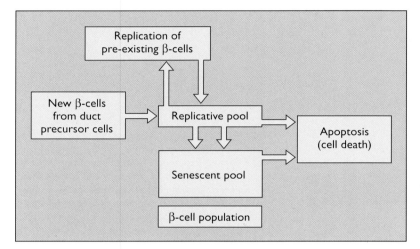

FIGURE 1-6. Mechanisms responsible for maintenance of β-cell mass. Both in normal development and in experimental studies it has become apparent that the population of β cells within an adult pancreas is dynamic and responds to metabolic demand with changes in mass and function in an effort to maintain euglycemia. The mass of β cells can change by cell number and/or cell size. Two mechanisms add new β cells: differentiation from precursor/stem cells in the ducts (often called neogenesis) and replication from pre-existing beta cells [8]. It has been suggested that most cell types have a limited number of replications after which the ability to respond to replication signals is lost, so they are then considered to be senescent cells (terminally differentiated). These senescent cells can be long-lived and functional, probably functioning in some ways differently than younger replicative cells. Additionally as with all cell types, β cells must have a finite lifespan and die by apoptosis [9]. The turnover of β cells implies that there are β cells of differing age at any stage of development. Adult β cells have only a low basal rate of replication but this rate coupled with birth of new β cells from ducts must be enough to counterbalance cell loss and to accommodate functional demand.

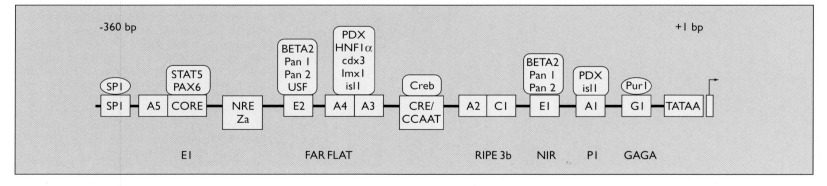

FIGURE 1-7. The promoter region of the insulin gene showing key enhancer elements and known binding transcription factors. Insulin gene expression is regulated by sequences at least 4 kb upstream from the transcription start site (represented by an arrow and designated as +1 bp) of the insulin gene. In adult mammals, insulin is selectively expressed in pancreatic β cells. A small (less than 400 bp) region of insulin promoter that is highly conserved in various mammalian species can regulate this selective expression and contains the major glucose control elements. This region can also recapitulate glucose responsive insulin gene expression.

In the figure the organization of the proximal portion (-360 to + 1 bp) of the insulin promoter is shown. Functionally conserved enhancer elements are illustrated as boxes. New names for these elements are shown within the boxes, while old names are shown below each box. Above the boxes are shown the names of cloned transcription factors that can bind corresponding elements are shown. Enhancer elements E1, A2-C1, A4-A3, and E2 have been implicated in β cell–specific

expression of the insulin gene. The cell-type-specific expression is mediated by the restricted cellular distribution of the transcription factors (such as BETA2 and PDX-1) that bind these elements. Furthermore these elements, along with element Za, are also responsible for glucose-regulated insulin gene expression. Other enhancer elements CRE/CCAAT and CORE regulate insulin gene expression in response to other signals such as cAMP (by regulating cAMP Regulatory Element Binding protein) and growth hormone or leptin (via Signal transducer and activator of transcription [STAT] factor 5).

In addition to their role in regulating cell-specific and glucose responsive expression, insulin gene transcription factors are involved in pancreatic development and differentiation of fl-cells. Lack of transcription factors such as PDX-1, BETA2, PAX6, HNF-1α and isl1 results in either complete absence of or abnormal pancreatic development. Interestingly, humans with a mutant allele for PDX-1, BETA2 or HNF-1α develop MODY, whereas individual with mutations in both pdx-1 alleles show pancreatic agenesis. (*Adapted from* Sander and German [10].)

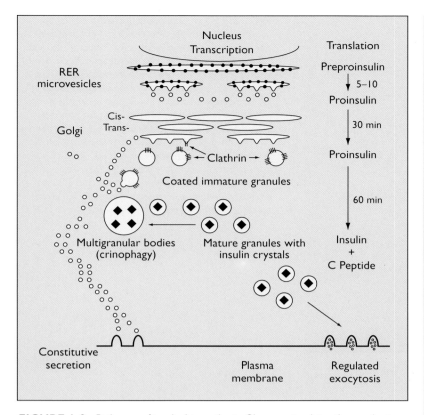

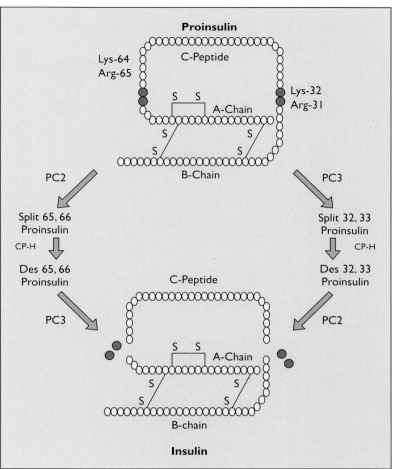

FIGURE 1-8. Pathways of insulin biosynthesis. Glucose stimulates the production of preproinsulin through effects on transcription and even stronger influences on translation. Shortly after its inception preproinsulin is cleaved to proinsulin which is then transported through the Golgi and packaged into clathrin-coated immature granules, where proinsulin is further processed to proinsulin-like peptides, insulin and c-peptide. Granules containing crystallized insulin can either remain in a storage compartment, be absorbed into multigranular bodies where they are degraded by the process of crinophagy, or be secreted via the regulated pathway of secretion with is final event of exocytosis. Although the vast majority of insulin is secreted through the regulated pathway, a small amount can be released from microvesicles through the pathway of constitutive secretion. (See references 11 and 12 for more details).

FIGURE 1-9. Proinsulin processing. Proinsulin is cleaved by endopeptidases contained in secretory granules which act at the two dibasic sites, Arg31, Arg32 and Lys64, Arg65. PC2 also is known as type II proinsulin-processing endopeptidase and PC3 is the type I endopeptidase. Following cleavage by either PC2 or PC3, the dibasic amino acids are removed by the exopeptidase carboxypeptidase H (CP-H). Insulin and C-peptide are usually released in equimolar amounts. Of the secreted insulin immunoreactivity, about 2-4% consists of proinsulin and proinsulin-related peptides. Because the clearance of these peptides in the circulation is considerably slower than insulin, they account for 10-40% of circulating insulin immunoreactivity. About one third of proinsulin-like immunoreactivity is accounted for by proinsulin and most of the rest by des 32-33 split proinsulin, with only small amounts of des 65-66 split proinsulin being present. In Type 2 diabetes the ratio of proinsulin-like peptides to insulin is increased, while in IGT this finding is less consistent. The increased proportion of secreted proinsulin-like peptides is thought to be due to depletion of mature granules from the increased secretory demand by hyperglycemia, leading to the release of the incompletely processed contents of the available immature granules [11,12]. (*Adapted from* Rhodes [11].)

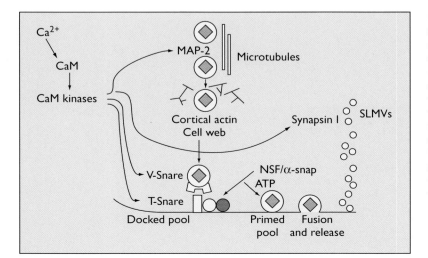

FIGURE 1-10. Distal steps of secretion. Insulin-containing secretory granules are associated with microtubules and the move to the cell surface via further interactions with the microfilaments of the cortical actin web. Increased cytosolic calcium plays a key roles in several distal steps. Initially calcium binds to calmodulin (CaM) which can the bind CaM kinases. CaM kinase II has been localized to insulin secretory granules. These kinases can then phosphorylate proteins such as microtubule-associated protein-2 (MAP-2) and synapsin I which may be involved in the exocytosis of synaptic-like microvesicles (SLMV). They may also regulate the key proteins involved in the docking of granules, v-SNARES (synaptobrevin (VAMP) and cellubrevin) and t-SNARES (SNAP-25 and syntaxin). The docking complex binds to α-SNAP (soluble NSF attachment protein) and NSF (N-ethyl-maleimide-sensitive fusion protein), the latter having ATPase activity which probably allows the formation of fusion competent granules that are primed for release as the first phase of insulin secretion. (*Adapted from* Easom [13].)

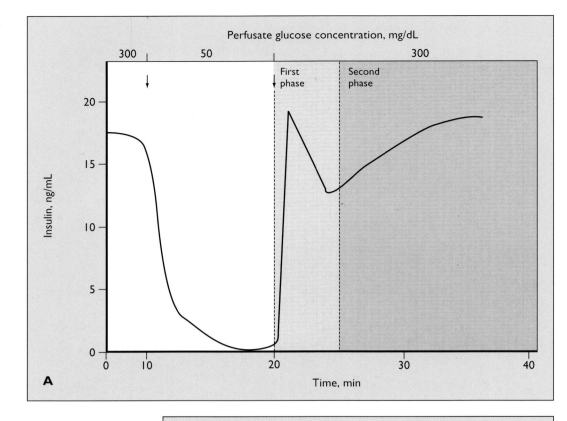

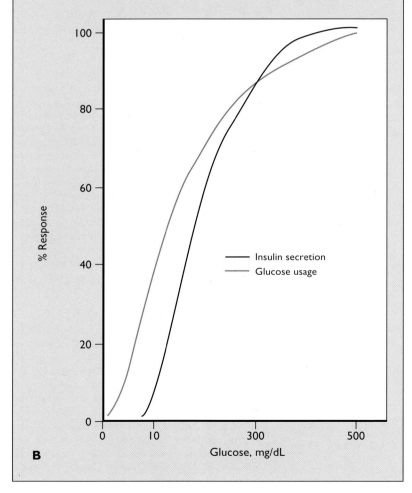

FIGURE 1-11. Glucose stimulation of insulin secretion. **A,** Insulin secretion from the isolated perfused rat pancreas. At glucose concentrations at 50 mg/dL or below, insulin secretory rates are very low. Challenge with a high concentration of glucose provokes a biphasic pattern of insulin response [14]. **B,** Comparative rates of insulin secretion and glucose utilization in isolated rat islets. Glucose utilization was measured by the conversion of 5-tritiated glucose to tritiated H_2O [15]. The curves show the close relationship between the two except at glucose concentrations below 4 mmol. Similar relationships are found between insulin secretion and glucose oxidation as measured by conversion labeled glucose to carbon dioxide. (*Adapted from* Leahy, *et al.* [12].)

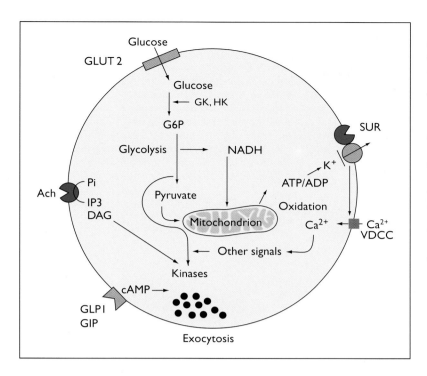

FIGURE 1-12. Mechanisms of β-cell secretion. Glucose enters the β-cell through a facultative glucose transporter that allows rapid equilibration between extra- and intracellular glucose concentrations. Although GLUT2 is dominant in many species, GLUT1 may be more important in humans. Glucose is phosphorylated mainly by glucokinase (GK), rather than hexokinase (HK). Metabolism increases the ATP/ADP ratio both through oxidation via pyruvate and by NADH that is brought by shuttles into mitochondria (14). The increases in the ATP/ADP ratio inhibit the ATP-sensitive potassium channel which leads to depolarization and opening of voltage-dependent calcium channels (VDCC), with a resultant major increase in cytosolic calcium which triggers exocytosis. Cytosolic calcium levels can also be increased by release of calcium from the endoplasmic reticulum. Glucose has stimulatory effects on insulin secretion that are separate from depolarization, but poorly understood. Insulin secretion can also be stimulated by agents such as acetylcholine (Ach) that via muscarinic receptors work through lipid mediators such as inositol 1, 4, 5-triphosphate (IP3) and diacylglycerol DAG. Glucagon-like peptide 1 (GLP-1) and gastric inhibitory peptide (GIP), hormones released from gut with meals that stimulates secretion via adenylate cyclase and cAMP. There are many other agents that influence insulin secretion.

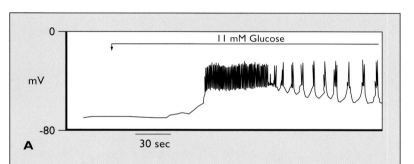

A

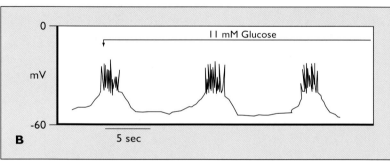

B

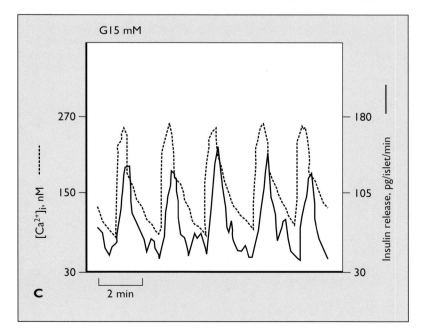

C

FIGURE 1-13. Glucose-induced electrical activity of the mouse beta cell. **A,** The electrical activity of a mouse β-cell contained in an isolated islet induced by stimulation with 11 mM glucose. When the membrane depolarizes to about -50 mV bursting occurs which is periodic electrical activity. Note the biphasic pattern of electrical activity which may be related to the first phase of insulin secretion but is shorter in duration and unlikely to be the full explanation. When depolarization reaches about -35 mV action potentials, or spikes occur, which are best seen in the expanded scale in **B**. When glucose levels are very high (> 22 mM), continuous spiking activity is observed. **C,** Comparison of the oscillations of insulin release and calcium in a single pancreatic mouse islet during steady state stimulation with 15 mM glucose, suggesting a cause and effect relationship. Calcium was measured with fluorescence of fura-2 loaded into islets. Increased calcium spikes come mainly from entrance of extracellular calcium through L-type voltage gated calcium channels. The depolarization is mainly caused by closure of ATP-regulated potassium channels [18]. (Part A and B *adapted from* Atwater, *et al.* [17]; part C *adapted from* Gilon, *et al.* [18].)

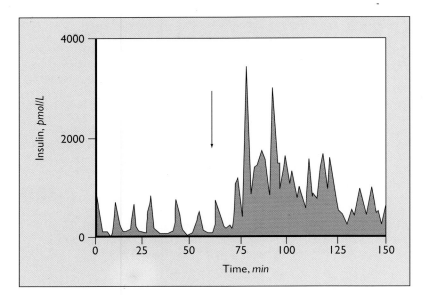

FIGURE 1-14. Pulsatile insulin secretion. Insulin is normally secreted in coordinated secretory bursts. In humans pulses occur about every 10 minutes. In dogs they occur somewhat more rapidly, at about 7-minute intervals in a basal state. Although the variations in peripheral insulin levels are modest, marked variations can be found in the portal vein [21]. Basal pulsation is depicted during the 60-minute period. After oral ingestion of glucose (arrow), which produces both a glucose stimulus and an incretin effect, an increase in the amplitude of the bursts is seen, as well as an increase in frequency, with intervals falling from about 7 to 5 minutes. The mechanisms controlling the oscillations are uncertain. Metabolic oscillation of glycolysis must play a key role, but there may also be some kind of neural network exists that can coordinate communication between islets in different parts of the pancreas. (Adapted from Porksen, et al. [19]; with permission.)

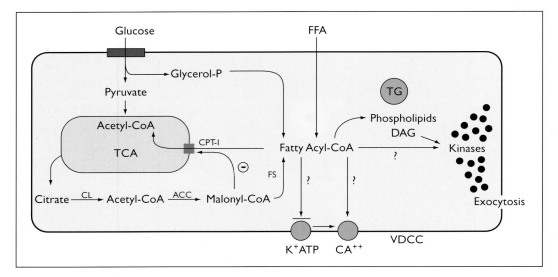

FIGURE 1-15. Fatty acid influence upon β-cell function. Fat metabolism is likely to have important influences upon insulin secretion, but the mechanisms responsible for these effects are still not well understood. It appears that the modest elevations of free fatty acids (FFAs) of obesity contribute the hyperinsulinemia of that state. Depletion of circulating FFAs during prolonged fasting when glucose levels are low and β-cell lipid stores depleted results in impairment of insulin secretion. Excessive elevations of FFAs can have an inhibitory influence upon insulin secretion.

Some of glucose-stimulated insulin secretion could be mediated not only by glucose metabolism, but also by fatty acid mediators. Thus, increases in glucose metabolism could produce increased cytosolic concentrations of citrate, which can be converted by citrate lyase (CL) to acetyl-CoA which can be turned into malonyl-CoA by acetyl-CoA carboxylase (ACC). Malonyl-CoA can inhibit carnitine palmitoyltransferase I (CPT I), which helps control the entrance of fatty acyl-CoA into the fatty acid oxidation pathways of mitochondria. By inhibiting the entrance of fatty acyl-CoA into mitochondria, fatty acid mediators could be generated in the cytoplasm that might influence insulin secretion.

Fatty acids that enter the β cell could be converted to fatty acid mediators which can act upon ion channels, kinases or through other mechanisms to stimulate the exocytosis of insulin. Some of the lipid mediators include the phospholipid inositol 1, 4, 5-triphosphate (IP3) and diacylglycerol (DAG) which can act via protein kinase C. Alternatively, fatty acids could be stored as triglycerides for use during times of fuel deprivation. Fatty acid oxidation may under some circumstances contribute to ATP formation and thus help close the ATP-sensitive potassium channel (K+ATP) resulting in depolarization and opening of the voltage dependent calcium channels (VDCC). (Adapted from reviews by McGarry and Dobbins [20] and Prentki and Corkey [21]. TG—triglycerides; TCA—tricarboxylic acid cycle.)

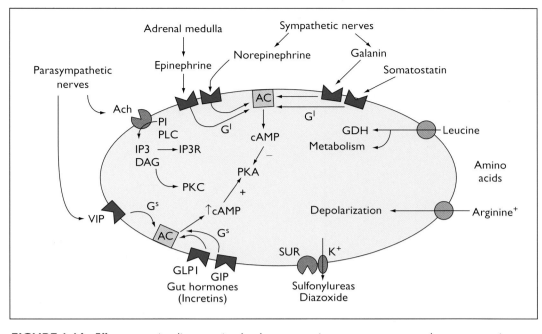

FIGURE 1-16. Effects upon insulin secretion by the autonomic nervous system, gut hormones, amino acids and drugs. The parasympathetic arm of the autonomic nervous system has a stimulatory influence upon insulin secretion exerted by acetylcholine acting mainly through phospholipase C (PLC) to generate inositol phosphate mediators and diacylglycerol (DAG). Parasympathetic stimulation also leads to release of the peptide mediator vasoactive intestinal peptide (VIP), which enhances secretion via stimulatory G proteins (G^S) acting through adenylate cyclase (AC). The sympathetic nervous system inhibits insulin secretion, with epinephrine and norepinephrine having a negative effect on AC through inhibitory G proteins (G^I). The sympathetic peptide mediator galanin and somatostatin have inhibitory effects on insulin secretion through similar mechanisms. The gut hormones GLP-1 and gastric inhibitory peptide (GIP) stimulate insulin secretion through cAMP and protein kinase A (PKA). Sulfonylureas stimulate insulin secretion by acting on the sulfonylurea receptor (SUR) to close the ATP-sensitive potassium channel which causes depolarization. Diazoxide has an opposite effect leading to hyperpolarization, which is inhibitory. Amino acids stimulate insulin secretion by several mechanisms. Arginine is positively charged, producing depolarization when transported into β cells, but this is not an important mechanism at physiologic concentrations of arginine. Leucine can influence insulin secretion by being oxidized via acetyl CoA or through a more complex metabolic effect mediated by glutamate dehydrogenase (GDH). IP3—inositol 3 phosphate; IP3R—inositol 3 phosphate receptor

Insulin Secretion in Type 2 Diabetes

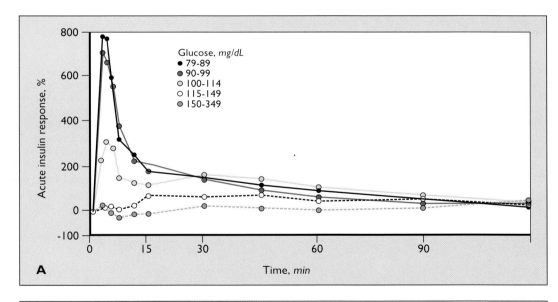

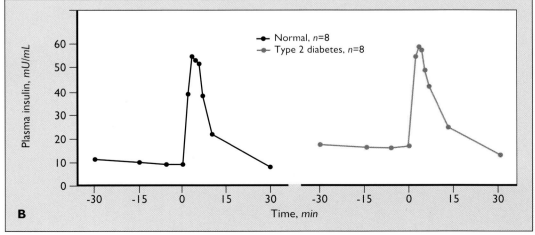

FIGURE 1-17. Insulin secretory characteristics in Type 2 diabetes. **A,** Loss of early insulin secretory response to an intravenous glucose challenge as fasting plasma glucose rises in subjects progressing from the normal state towards Type 2 diabetes [22]. It should be noted that impaired insulin responses to glucoses can even be seen before glucose levels rise to levels required for the diagnosis of impaired glucose tolerance (fasting glucose levels 110 mg/dL or above).

B, Preservation of acute insulin secretion in response to an intravenous pulse of arginine in Type 2 diabetes [23]. The acute insulin responses to glucose were lost in these subjects. Insulin responses are also be preserved for a variety of other secretagogues including isoproterenol, sulfonylureas, and the gut hormones glucagon-like peptide 1 and GIP.

(Continued on next page)

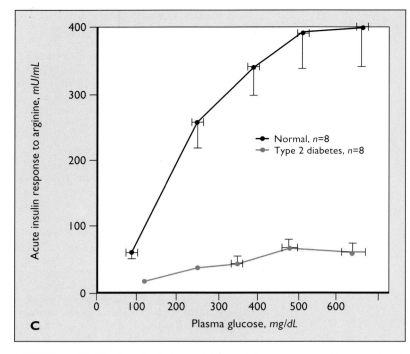

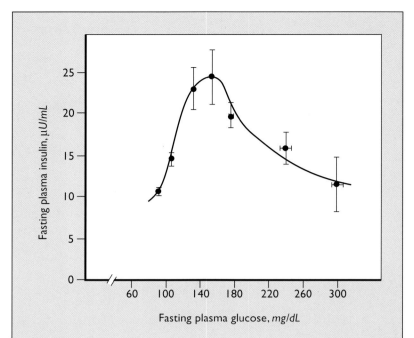

FIGURE 1-17. (*Continued*) **C,** Loss of glucose influence upon arginine-stimulated insulin secretion in type 2 diabetes [24]. The insulin secretory responses to a 350 mg/dL glucose concentration in subjects with type 2 diabetes were similar to the responses to an 80 mg/dL glucose concentration in control subjects. However, when the glucose concentrations in control subjects were raised with glucose infusions, the insulin responses far exceeded those of subjects with type 2 diabetes. Because individuals with type 2 diabetes have been found to have a β-cell mass approximately 50% of normal, the response in these subjects which is only about 15% of controls suggests that the secretory capacity for a given beta cell mass is severely impaired. (*Adapted from* Ward, *et al.* [24]; with permission.)

FIGURE 1-18. Inverted U-shaped curve of insulin secretion during progression from normal state to type 2 diabetes. Fasting plasma insulin levels rise as fasting glucose levels climb into the range of impaired glucose tolerance but then fall as diabetes develops and worsens. A similar pattern can be seen for plasma insulin levels obtained after an oral glucose or meal challenge. The rising insulin levels are likely to reflect a compensatory response to increasing insulin resistance, while the falling levels are indicative of beta-cell failure, probably through a combination of impaired function of individual beta-cell mass. (*Adapted from* DeFronzo *et al.* [25]; with permission.)

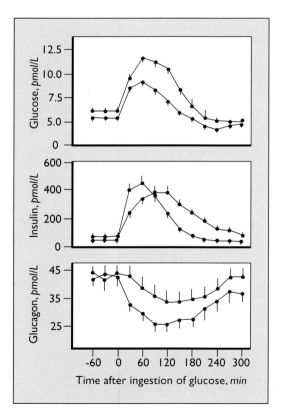

FIGURE 1-19. Insulin secretory profiles in the state of impaired glucose tolerance (IGT) during an oral glucose tolerance test (OGTT). The insulin responses at 60 and 90 minutes may be higher than those found in normal subjects, which probably reflects the combined influence of higher glucose levels at these time points and insulin resistance. Importantly, the insulin responses at 30 minutes in IGT are typically lower than normal, indicating the presence of a reduction in early impairment of glucagon suppression lead to an inefficient suppression of hepatic glucose output, which contributes to the higher glucose levels found in the latter stages of OGTT. Note that the early insulin responses found after oral glucose are much higher than those seen after an intravenous glucose challenge (Fig. 1-17.) This is thought to be due to the insulinotropic effects of the gut peptides GLP-1 and GIP, and possibly to some influence from activation of the parasympathetic nervous system. (*Adapted from* Mitrakou, *et al.* [26]; with permission.)

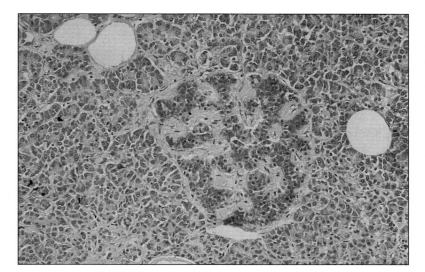

FIGURE 1-20. (*see* Color Plate) Amyloid deposits in islets in type 2 diabetes. In this photomicrograph of an islet, insulin containing cells are immunostained and amyloid deposition can be seen in the pericapillary space. The amyloid found in a high proportion of the islets of people with type 2 diabetes consists of β-pleated sheets of the peptide islet-associated polypeptide (IAPP, amylin), which consists of 37 amino acids. The sequence between positions 20 and 29 is important for the ability of this peptide to form amyloid. Production of IAPP is restricted to β cells and its content is only about 1% that of insulin. Amyloid deposition adjacent to β cells is found in diabetes and some insulinomas, but not in the normal state or in obesity with its insulin resistance and high rates of insulin secretion [27]. The mechanisms responsible for its deposition are not known. It is also unclear whether this amyloid formation contributes to the pathogenesis of type 2 diabetes, but it has been shown that human IAPP fibrils have a toxic effect on islet cells [28].

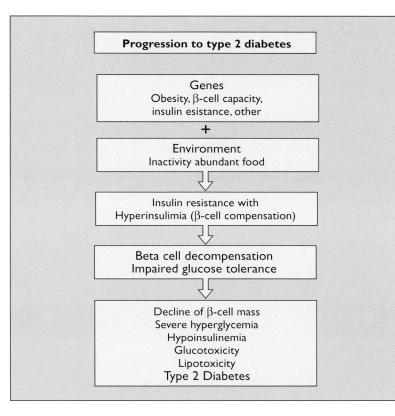

FIGURE 1-21. Pathogenesis of type 2 diabetes. This schema shows the various factors that contribute to the pathogenesis of type 2 diabetes [29]. Genes are likely to determine how well β-cells can function over a lifetime. For example, most of the gene defects of MODY (MODY 1,3 and 4) and some mutations of mitochondrial DNA lead to diabetes which often does not become manifest until middle age. There are probably genes which limit the ability of β-cell mass to compensate for insulin resistance over decades and even lead to a critical reduction in β-cell mass. Everything is made worse by the challenges of Western life style with its plentiful food and lack of exercise. Once hyperglycemia develops, glucose toxicity can produce further impairment of β-cell function and worsen insulin resistance. Lipotoxicity also appears to have adverse effects on the same two sites.

STAGES OF β-CELL DECOMPENSATION IN DIABETES

Compensation for Insulin Resistance

β cell hypertrophy

β cell hyperplasia

Shift to the left of glucose dose-response curve

(Increased secretion per cell at given glucose level)

"Normal" or increased glucose-induced insulin secretion

Decompensation: mild hyperglycemia

Loss of glucose-induced insulin secretion

Preservation of responses to non-glucose secretagogues (arginine, etc.)

Normal insulin stores

Early β cell dedifferentiation

Decreased gene expression of GLUT2, Glucokinase, mGAPDH,

Pyruvate carboxylase, VDCC, SERCA3, IP3R-II and transcription factors (PDX-1, HNFs, Nkx6.1, Pax6)

Increased gene expression of LDH, Hexokinase, Glucose-6-phosphatase, and the transcription factor c-myc.

Decompensation: severe hyperglycemia

Loss of glucose-induced insulin secretion

Impairment of responses to non-glucose secretagogues (arginine, etc.)

Increased ratio of secreted proinsulin to insulin

Reduced insulin stores (degranulation)

More severe β cell dedifferentiation

Decrease gene expression of insulin, IAPP, glucokinase, Kir6.2, SERCA2B, and transcription factor Beta 2.

Increased gene expression of glucose-6-phosphatase, 12-lipoxygenase, fatty acid synthase, and the transcription factor C/EBPβ

FIGURE 1-22. Stages of β-cell decomposition in diabetes [3,22,30].

β-CELL GLUCOTOXICITY AND LIPOTOXICITY

Abnormal β cell function in diabetes: β-cell function in diabetes is abnormal, whether in type 2 diabetes, early type 1 diabetes or with an inadequate number of transplanted islets. A variety of secretory abnormalities have been identified, most notably loss of glucose-induced insulin secretion (GIIS), thought to be caused by exposure of β cells to the diabetic milieu.

Definition problem: Descriptive terms include: glucotoxicity, lipotoxicity, exhaustion, excess demand, decreased reserve, fatigue, overwork, desensitization, stress, dysfunction, and others.

Glucotoxicity

Loss of GIIS tightly tied to modest climb of glucose levels.

Reduction of GIIS can be seen with fasting plasma glucose (FPG) of 100 mg/dL.

Complete loss usually when FPG above 115 mg/dL

Abnormal GIIS in a diabetic state can be seen in absence of FFA increase.

Lipotoxicity

Free fatty acids (FFAs) important for β-cell function, at least as permissive factor.

Increased FFAs of obesity associated with high GIIS

Close correlation between FFAs of mild diabetes and loss of GIIS not well established.

Very high FFAs inhibit GIIS

Synergy between FFAs and hyperglycemia not yet understood

FFAs important for maintaining insulin secretion during a prolonged fast

FIGURE 1-23. β-cell glucotoxicity and lipotoxicity [20,22,29].

References

1. Edlund H: Transcribing pancreas. *Diabetes* 1998, 47:1817–1823.

2. Jonas J-C, Sharma A, Hasenkamp W, *et al.*: Chronic hyperglycemia and loss of β-cell differentiation. *J Biol Chem* 1999, (In Press)

3. Weir GC, Sharma A, Zangen DH, Bonner-Weir S: Transcription factor abnormalities as a cause of beta cell dysfunction in diabetes: a hypothesis. *Acta Diabetol* 1997, 34:177–184.

4. Bonner-Weir S, Orci L: New perspectives on the microvasculature of the islets of Langerhans in the rat. *Diabetes* 1982, 31:883–939.

5. Weir GC, Bonner-Weir S: Islets of Langerhans: the puzzle of intraislet interactions and their relevance to diabetes. *J Clin Inves* 1990, 85:983–987.

6. Orci L: The insulin factory: A tour of the plant surroundings and a visit to the assembly line. *Diabetologia* 1985, 28:528–546.

7. Guest PC, Bailyes EM, Rutherford NG, Hutton JC: Insulin secretory granule biogenesis. *Biochem J* 1991, 274:73–78.

8. Bonner-Weir S, Baxter LA, Schuppin GT, Smith FE: A second pathway for regeneration of the adult exocrine and endocrine pancreas: A possible recapitulation of embryonic development. *Diabetes* 1993, 42:1715–1720.

9. Finegood DT, Scaglia L, Bonner-Weir S: (Perspective) Dynamics of B-cell mass in the growing rat pancreas: estimation with a simple mathematical model. *Diabetes* 1995, 44:249–256.

10. Sander M, German MS: The β-cell transcription factors and development of the pancreas. *J Mol Med* 1997, 75:327–340.

11. Rhodes, CJ: Processing of the insulin molecule. *In Diabetes Mellitus* Edited by LeRoith, D Taylor, SI and Olefsky, JM. Philadelphia: Lippincott-Raven; 1996:27–41.

12. Rhodes CJ Alarcon C: What β-cell defect could lead to hyperproinsulinemia in NIDDM: Some clues from recent advances made in understanding the proinsulin conversion mechanism. *Diabetes* 1994, 43:511–517.

13. Easom RA: CaM Kinase II: A protein kinase with extraordinary talents germane to insulin exocytosis. *Diabetes* 1999, (In Press)

14. Leahy JL, Cooper HE, Deal DA Weir GC: Chronic hyperglycemia is associated with impaired glucose influence on insulin secretion: a study in normal rats using chronic in vivo glucose infusions. *J Clin Invest* 1986, 77:908–915.

15. Meglasson MD Matschinsky FM: New perspectives on pancreatic islet glucokinase. *Am J Physiol* 1984, 246:E1–E13.

16. Eto K, Tsubamoto Y, Terauchi Y, et al: Role of NADH shuttle system in glucose-induced activation of mitochondrial metabolism and insulin secretion. *Science* 1999, 283:981–985.

17. Atwater I, Mears D Rojas E: Electrophysiology of the pancreatic β-cell. *In Diabetes Mellitus.* Edited by LeRoith, D Taylor, SI and Olefsky, JM. Philadelphia: Lippincott-Raven; 1996:78–102.

18. Gilon P, Shepherd RM Henquin JC: Oscillations of secretion driven by oscillations of cytoplasmic Ca2 as evidenced in single pancreatic islets. *J Biol Chem* 1993, 268:22265–22268.

19. Porksen N, Munn S, Steers J, *et al.*: Effects of glucose ingestion versus infusion on pulsatile insulin secretion. *Diabetes* 1996, 45:1317–1323.

20. McGarry JD Dobbins RL: Fatty acids, lipotoxicity and insulin secretion. *Diabetolgia* 1999, 42:128–138.

21. Prentki M Corkey BE: Are the β-cell signaling molecules malonyl-CoA and cytosolic long-chain acyl-CoA implicated in multiple tissue defects of obesity and NIDDM? *Diabetes* 1996, 45:273–283.

22. Brunzell JD, Robertson RP, Lerner RL, et al.: Relationships between fasting plasma glucose levels and insulin secretion during intravenous glucose tolerance tests. *J Clin Endocrinol Metab* 1976, 42:222–229.

23. Ward WK, Beard JC, Halter JB, *et al.*: Pathophysiology of insulin secretion in non-insulin-dependent diabetes mellitus. *Diabetes Care* 1984, 7:491–502.

24. Ward WK, Bolgiano DC, McKnight B, *et al.*: Diminished β-cell secretory capacity in patients with noninsulin-dependent diabetes mellitus. *J Clin Invest* 1984, 74:1318–1328.

25. DeFronzo RA, Ferrannini E, Simonson DC: fasting hyperglycemia in noninsulin-dependent diabetes mellitus: contributions of excessive hepatic glucose production and impaired tissue glucose uptake. *Metabolism* 1989, 38:387–395.

26. Mitrakou A, Kelley D, Mokan M, *et al.*: role of suppression of glucose production and diminished early insulin release in impaired glucose tolerance. *N Engl J Med* 1992, 326:22–29.

27. Kahn SE, Andrikopoulos S Verchere CB: Islet amyloid: A long-recognized but underappreciated pathological feature of type 2 diabetes. *Diabetes* 1999, 48:241–253.

28. Lorenzo A, Bronwyn R, Weir GC Yankner BA: Pancreatic islet cell toxicity of amylin associated with type-2 diabetes mellitus. *Nature* 1994, 368:756–760.

29. Weir, GC and Bonner-Weir, S: Insulin secretion in non-insulin-dependent diabetes mellitus. *In Diabetes Mellitus*. Edited by LeRoith, D Taylor, SI and Olefsky, JM. Philadelphia: Lippincott-Raven; 1996:503–508.

30. Tokuyama Y, Sturis J, Depaoli AM, *et al.*: Evolution of β cell dysfunction in the male Zucker diabetic fatty rat. *Diabetes* 1995, 44:1447–1457.

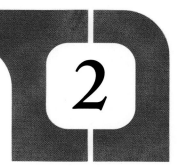

THE MECHANISMS OF INSULIN ACTION

Domenico Accili and Hiroko Kanno

Insulin promotes a wide range of metabolic and growth-promoting functions in multiple target cells such as liver, muscle, and fat, and to a lesser extent in other tissues. The mechanism by which insulin regulates energy metabolism and promotes cell growth has been studied extensively. Almost 50 years ago, the pioneering work of Levine and coworkers led to the hypothesis that the effect of insulin on glucose utilization was due to increased glucose transport across the plasma membrane. In 1971, Roth and colleagues discovered the insulin receptor. This discovery ushered in a new era of investigations that led to identification of the tyrosine kinase activity of the insulin receptor a decade later and, ultimately, to the discovery and characterization of intracellular mediators of insulin action.

Insulin exerts its diverse actions by inducing tyrosine phosphorylation, that is, the transfer of a phosphate group from ATP to a tyrosine residue, in its cell surface receptor [1]. Autophosphorylation further activates the receptor as a tyrosine-specific protein kinase, allowing the activated receptor to phosphorylate a host of cytosolic and membrane-bound proteins. Phosphorylation of protein substrates is required to mediate insulin action. The proximal effectors of insulin action have been identi-fied convincingly; they include insulin receptor substrate (IRS) proteins and several others [2]. IRS proteins serve an important function as "docking" molecules, favoring the assembly of multiprotein complexes and generation of intracellular signals. Much work remains to be done to understand how these intracellular signals eventuate in biologic effects. For example, it is clear that insulin stimulation of glucose transport requires synthesis of a lipid mediator, phosphatidylinositol 3-phosphate. However, the same signaling pathway is used by different agents that do not stimulate glucose transport. Thus, elements that account for the specificity of insulin signaling have not yet been identified entirely.

Understanding the molecular basis of insulin action is especially relevant to uncovering the pathophysiology of human diabetes. It is firmly established that patients with type II diabetes have defects of insulin action, commonly referred to as insulin resistance. However, the nature of the fundamental defect in type II diabetes remains unclear. It is widely held that a defect at an early postreceptor step in insulin action could provide a unifying mechanism for insulin resistance. A thorough understanding of the steps involved in regulation of fuel homeostasis by insulin undoubtedly will lead to better strategies for prevention and cure of type II diabetes [3].

Insulin Receptor

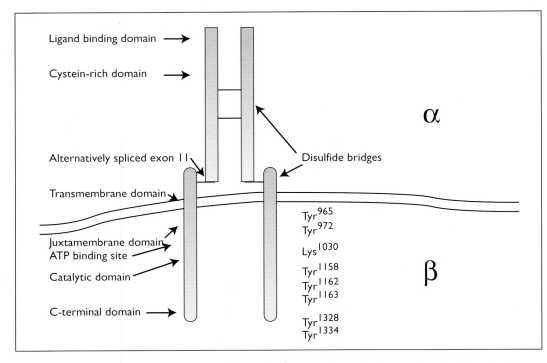

FIGURE 2-1. Insulin receptor structure. The insulin receptor is required to mediate insulin action. The product of a single copy gene located on the short arm of chromosome 19 (cytogenetic band 19p13), the insulin receptor initially is synthesized as a single-chain polypeptide precursor. This precursor undergoes post-translational cleavage into separate α and β subunits, followed by dimerization and export to the plasma membrane. On route to its plasma membrane localization, the receptor also is glycosylated and acylated. The mature receptor is a homodimer composed of two α and two β subunits (α_2-β_2). The α subunit is completely extracellular and contains the ligand binding domain located near the amino-terminal end of the protein. The β subunit spans the plasma membrane once and is linked to the α subunit by way of disulfide bridges and noncovalent interactions. The intracellular part of the β subunit contains a tyrosine-specific protein kinase domain. Insulin binding to the extracellular domain causes a conformational modification in the intracellular domain such that the receptor undergoes autophyosphorylation and can bind adenosine triphosphate (ATP). Several tyrosine residues are phosphorylated: a residue in the juxtamembrane domain of the receptor (tyrosine 972) plays a crucial role in substrate binding and phosphorylation. The residues in the catalytic domain (tyrosines 1158, 1162, and 1163) are essential to promote the kinase activity of the receptor toward other protein substrates. The role of the carboxy-terminal phosphorylation sites (tyrosines 1328 and 1334) is more controversial, with some investigations suggesting these sites may play a role in stimulating the mitogenic activity of the receptor.

The insulin receptor is expressed as two variably spliced isoforms, resulting from inclusion (isoform B) or exclusion (isoform A) of exon 11 during processing of messenger RNA (mRNA). The additional exon encodes a peptide with 12 amino acids located at the carboxy-terminal end of the α subunit of the receptor. The role of alternative splicing in receptor function is not clear; however, it has been shown that the long isoform binds insulin with lower affinity than does the short isoform [4].

Overview of Insulin Effects

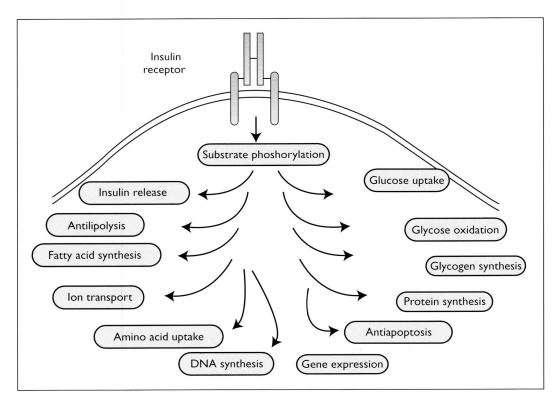

FIGURE 2-2. Insulin actions in peripheral tissues. Protein phosphorylation is required to mediate insulin action. After receptor autophosphorylation, the β subunit becomes active as a tyrosine-specific kinase and catalyzes phosphorylation of several intracellular proteins. This event provides the underpinning for the multifaceted actions of insulin. Insulin stimulates glucose turnover by favoring its transport across the plasma membrane, followed either by oxidative or nonoxidative disposal, the latter being associated with glycogen synthesis. The effect of insulin on glucose transport is observed only in skeletal muscle, adipose cells, and heart. Insulin promotes protein synthesis in almost all tissues, by virtue of a combined effect on gene transcription, messenger RNA translation, and amino acid uptake. Insulin also has a mitogenic effect that is mediated through increased DNA synthesis and prevention of programmed cell death, or *apoptosis*. In addition, insulin stimulates ion transport across the plasma membrane of multiple tissues. Finally, insulin stimulates lipid synthesis in fat cells, skeletal muscle, and liver; and insulin prevents lipolysis by inhibiting hormone-sensitive lipase. There is increasing evidence for a direct role of insulin, acting through the insulin receptor, to regulate insulin release from the pancreatic β cell [5].

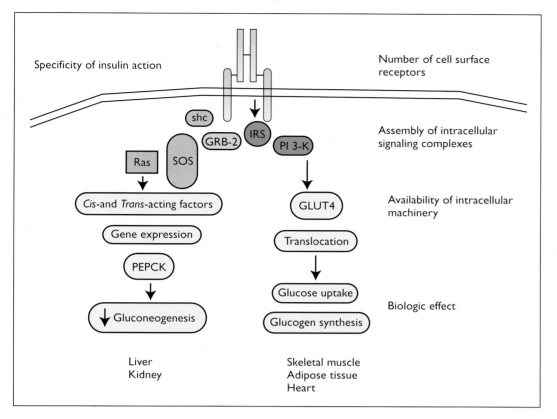

FIGURE 2-3. Tissue-specific effects of insulin. Different tissues are known to respond differently to insulin. Tissue sensitivity to insulin correlates with the levels of insulin receptors expressed on the plasma membrane. However, it has become clear that the assembly of different components of the insulin signaling pathway also is responsible for bestowing specificity of insulin signaling on target cells. Thus, insulin-dependent glucose transport is only observed in skeletal muscle and adipose cells because these cells possess the insulin-dependent glucose transporter GLUT4 (*see* Figs. 2-16 to 2-18). Likewise, the effect of insulin to inhibit gluconeogenesis is specific to liver and kidney. In contrast, the effects on ion transport, DNA synthesis, and protein synthesis appear to be ubiquitous. GLUT4—glucose transporter 4; GRB-2—growth factor receptor binding protein 2; IRS—insulin receptor substrate; PEPCK— phosphoenol-pyruvate carboxy-kinase; PI 3-K—phosphatidylinositol 3-kinase; shc—*src* homology 2/collagen homology containing protein; SOS—son-of-sevenless.

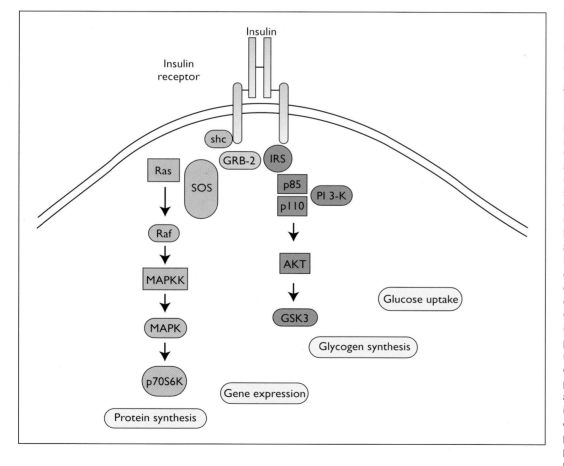

FIGURE 2-4. Activation of several intracellular signaling pathways by insulin. The diversity of insulin action in different tissues is partly explained by the different signaling pathways activated by the hormone. There are two main limbs that propagate the signal generated through the insulin receptor: the insulin receptor substrate/phosphatidylinositol 3-kinase (IRS/PI 3-K) pathway, and the Ras/mitogen-activated protein kinase (MAPK) pathway. The IRS/PI 3-K pathway leads to generation of PI 3-phosphate and consequent activation of PI-dependent kinases such as PDK1, PDK2, and PKC. Some of these kinases may be required to activate downstream kinases such as the serine/threonine kinase AKT [6]. It is thought that AKT may directly phosphorylate and inactivate glycogen synthase kinase 3 (GSK3), thus leading to dephosphorylation and activation of GS and increased glycogen synthesis (*see* Fig. 2-20) [7]. Evidence also exists linking AKT to translocation of glucose transporters [8]. The Ras/MAPK pathway can be activated by insulin through formation of complexes between the exchange factor SOS and GRB-2 [9]. GRB-2 can be activated by IRS or shc (*src* homology 2/collagen homology containing protein), which are direct substrates of the insulin receptor kinase. It appears that the acute metabolic effects of insulin require activation of the IRS/PI 3-K pathway, whereas the Ras/MAPK pathway may play a role in certain tissues to stimulate the actions of insulin on growth and proliferation. AKT—product of the *akt* proto-oncogene; GAP—guanosine triphosphatase–associated protein; GLUT4—glucose transporter 4; GRB-2—growth factor receptor binding protein 2; GSK3—glycogen synthase kinase 3; MAPKK—MAPK kinase; PDK—PI-dependent protein kinase; PKC—protein kinase C; SOS—son-of-sevenless.

Role of Insulin Receptor Substrate Proteins in Insulin Signaling

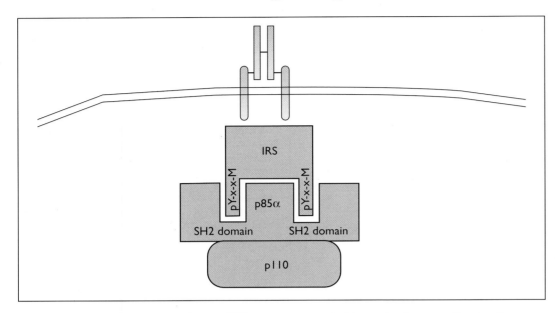

FIGURE 2-5. Insulin receptor substrate (IRS) proteins act as docking molecules to mediate insulin signaling. Initially, IRSs were identified as tyrosine-phosphorylated proteins in cells treated with insulin. In addition to insulin, other agents such as insulin-like growth factors and interleukins can stimulate IRS phos-

phorylation. Tyrosine phosphorylation occurs at signature Y-x-x-M motifs (where x is any amino acid and M is methionine). The phosphorylated tyrosines become binding sites for so-called SH2 (for *src* homology 2) motifs [2]. SH2 motifs are 50 to 100 amino acids long; they act as high-affinity phospho-tyrosine binding sites and are found in many intra-cellular signaling molecules [10]. Binding of phos-photyrosine to SH2 domains leads to formation of signaling complexes. A key signaling complex in insulin action is formed between IRS and the regu-latory subunit (p85) of the enzyme phosphatidyli-nositol 3-kinase (PI 3-K). There are two SH2 domains in the structure of p85. Binding of IRS to the two SH2 domains of p85 leads to activation of the p110 (catalytic) subunit of PI 3-K. The catalytic activity of p110 stimulates phosphorylation of PI on the D3 position of the inositol ring, leading to the generation of PI 3-phosphate from PI, PI 3,4-bispho-sphate from PI 4-phosphate, and PI 3,4,5-trisphos-phate from PI 4,5-bisphosphate. There is increasing evidence that 3-phosphorylated inositides act as intracellular messengers, leading to activation of PI-dependent kinases, changes in intracellular traf-ficking, and growth stimulation [11].

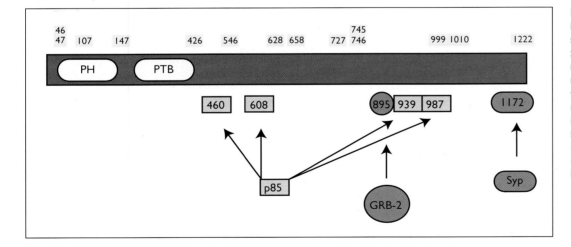

FIGURE 2-6. Different phosphorylation sites of insulin receptor substrate-1 (IRS-1) engage different signaling molecules. Different Y-x-x-M motifs (where x is any amino acid and M is methionine) of IRS molecules are able to engage different signaling molecules. This schematic diagram of IRS-1 indicates the preferred binding site of each of the main molecules that form complexes with IRS-1 after insulin stimulation. The boxed areas indicate two structural motifs of IRS, the pleckstrin homology (PH) and phosphotyrosine binding (PTB) domains (*see* Fig. 2-8) [2]. GRB-2—growth factor receptor binding protein 2; Syp—tyrosine phosphatase.

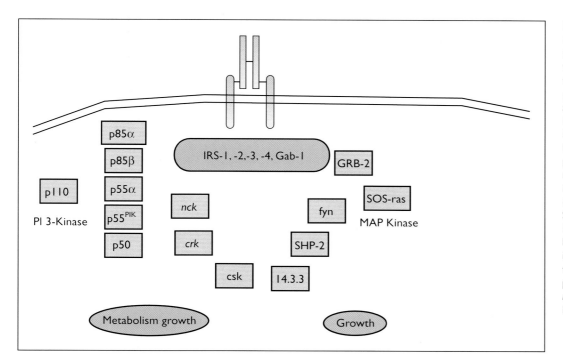

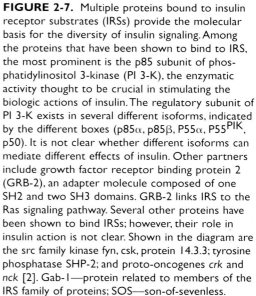

FIGURE 2-7. Multiple proteins bound to insulin receptor substrates (IRSs) provide the molecular basis for the diversity of insulin signaling. Among the proteins that have been shown to bind to IRS, the most prominent is the p85 subunit of phosphatidylinositol 3-kinase (PI 3-K), the enzymatic activity thought to be crucial in stimulating the biologic actions of insulin. The regulatory subunit of PI 3-K exists in several different isoforms, indicated by the different boxes (p85α, p85β, P55α, P55PIK, p50). It is not clear whether different isoforms can mediate different effects of insulin. Other partners include growth factor receptor binding protein 2 (GRB-2), an adapter molecule composed of one SH2 and two SH3 domains. GRB-2 links IRS to the Ras signaling pathway. Several other proteins have been shown to bind IRSs; however, their role in insulin action is not clear. Shown in the diagram are the src family kinase fyn, csk, protein 14.3.3; tyrosine phosphatase SHP-2; and proto-oncogenes crk and nck [2]. Gab-1—protein related to members of the IRS family of proteins; SOS—son-of-sevenless.

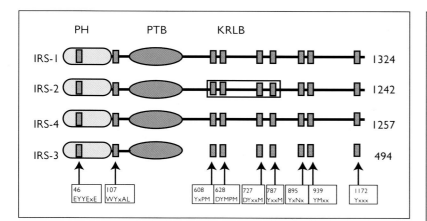

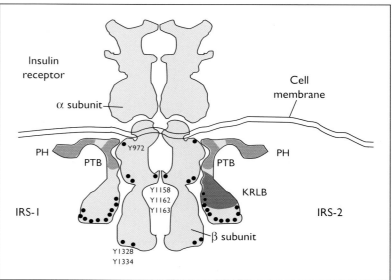

FIGURE 2-8. Multiple members of the insulin receptor substrate (IRS) family of proteins. There are four cloned members of the IRS family of proteins and a related protein called Gab-1. An alignment of the four cloned IRSs is shown. The length of the polypeptide chain is shown to the right of the bar graph. The main structural motifs of the IRS molecules are indicated by boxes: the pleckstrin homology (PH) domain, phosphotyrosine binding domain (PTB), and kinase regulatory loop binding (KRLB) domain. The conserved phosphorylation sites are indicated by boxes. In addition to these, each molecule contains unique phosphorylation sites. It is conceivable that the presence of a unique assortment of sites in each molecule would allow for the recruitment of different signaling molecules and lead to the formation of unique signaling complexes. In addition, distinctive patterns of tissue expression exist such that each IRS protein may play a different role in different tissues [2].

FIGURE 2-9. Model for the interaction of insulin receptors and insulin receptor substrate (IRS) molecules. After activation of the insulin receptor kinase, the phosphotyrosine binding (PTB) domain of IRS becomes closely associated with the juxtamembrane region of the insulin receptor. This interaction requires phosphorylation of tyrosine 972 in the insulin receptor. In addition, it is possible that the pleckstrin homology (PH) domain would further stabilize this conformation. The PH domain is located at the N-terminal end and is thought to play a role in the interaction between IRS and the membrane bilayer. It is possible that the PH domain binds phospholipids. In addition, there exists at least one additional domain that plays a role in the interaction between IRS-2 and the insulin receptor. This domain is the kinase regulatory loop binding (KRLB) domain. Its interaction with the insulin receptor requires phosphorylation of tyrosine residues in the catalytic domain of the receptor (tyrosines 1158, 1162, and 1163). Interestingly, this motif is present in IRS-2 but not in IRS-1, providing an additional determinant exists for the specificity of the interaction between the insulin receptor and its substrates [12,13]. Gene ablation experiments in mice indicate that the roles of different IRS molecules are not interchangeable. Mice lacking IRS-1 are growth-retarded and mildly insulin resistant, suggesting that IRS-1 plays an important role in both insulin and insulin-like growth factor I receptor function [14,15]. Mice lacking IRS-2 develop diabetic ketoacidosis owing to a combination of insulin resistance and impaired β cell development, suggesting that IRS-2 is important for metabolic regulation in response to insulin [16].

Effectors of Insulin Action Downstream from Insulin Receptor Substrate

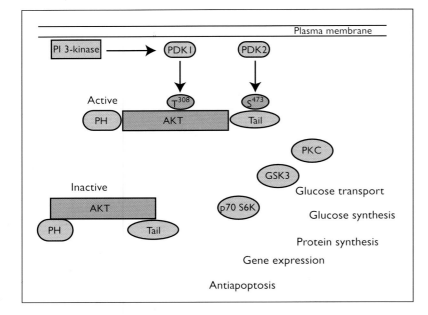

FIGURE 2-10. Downstream effectors of insulin action: the AKT (product of the *akt* proto-oncogene) kinase. The rapid increase in intracellular concentrations of phosphatidylinositol (PI) 3-phosphate after activation of the insulin receptor has led to the hypothesis that inositol 3-phosphate may act as an intracellular mediator. Several kinases are activated by the increase in PI 3-phosphate. The PI-dependent kinases 1 and 2 (PDK1 and PDK2) are two members of this family that may be involved in mediating some insulin actions. PDK1 and PDK2 phosphorylate residues threonine 308 and serine 473, respectively, in the primary sequence of the AKT serine/threonine kinase. The AKT kinase has been linked to insulin stimulation of glycogen synthesis and glucose transport [7,8]. The enzyme is composed of a pleckstrin homology (PH) domain and a kinase domain with the two PI-dependent phosphorylation sites. Maximal enzyme activity requires that both sites be phosphorylated. The role of the PH domain is as yet unclear; however, it may provide a targeting sequence for membrane translocation or for PI 3-phosphate binding. In addition to its role in glucose turnover, the serine/threonine kinase AKT has been involved in insulin-like growth factor I–mediated protection from apoptosis, as well as the activation of the enzyme p70 S6 kinase with attendant protein synthesis, regulation of entry into the cell cycle, and cellular differentiation [17,18]. GSK3—glycogen synthase kinase 3; PKC—protein kinase C; PIP₃—phosphatidylinositol 3,4,5-trisphosphate.

FIGURE 2-11. Downstream effectors of insulin action: protein kinase C (PKCs). Members of the PKC family of serine/threonine kinases have been implicated in several insulin actions. There are four subgroups of PKCs. The "classic" ones require calcium binding for activation; whereas the other three groups can be activated by diacylglycerol (DAG) binding, or by other phospholipids such as phosphatidylinositol 3,4,5-trisphosphate (PIP₃) (atypical PKCs). Insulin can activate different members of this kinase family through formation of DAG and PIP₃. Insulin stimulates DAG formation through phosphatidylcholine (PC) hydrolysis into DAG and phosphatidic acid (PA), or through activity of a glycosyl-phosphatidylinositol-specific phospholipase C (GPI-PLC), leading to the formation of DAG and inositol-phospho-glycan (IPG). Different isoforms of PKC have been shown to undergo translocation from the cytosol to the membrane in response to insulin stimulation in different tissues. Evidence exits that this process may be important for the biologic activity of PKCs [19]. It is known that PKCs can directly activate the MAP kinase pathway and the transcription factor NF-κB, leading to increased gene expression and protein synthesis. More recently, evidence has emerged that activation of atypical PKCs by PIP₃ may be important in the process of insulin-dependent glucose transport [20]. AKT—product of the *akt* proto-oncogene; GLUT4—glucose transporter 4; IRS—insulin receptor substrate; MAPK—mitogen-activated protein kinase; PI 3-K—phosphatidylinositol 3-kinase; PLD—phospholipase D; PKD—protein kinase D.

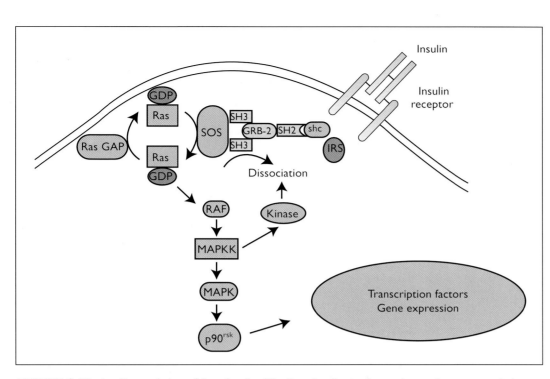

FIGURE 2-12. Insulin regulation of Ras signaling. The Ras signaling pathway plays an important role in cellular growth and transformation. Insulin can activate the Ras pathway, leading to increased protein

synthesis and mitogenesis. Activation of Ras in response to insulin requires formation of a signaling complex between insulin receptor substrate (IRS) or shc (*src* homology 2/collagen homology–containing protein) and the adapter protein, growth factor receptor binding protein 2 (GRB-2). GRB-2 consists of one SH2 domain that binds the phosphorylated tyrosine residues in IRS or shc, and two SH3 (a *src* homology 3 motif) domains that recognize proline-rich motifs of the exchange factor son-of-sevenless (SOS). SOS catalyzes the conversion of Ras from an inactive form (guanosine diphosphate [GDP–] bound) to an active form (guanosine triphosphate [GDT–] bound). The guanosine triphosphatase protein (GTPase) Ras-GTPase (GAP–) associated protein catalyzes the reverse reaction, with formation of inactive Ras. Ras-GTP activates the Raf kinase that, in turn, phosphorylates mitogen-activated protein kinase kinase (MAPKK), leading to increased MAPK activity and effects on protein synthesis and gene expression through the p90^{rsk} kinase. On activation, MAPKK also is able to activate an additional pathway that catalyzes the dissociation of GRB-2 from SOS, thus effectively terminating insulin action through Ras. It appears that the relative roles of IRS and SHC in activating SOS through GRB-2 vary in different tissues [21].

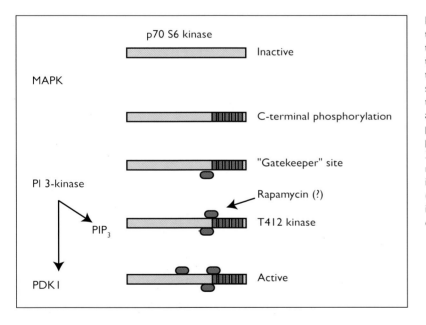

FIGURE 2-13. Regulation of p70 S6 kinase. Many effects of insulin are mediated through protein serine/threonine kinases. The enzyme p70 S6 kinase is a prototypic member of the family of insulin-activated serine/threonine kinases. It is thought that p70 may affect cell proliferation and protein synthesis in response to insulin. The enzyme is subject to a complex multisite regulation. The initial step in the activation of p70 is phosphorylation of several residues at the carboxy-terminal end. This step is mediated by mitogen-activated protein kinases (MAPKs) and stress-activated protein kinases (SAPKs). After this step, p70 undergoes further phosphorylation at its threonine 394 site, which is a requirement for additional phosphorylation. Next, the enzyme is phosphorylated in a phosphatidylinositol 3-kinase (PI 3-K–) dependent manner at threonine 412 and 252. The enzymes responsible for this phosphorylation are PIP-dependent kinases. Threonine 252 is phosphorylated by the same phosphatidylinositol-dependent protein kinase 1 (PDK1) enzyme that phosphorylates threonine 308 in AKT. Full enzyme activity is achieved only when all sites are phosphorylated [22]. AKT—product of the *akt* proto-oncogene; PIP$_3$—phosphatidylinositol 3,4,5-trisphosphate.

Alternative Signaling Pathways

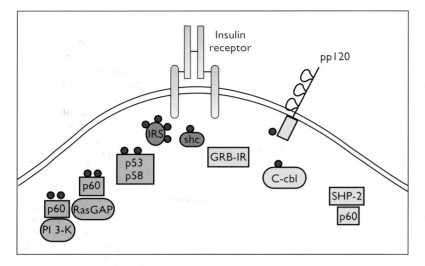

FIGURE 2-14. Alternative substrates of the insulin receptor kinase (IRS). In addition to the growing interest in IRS proteins as the main mediators of

insulin action, substantial evidence exists that insulin receptors activate an entire host of cytosolic and membrane-bound proteins. Some of these proteins appear to be specific substrates of the insulin receptor, raising the possibility that they may be involved in mediating some actions of insulin. For example, pp120 is a liver-specific glycoprotein that may regulate insulin receptor recycling, and it is phosphorylated specifically by insulin receptors but not by insulin-like growth factor I (IGF-I) receptors [23]. Likewise, growth factor receptor binding protein–insulin receptor (GRB-IR) is an adapter protein that binds to the insulin but not the IGF-I receptor, is weakly tyrosine-phosphorylated in response to insulin, and has been shown to dampen insulin signaling [24]. C-cbl also is a substrate of the insulin receptor in adipocytes, where it has been shown to direct insulin-dependent phosphorylation of caveolin [25]. Several substrates for phosphorylation by the insulin receptor in the range of 53 to 60 kD also have been cloned. Some are associated with molecules that play an important role in insulin action, such as phosphatidylinositol 3-kinase (PI 3-K) (p85), the tyrosine phosphatase SHP-2, and Ras–guanosine triphosphatase-associated protein. Thus, it is possible that phosphorylation of these substrates may affect insulin signaling in different tissues. Like IRS proteins, there is evidence that substrate phosphorylation requires phosphorylation of tyrosine 972 in the juxtamembrane domain of the insulin receptor [26]. shc—src homology 2/collagen homology–containing protein.

Insulin Action on Glucose Metabolism

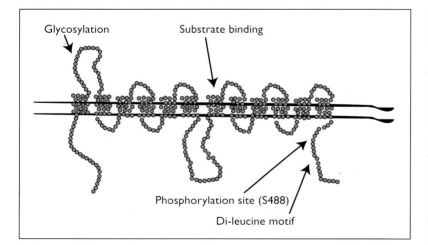

FIGURE 2-15. Insulin action on glucose transport: glucose transporter structure. Glucose transport is mediated by a family of facilitative glucose carriers, or glucose transporters. These proteins have a typical structure with a cytoplasmic amino-terminus followed by 12 membrane-spanning domains and a cytoplasmic tail. As an example, the proposed structure of the insulin-responsive transporter glucose transporter 4 (GLUT4) is shown. The first exofacial loop contains glycosylation sites, whereas the cytoplasmic carboxy-terminal domain contains

a putative phosphorylation site (serine 488) and a di-leucine motif thought to play a role in the rapid endocytosis of GLUT4. The proposed substrate binding site also is shown [27].

There is evidence for eight different members of the glucose transporter gene family. GLUT1 is expressed in all tissues and cell lines, and accounts for most basal (insulin-independent) glucose uptake. GLUT2 is mainly expressed in liver and pancreatic β cells; because of its relatively low affinity for glucose and high capacitance, it serves to provide a constant flux of glucose into these organs at physiologic plasma glucose concentrations ($\approx$5 mM). In the β cell, this mechanism couples glucose transport to glucose phosphorylation by the low-affinity β cell/liver glucokinase. The resulting change in adenosine triphosphate:adenosine diphosphate (ATP:ADP) ratio causes calcium ion mobilization and closure of ATP-sensitive potassium ion channels, with consequent insulin release. GLUT3 is expressed rather ubiquitously and possesses a relatively high affinity for glucose. Interestingly, GLUT3 is abundant in the central nervous system, where glucose concentrations are lower than in the bloodstream and the presence of a high-affinity glucose transporter provides a mechanism for maximally efficient glucose uptake by neurons. GLUT4 is the prototypical insulin-responsive glucose transporter. GLUT4 is found in specialized intracellular organelles, the GLUT4 vesicles, found in insulin-responsive tissues: skeletal muscle, adipose cells, and heart. Evidence now exists for the presence of an additional insulin responsive glucose transporter, GLUT8. GLUT5 is a fructose transporter expressed in the intestinal epithelial membrane and kidney. GLUT6 is a nonfunctional pseudogene. GLUT7 is a microsomal glucose transporter. It is part of the glucose-6-phosphatase complex thought to play a role in glucose release from the endoplasmic reticulum [27].

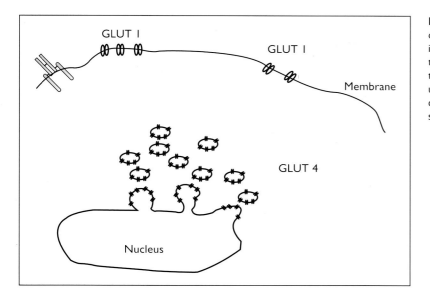

FIGURE 2-16. Insulin action on glucose transport: basal state. Under basal conditions, glucose transport across the plasma membrane occurs in an insulin-independent fashion. Glucose transporter 1 (GLUT1) catalyzes glucose flux across the plasma membrane under these conditions. In most tissues, this pathway is the only one for glucose uptake. In tissues that are insulin-responsive for glucose uptake there exists a second pool of glucose transporters, which under basal conditions is located intracellularly. These glucose transporters are located in specialized intracellular organelles, the GLUT4-containing vesicles [28].

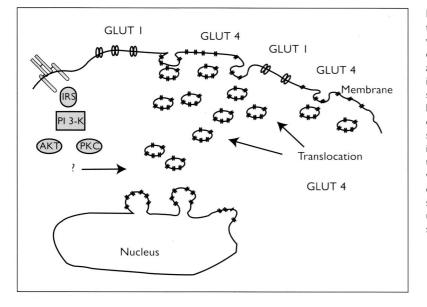

FIGURE 2-17. Insulin action on glucose transport: stimulation of glucose transporter 4 (GLUT4) translocation. On insulin stimulation, GLUT4-containing vesicles are released from an intracellular storage compartment and reach the cell surface, where they mediate glucose uptake. First recognized by Cushman and Kono, the mechanism of insulin-induced redistribution of glucose transporters is referred to as *translocation*. It is not clear whether the effect of insulin to stimulate glucose uptake in muscle and fat can be accounted for in its entirety by the translocation hypothesis. Other factors, such as an increase in the activity of glucose transporters, may also play a role. Substantial evidence exists to suggest that phosphatidylinositol 3-kinase (PI 3-K) activity and increases in intracellular phosphatidylinositol 3,4,5-trisphosphate (PIP_3) levels are necessary to mediate the effect of insulin on glucose transport. However, it is not clear whether PI 3-K activity also is sufficient for this purpose. Notably, many agents exist that can cause increases in PI 3-K activity to an extent comparable or superior to that of insulin; however, they do not cause significant glucose uptake [28]. AKT—product of the *akt* proto-oncogene; IRS—insulin receptor substrate; PKC—protein kinase C.

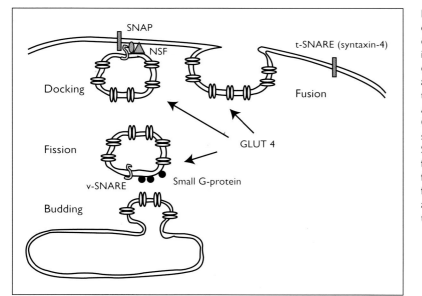

FIGURE 2-18. Formation of glucose transporter 4 (GLUT4) vesicles. Because of its central role in insulin action, glucose transport has been investigated in great detail. The insulin-responsive glucose transporter is contained in a specialized intracellular compartment, the GLUT4 vesicle. Four main steps can be identified during the formation of GLUT4-containing vesicles: budding, fission, docking, and fusion with the plasma membrane. Many of the accessory components of the GLUT4 vesicles have now been identified. Small (≈20 kD) G proteins of the Arf family are thought to be important for both the fission and fusion processes. Other components of the docking and fusion processes are *N*-ethylmaleimide sensitive fusion (NSF) proteins, soluble NSF attachment proteins (SNAPs), and SNAP receptor (SNARE) proteins. The two members of the SNARE family found in GLUT4 vesicles are synaptobrevin-2 and cellubrevin. These proteins form complexes with NSF, SNAP, and syntaxin-4, a member of the t-SNARE family found in the plasma membrane of insulin-sensitive tissues. There is general agreement that phosphatidylinositol 3-kinase (PI 3-K) activity is important for these steps; however, the exact site or sites of action of PI 3-K are not known [28].

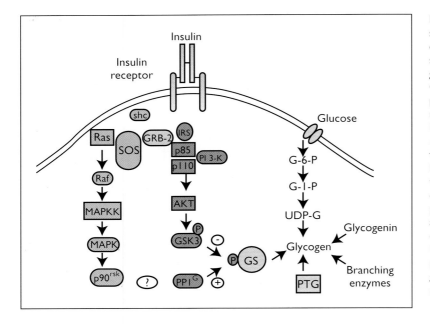

FIGURE 2-19. Insulin stimulation of glycogen synthesis. Insulin plays a key role in stimulating glycogen synthesis in many tissues. This process involves the regulation of multiple enzymatic activities. An important site of insulin action is glycogen synthase kinase-3 (GSK3), the enzyme that catalyzes the phosphorylation of glycogen synthase at several sites. It has been proposed that insulin affects GSK3 phosphorylation through activation of the AKT kinase (product of the *akt* proto-oncogene kinase). AKT is phosphorylated in response to phosphatidyli-nositol 3-kinase (PI 3-K) through PI-dependent kinases 1 and 2 (PDK1 and PDK2). AKT can phosphorylate and inactivate GSK3, thus decreasing the net rate of GS phosphorylation. Whether this effect on GSK3 is sufficient to account for the effect of insulin on glycogen synthesis is not clear. Moreover, insulin has been shown to increase the activity of the glycogen-bound form of the serine/threonine protein phosphatase-1 (PPI$_G$), although the exact mechanism of this effect is unknown [29]. Glycogen synthesis requires the assembly of a complex of proteins, including glycogenin to provide a molecular scaffold, branching enzymes, and protein targeted to glycogen (PTG), a novel protein that is specifically expressed in insulin-sensitive tissues [30]. GRB-2—growth factor receptor binding protein 2; IRS—insulin receptor substrate; MAPK—mitogen-activated protein kinase; MAPKK—MAPK kinase; G-6-P—glucose-6-phosphate; G-1-P—glucose-1-phosphate; shc—*src* homology 2/collagen homology–containing protein; SOS—son-of-sevenless; UDP-G—uridine diphosphate-glucose.

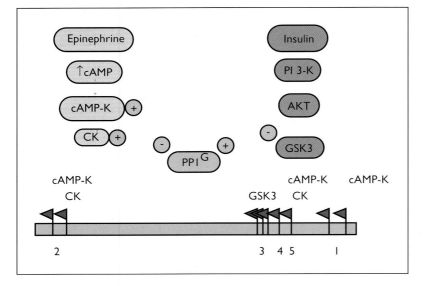

FIGURE 2-20. Opposing effects of insulin and cyclic adenosine monophosphate (cAMP) on glycogen synthase (GS).

GS plays a key role in the regulation of glycogen synthesis. The enzymatic activity of the protein is affected by the phosphorylation of several sites clustered at the amino- (site 2) and carboxy-terminal (sites 1, 3, 4, and 5) ends of the protein. Multiple kinases are known to affect the phosphorylation of these sites, resulting in decreased synthase activity. In addition, the glycogen-bound form of the serine/threonine protein phosphatase-1 (PPI$_G$) dephosphorylates and activates GS.

In the model depicted, glycogenolytic agents such as epinephrine act by raising intracellular cAMP levels. In turn, this increase activates the cAMP-dependent kinase (cAMP-K) that phosphorylates N- and C-terminal sites of GS. In addition, casein kinase I and II (CK) also are activated and result in further phosphorylation of GS at sites 2 and 5. cAMP also causes the phosphorylation of PPI$_G$, with a resulting decrease in enzyme activity. The net effect of these changes is to increase GS phosphorylation and inhibit glycogen synthesis. Opposite changes are effected by insulin, mostly through inactivation of GS kinase 3 (GSK3) and activation of PPI$_G$. It should be emphasized that numerous other kinases are known to phosphorylate various sites of GS [29]. AKT—product of the *akt* proto-oncogene; PI 3-K—phosphatidylinositol 3-kinase.

Other Actions of Insulin

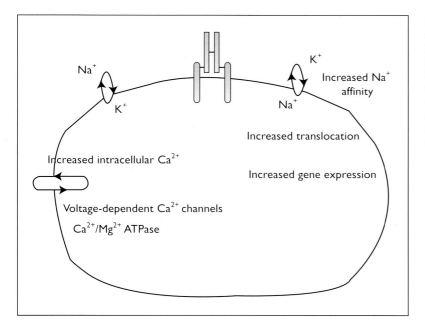

FIGURE 2-21. Regulation of ion transport by insulin. Insulin exerts a ubiquitous effect to promote ion transport across the plasma membrane. There are several levels at which insulin action can affect ion transport: (1) by stimulating sodium ion–hydrogen ion (Na^+/H^+) exchange to cause Na^+ influx and H^+ efflux, either by affecting subcellular localization of the transporter or increasing its affinity for Na^+; (2) by increasing the activity of the sodium ion–potassion ion (Na^+/K^+) transporter, favoring Na^+ efflux and K^+ influx; (3) by increasing intracellular calcium through an effect on the calcium ion–magnesium ion adenosine triphosphatase (Ca^{2+}/Mg^{2+} ATPase) transporter, or by activating voltage-dependent Ca^{2+} channels. Some of these effects are tissue-specific [31].

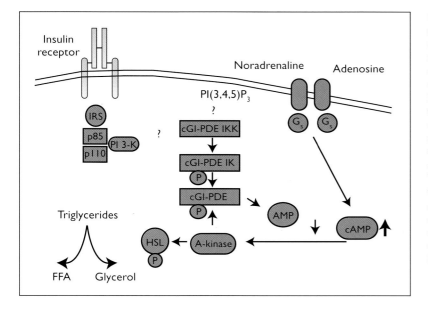

FIGURE 2-22. Regulation of antilipolysis by insulin. Insulin is a potent antilipolytic agent. An important mechanism for the antilipolytic action of insulin is the inhibition of hormone-sensitive lipase (HSL) through the activation of the cyclic guanosine monophosphate–inhibited phosphodiesterase (cGI-PDE). This enzyme decreases cyclic adenosine monophosphate (cAMP) levels, resulting in inhibition of cAMP-dependent protein kinase (A-kinase) and a consequent reduction in phosphorylation of HSL and a reduction of lipolysis of triglycerides into glycerol and free fatty acids (FFA). The exact mechanism leading to increased cGI-PDE activity is not known but has been demonstrated to involve the activity of at least two separate kinases (cGI-PDE insulin-dependent kinase kinase [cGI-PDE IKK] and cGI-PDE insulin-dependent kinase [cGI-PDE IK], respectively) that phosphorylate cGI-PDE in a phosphatidylinositol 3,4,5-trisphosphate (PIP_3–) dependent manner. Thus, it appears that phosphatidylinositol 3-kinase (PI 3-K) activity is required for this insulin effect. The mediators of this process have not been determined. As for many other effects of insulin, agents that raise intracellular cAMP concentrations, such as noradrenaline and adenosine, have the opposite effect of stimulating A-kinase and lipid breakdown [32]. G_i—inhibitory G protein subunit; G_s—stimulatory G protein subunit; IRS—insulin receptor substrate; P—phosphate moiety.

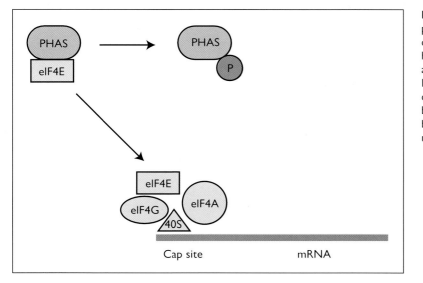

FIGURE 2-23. Regulation of messenger (mRNA) translation by insulin. Insulin promotes mRNA translation by affecting formation of the translation initiation complex. In the basal state, PHAS (thus designated because of its properties of heat and acid stability) is bound to the eukaryotic initiation factor 4E (eIF4E), and translation of mRNA containing a 5' untranslated region occurs slowly. Insulin stimulates phosphorylation of PHAS, and dissociation of the PHAS/eIF4E complex. The released eIF4E then can bind to eIF4G and eIF4A (helicase). This binding allows for melting of the secondary structure of the mRNA, with binding of 40S ribosomal subunit to the mRNA cap site and scanning of the mRNA molecule [33]. P—phosphate.

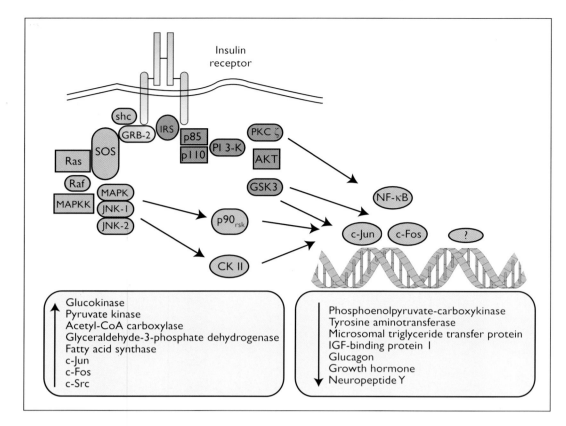

FIGURE 2-24. Regulation of gene expression by insulin. Insulin affects target gene expression in a variety of cells and organs. Both the insulin receptor substrate/phosphatidylinositol 3-kinase (IRS/PI 3-K) and the Ras/mitogen-activated protein kinase (MAPK) signaling pathways have been shown to mediate insulin action on gene transcription in different tissues. The IRS/PI 3-K pathway activates AKT (product of the *akt* proto-oncogene) and glycogen synthase kinase 3 (GSK3), both of which can potentially phosphorylate transcription factors and regulate their function. Moreover, atypical forms of protein kinase C (PKC), such as PKC, have been shown to phosphorylate NF-κB, altering its nuclear translocation. It also has been shown that inhibitors of the PI 3-K pathway can abolish the effect of insulin on the transcription of a variety of genes. The Ras/MAPK pathway has been shown to activate p90^{rsk} and casein kinase II, both of which are able to phosphorylate transcription factors of the Jun/Fos/AP-1 family. A list of genes, expression of which is up- or downregulated by insulin, is shown [34]. GRB-2—growth factor receptor binding protein 2; IGF—insulin-like growth factor; JNK-1—Janus kinase 1; JNK-2—Janus kinase 2; MAPKK—MAPK kinase; shc—*src* homology 2/collagen homology–containing protein; SOS—son-of-sevenless.

Modulation of Insulin Action

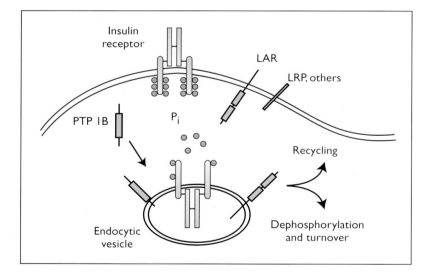

FIGURE 2-25. Role of protein tyrosine phosphatases (PTPs) as modulators of insulin action. PTPs may play an important role in deactivating the insulin receptor, providing a mechanism for fine-tuning the insulin response. There are two major classes of tyrosine phosphatases: receptor-type (membrane-bound) and nonreceptor-type (cytosolic). Several tyrosine phosphatases have been identified as insulin receptor phosphatases: among the receptor type, LAR and LRP; and among the cytosolic ones, PTP 1B. The latter also may play a role to dephosphorylate insulin receptor substrates, such as insulin receptor substrate, or pp120 (*see* Fig. 2-14). Another important step that could result in receptor dephosphorylation is the endocytic step that follows insulin binding, with internalization of the ligand/receptor complex into clathrin-coated vesicles. Deactivation of the receptor at this stage also may be physiologically important, because the internalized receptor may have access to different intracellular compartments [35]. LAR—leukocyte common antigen-related, receptor-type phospatase; LRP—LAR-related phosphatase.

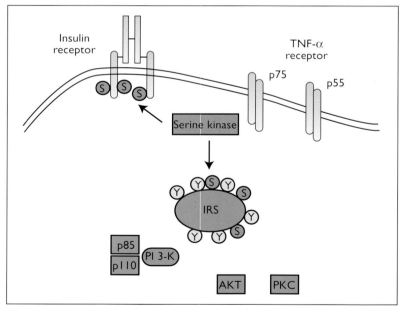

FIGURE 2-26. Tumor necrosis factor α (TNF-α) as modulator of insulin action. An important emerging area of investigation of insulin action is the role of serine/threonine phosphorylation in modulating the kinase activity of the insulin receptor and the subsequent biologic response. An interesting paradigm has surfaced from studies of TNFα-induced insulin resistance. It has been known for several years that TNFα can induce insulin resistance *in vitro*. Activation of the p75 and p55 isoforms of the TNFα receptor stimulates a serine/threonine kinase that can phosphorylate insulin receptor substrate-1 (IRS-1) and prevent its association with phosphatidylinositol 3-kinase (PI 3-K), thus leading to an effective dampening of the insulin signal. Presumably, a similar activity also can phosphorylate serine/threonine residues of the insulin receptor, and thus reduce the tyrosine kinase activity of the receptor toward intracellular substrates [36]. AKT—product of the *akt* proto-oncogene; PKC—protein kinase C; S—serine; Y—tyrosine.

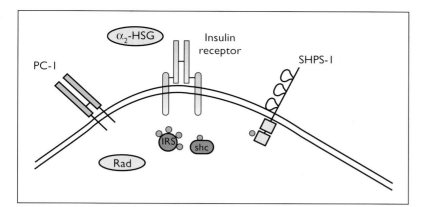

FIGURE 2-27. Other modulators of insulin action. Multiple signals converge on the insulin receptor to modulate its function. The membrane glycoprotein PC-1 has been proposed to exert a negative effect on insulin receptor function by dampening its kinase activity [37]. A correlation between PC-1 expression and insulin resistance has been established in patients with type II diabetes. Another inhibitor of the insulin receptor kinase is the serum glycoprotein α2-HSG. This 63-kD protein has been reported to inhibit insulin-induced receptor autophosphorylation and phosphorylation of insulin receptor substrate-1 and insulin receptor substrate SHC, with an associated decrease of the mitogenic actions of insulin. No effect of α2-HSG has been reported on the metabolic functions of insulin [38]. The raslike molecule Rad (raslike protein associated with diabetes) originally was identified by subtractive hybridization as a gene overexpressed in patients with diabetes. Although subsequent studies have failed to confirm this association, it is interesting that overexpression of Rad in transfected cells impairs insulin-dependent glucose uptake [39]. The transmembrane glycoprotein SHPS-1 is a 115-kD protein expressed in many tissues, and is phosphorylated in response to insulin. Cloning studies have demonstrated that SHPS-1 is a substrate for the phosphatase activity of SH-PTP1, a tyrosine phosphatase. The role of SHPS-1 in insulin action is not clear [40]. shc—*src* homology 2/collagen homology–containing protein.

References

1. Kahn CR: Banting Lecture. Insulin action, diabetogenes, and the cause of type II diabetes. *Diabetes* 1994, 43:1066–1084.

2. White MF: The IRS-signalling system: a network of docking proteins that mediate. *Mol Cell Biochem* 1998, 182:3–11.

3. Kahn CR: New concepts in the pathogenesis of diabetes mellitus. *Adv Intern Med* 1996, 41:285–321.

4. Tavare JM, Siddle K: Mutational analysis of insulin receptor function: consensus and controversy. *Biochim Biophys Acta* 1993, 1178:21–39.

5. Flakoll P, Carlson M, Cherrington A: Physiologic action of insulin. *In* Diabetes Mellitus. A Fundamental and Clinical Text. Edited by LeRoith D, Taylor SI, Olefsky JM. Philadelphia, New York: Lippincott-Raven; 1996:121–132.

6. Burgering BM, Coffer PJ: Protein kinase B (c-Akt) in phosphatidylinositol-3-OH kinase signal transduction. *Nature* 1995, 376:599–602.

7. Cross DA, Alessi DR, Cohen P, *et al.*: Inhibition of glycogen synthase kinase-3 by insulin mediated by protein kinase B. *Nature* 1995, 378:785–789.

8. Kohn AD, Summers SA, Birnbaum MJ, Roth RA: Expression of a constitutively active Akt Ser/Thr kinase in 3T3-L1 adipocytes stimulates glucose uptake and glucose transporter 4 translocation. *J Biol Chem* 1996, 271:31372–31378.

9. Skolnik EY, Batzer A, Li N, *et al.*: The function of GRB2 in linking the insulin receptor to Ras signaling pathways. *Science* 1993, 260:1953–1955.

10. Pawson T, Scott JD: Signaling through scaffold, anchoring, and adaptor proteins. *Science* 1997, 278:2075–2080.

11. Toker A, Cantley LC: Signalling through the lipid products of phospho-inositide-3-OH kinase. *Nature* 1997, 387:673–676.

12. He W, Craparo A, Zhu Y, *et al.*: Interaction of insulin receptor substrate-2 (IRS-2) with the insulin and insulin-like growth factor I receptors. Evidence for two distinct phosphotyrosine-dependent interaction domains within IRS-2. *J Biol Chem* 1996, 271:11641–11645.

13. Sawka-Verhelle D, Tartare-Deckert S, White MF, Van Obberghen E: Insulin receptor substrate-2 binds to the insulin receptor through its phospho-tyrosine-binding domain and through a newly identified domain comprising amino acids 591-786. *J Biol Chem* 1996, 271:5980–5983.

14. Tamemoto H, Kadowaki T, Tobe K, *et al.*: Insulin resistance and growth retardation in mice lacking insulin receptor substrate-1. *Nature* 1994, 372:182–186.

15. Araki E, Lipes MA, Patti ME, *et al.*: Alternative pathway of insulin signalling in mice with targeted disruption of the IRS-1 gene. *Nature* 1994, 372:186–190.

16. Withers DJ, Sanchez-Gutierrez J, Towery H, *et al.*: Disruption of IRS-2 causes type 2 diabetes in mice. *Nature* 1998, 391:900–904.

17. Kohn AD, Barthel A, Kovacina KS, *et al.*: Construction and characterization of a conditionally active version of the serine/threonine kinase Akt. *J Biol Chem* 1998, 273:11937–11943.

18. Kitamura T, Ogawa W, Sakaue H, *et al.*: Requirement for activation of the serine-threonine kinase Akt (protein kinase B) in insulin stimulation of protein synthesis but not of glucose transport. *Mol Cell Biol* 1998, 18:3708–3717.

19. Farese RV: Protein kinase C. In Diabetes Mellitus. A Fundamental and Clinical Text. Edited by LeRoith D, Taylor SI, Olefsky JM. Philadelphia, New York: Lippincott-Raven; 1996:187–197.

20. Standaert ML, Galloway L, Karnam P, *et al.*: Protein kinase C-zeta as a downstream effector of phosphatidylinositol 3-kinase during insulin stimulation in rat adipocytes. Potential role in glucose transport. *J Biol Chem* 1997, 272:30075–30082.

21. Ceresa BP, Pessin JE: Insulin regulation of the Ras activation/inactivation cycle. *Mol Cell Biochem* 1998, 182:23–29.

22. Avruch J: Insulin signal transduction through protein kinase cascades. *Mol Cell Biochem* 1998, 182:31–48.

23. Najjar SM, Blakesley VA, Calzi SL, *et al.*: Differential phosphorylation of pp120 by insulin and insulin-like growth factor-1 receptors: role for the C-terminal domain of the beta-subunit. *Biochemistry* 1997, 36:6827–6834.

24. Liu F, Roth RA: Grb-IR: a SH2-domain-containing protein that binds to the insulin receptor and inhibits its function. *Proc Natl Acad Sci USA* 1995, 92:10287–10291.

25. Ribon V, Saltiel AR: Insulin stimulates tyrosine phosphorylation of the proto-oncogene product of c-Cbl in 3T3-L1 adipocytes. *Biochem J* 1997, 324:839–845.

26. Danielsen AG, Roth RA: Role of the juxtamembrane tyrosine in insulin receptor-mediated tyrosine phosphorylation of p60 endogenous substrates. *Endocrinology* 1996, 137:5326–5331.

27. Czech MP: Molecular actions of insulin on glucose transport. *Ann Rev Nutr* 1995, 15:441–471.

28. Holman GD, Kasuga M: From receptor to transporter: insulin signalling to glucose transport. *Diabetologia* 1997, 40:991–1003.

29. Lawrence JC Jr, Roach PJ: New insights into the role and mechanism of glycogen synthase. *Diabetes* 1997, 46:541–547.

30. Printen JA, Brady MJ, Saltiel AR: PTG, a protein phosphatase 1-binding protein with a role in glycogen metabolism. *Science* 1997, 275:1475–1478.

31. Sweeney G, Klip A: Regulation of the Na^+/K^+-ATPase by insulin: Why and how? *Mol Cell Biochem* 1998, 182:121–133.

32. Degerman E, Leroy MJ, Taira M, et al.: A role for insulin-mediated regulation of cyclic guanosine monophosphate (cGMP)-inhibited phosphodiesterase in the antilipolytic action of insulin. In *Diabetes Mellitus. A Fundamental and Clinical Text*. LeRoith D, Taylor SI, Olefsky JM. Philadelphia, New York: Lippincott-Raven; 1996:197–205.

33. Lawrence JC Jr, Abraham RT: PHAS/4E-BPs as regulators of mRNA translation and cell proliferation. *Trends Biochem Sci* 1997, 22:345–349.

34. O'Brien RM, Granner DK: Regulation of gene expression by insulin. *Physiol Rev* 1996, 76:1109–1161.

35. Goldstein BJ, Ahmad F, Ding W, et al.: Regulation of the insulin signalling pathway by cellular protein-tyrosine phosphatases. *Mol Cell Biochem* 1998, 182:91–99.

36. Hotamisligil GS, Peraldi P, Budavari A, et al.: IRS-1-mediated inhibition of insulin receptor tyrosine kinase activity in TNF-α and obesity-induced insulin resistance. *Science* 1996, 271:665–668.

37. Goldfine ID, Maddux BA, Youngren JF, et al.: Membrane glycoprotein PC-1 and insulin resistance. *Mol Cell Biochem* 1998, 182:177–184.

38. Srinivas PR, Deutsch DD, Mathews ST, et al.: Recombinant human α 2-HS glycoprotein inhibits insulin-stimulated mitogenic pathway without affecting metabolic signalling in Chinese hamster ovary cells overexpressing the human insulin receptor. *Cell Signal* 1996, 8:567–573.

39. Moyers JS, Bilan PJ, Reynet C, Kahn CR: Overexpression of Rad inhibits glucose uptake in cultured muscle and fat cells. *J Biol Chem* 1996, 271:23111–23116.

40. Fujioka Y, Matozaki T, Noguchi T, et al.: A novel membrane glycoprotein, SHPS-1, that binds the SH2-domain-containing protein tyrosine phosphatase SHP-2 in response to mitogens and cell adhesion. *Mol Cell Biol* 1996, 16:6887–6899.

CONSEQUENCES OF INSULIN DEFICIENCY

Abbas E Kitabchi

Diabetes [Mellitus] is a remarkable disorder, and not one very common to man...The disease is chronic in its character, and is slowly engendered, though the patient does not survive long when it is completely established, for the marasmus produced is rapid, and death speedy. Life too is odious and painful, the thirst is ungovernable, and the copious potations are more than equaled by the profuse urinary discharge; for more urine flows away, and it is impossible to put any restraint to the patient's drinking or making water. For if he stop for a very brief period, and leave off drinking, the mouth becomes parched, the body dry; the bowels seem on fire, he is wretched and uneasy, and soon dies, tormented with burning thirst.

Aretaeus of Cappodocia (ea. 120 A.D. - 200 AD) [1]

Diabetes mellitus (Type 1 or Type 2) is the result of absolute or relative insulin deficient state that, if not corrected, gives rise to the acute metabolic decompensation of hyperglycemic crises so poignantly described above by Aretaeus of Cappodocia for more than 1800 years ago. The two major hyperglycemic crises are diabetic ketoacidosis (DKA) and hyperglycemic hyperosmolar state (HHS). Therefore, these two syndromes are the hallmark of insulin deficient states. These crises continue to be important causes of mortality and morbidity among diabetic patients. The annual incidence of DKA admission ranges from 4.6 - 8 episodes per 1000 patients with diabetes. It is estimated that DKA accounts for 4 - 9% of all hospital admissions for patients with diagnosis of diabetes whereas this figure for HHS is less than 1% [2, 3].

The most common precipitating causes for these hyperglycemic causes are a) infection, b) under treatment with or omission of insulin, c) previously undiagnosed diabetes, and d) presence of other comorbid conditions [4]. In addition, contributing factors for development of HHS include decreased intake of fluid and electrolytes and excessive use of such drugs as glucocorticoids, diuretics, β-blockers as well as use of immunosuppressive agents and diazoxide [4]. Although DKA is most frequently seen in type 1 diabetes and HHS is often associated with type 2 diabetes, each of these conditions can be seen in both types as DKA and HHS have common underlying causes, i.e., ineffective insulin concentration, dehydration and increased counterregulatory (stress) hormones, but at different levels. DKA can also occur in young, obese type 2 African-Americans, in whom a large percent had not had diagnosis of diabetes [5].

It is important to note that some patients may present with overlapping metabolic picture of both DKA and HHS and the incidence of HHS in DKA in some series may be as high as 30% [6]. HHS and DKA each can also occur in relatively pure form. In general in DKA, the insulin deficiency is absolute whereas in HHS, the insulin may be insufficient relative to the excessive levels of stress hormones (cortisol, glucagon, catecholamines and growth hormone).

With better understanding of the pathogenesis of insulin deficient states, the use of more physiological doses of insulin and frequent monitoring of such patients in the hospital, the mortality rate for DKA has been reduced to less than 5% and for HHS about 15% [3, 4, 7, 8]. Poor prognostic signs for these crises include advancing age, lower degree of consciousness and lower blood pressure. The cost of such crises in one study was estimated to be about $13,000 per episode [9]. The annual hospital cost for patients in hyperglycemic crisis may exceed billions of dollars per year [9]. Prevention of such crises, therefore, constitutes an important medical care endeavor. Preventive procedures should include extensive educational programs which should review steps to be taken during sick days in patients with diabetes. This should include frequent monitoring of blood glucose and urine ketones. The use of liquid diet, containing salt and carbohydrates, as well as close contact with health care providers and, above all, the use of short acting insulin are important precautionary measures for prevention of recurrence of these crises. Injection of short acting insulin should not be stopped in type 1 diabetic patients during sick days. Beyond these important educational programs, improvement in access to health care delivery system and medication in the less affluent segments of the society is one of the most effective methods for prevention of such crises. Indication for hospitalization include >5% loss of body weight during the crisis, respiration rate of >35/minute, intractable elevation of blood glucose, changes in mental status, uncontrolled fever and unresolved nausea and vomiting [4].

Structure of the Islets of Langerhans

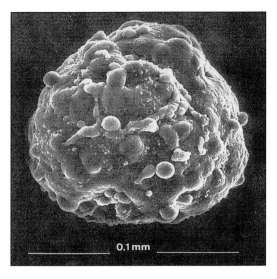

FIGURE 3-1. Very good insight into the surface topography of the periphery of the islet. ($\times$ 900) (From Orci [10]; with permission.)

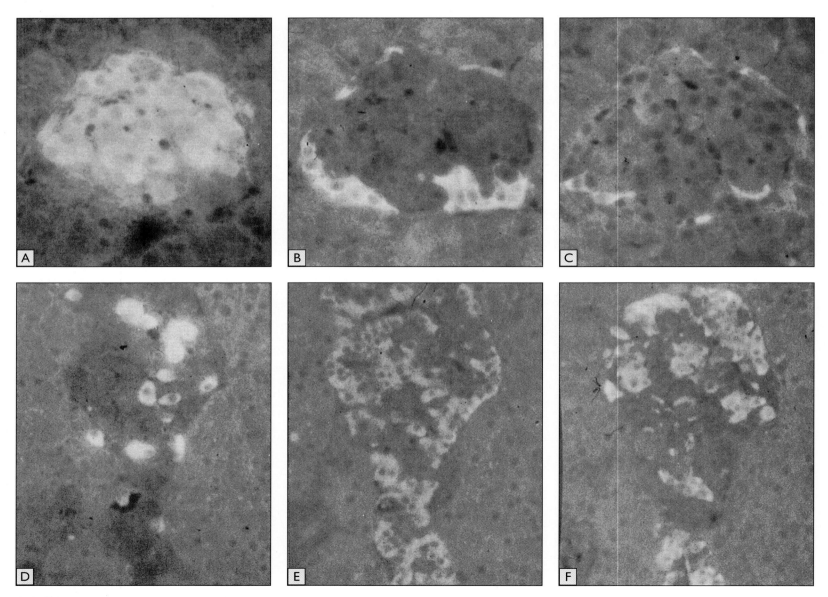

FIGURE 3-2. (*see* Color Plate) Consecutive serial section is of islets of Langerhans processed for indirect immunofluorescence. **A–C,** The location of insulin-, glucagon-, and somatostatin-containing cells, respectively, in the islet of a control rat. **D–F,** The profound perturbation of this normal distribution in the islet of a rat rendered experimentally diabetic for 17 months after a single IV injection of 45mg/kg streptozotocin. Note that the number of insulin-containing cells is strikingly reduced while that of glucagon and of somatostatin-containing cells is greatly increased. (*From* Orci, *et al.* [11]; with permission.)

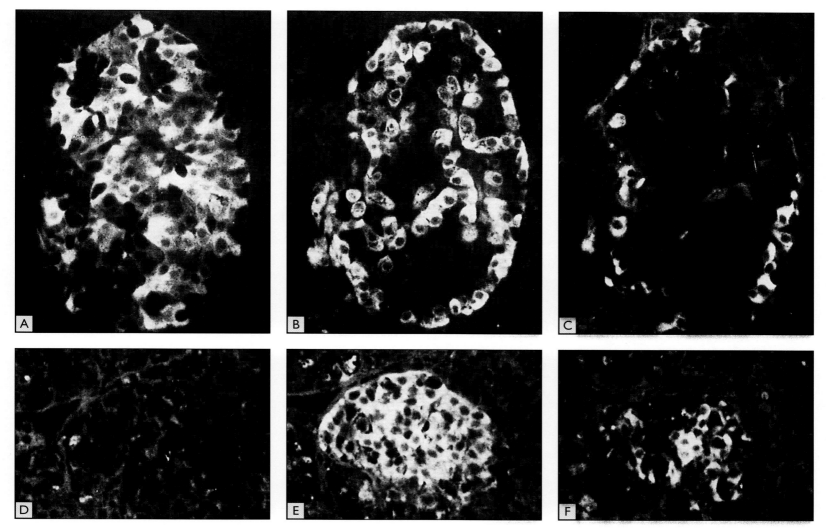

FIGURE 3-3. Distribution of B-, A-, and D-cells on serial sections of an islet from an adult nondiabetic subject, determined by the indirect immunofluorescent technique against insulin (**A**), glucagon (**B**), and somatostatin (**C**). **D–F**, Serial sections of the Islet of Langerhans in a chronic juvenile diabetic patient treated with the indirect immunofluorescent technique against insulin, glucagon, and somatostatin, respectively. The only detectable immunofluorescent cells within the islet are the numerous glucagon- and somatostatin-containing cells. (× 200) (*From* Orci, *et al.* [11]; with permission.).

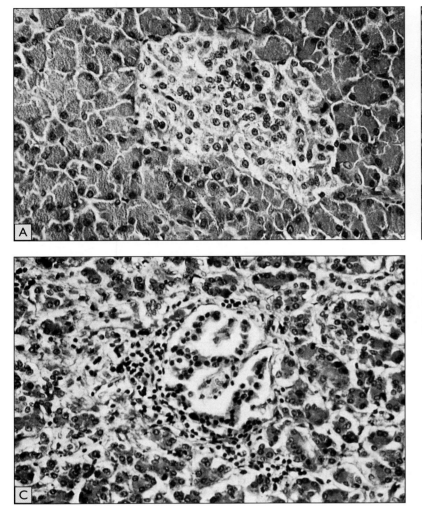

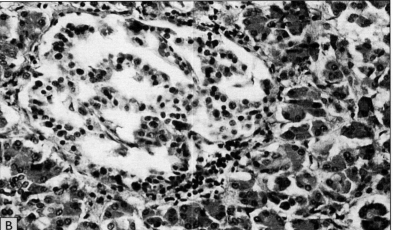

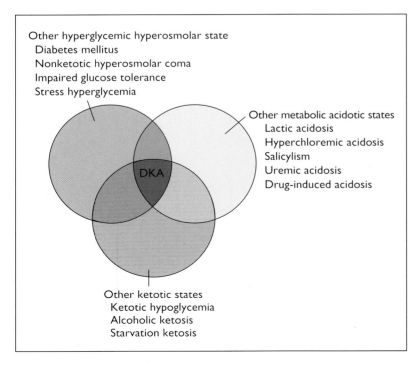

FIGURE 3-4. (*see* Color Plate) Islet cell necrosis and lymphocyte infiltration. **A**, Pancreatic islet section from normal, nondiabetic control subject. **B**, Pancreatic islet section from type 1 diabetes patient. Lymphocytic infiltration can be seen throughout the pancreatic islets with residual islet cells. **C**, Pancreatic islet section from type 1 diabetes patient, showing lymphocytic infiltration in the pancreatic islets, particularly the peripheral islets. (*From* Yoon, *et al.* [12]; with permission.)

Definition and Criteria for Insulin-Deficient State

Other hyperglycemic hyperosmolar state
  Diabetes mellitus
  Nonketotic hyperosmolar coma
  Impaired glucose tolerance
  Stress hyperglycemia

Other metabolic acidotic states
  Lactic acidosis
  Hyperchloremic acidosis
  Salicylism
  Uremic acidosis
  Drug-induced acidosis

DKA

Other ketotic states
  Ketotic hypoglycemia
  Alcoholic ketosis
  Starvation ketosis

FIGURE 3-5. Other conditions in which the components of the diagnostic triad for DKA (hyperglycemia, ketosis, and acidosis) may be found. (*From* Kitabchi and Wall [13]; with permission.)

DIAGNOSTIC CRITERIA AND TYPICAL TOTAL BODY DEFICITS OF WATER AND ELECTROLYTES IN DKA AND HHS

Factor Studied	DKA			HHS
	Mild	Moderate	Severe	
Diagnostic Criteria and Classification				
Plasma glucose, *mg/dL*	> 250	> 250	> 250	>600
Arterial pH	7.25–7.30	7.00– <7.24	<7.00	>7.30
Serum bicarbonate, *mEq/L*	15–18	10– <15	<10	>15
Urine ketone*	Positive	Positive	Positive	Small
Serum ketone*	Positive	Positive	Positive	Small
Effective serum osmolality[†]	Variable	Variable	Variable	>320 mOsm/kg
Anion gap[‡]	Wide (>14)	Wide (>14)	Wide (>14)	Normal to slightly wide (<14)
Alteration in sensorium or mental obtundation	Alert	Alert/Drowsy	Stupor/Coma	Stupor/Coma
Typical Deficit				
Total Water, *L*		6		9
Water, *mL/kg*[§]		100		100–200
Na+, *mEq/kg*		7–10		5–13
Cl-, *mEq/kg*		3–5		5–15
K+, *mEq/kg*		3–5		4–6
PO4, *mmol/kg*		5–7		3–7
Mg++, *mEq/kg*		1–2		1–2
Ca++, *mEq/kg*		1–2		1–2

*Nitroprusside reaction method
[†]*Calculation: Effective serum osmolality: 2[measure Na (mEq/L)] + glucose (mg/dL)/18*
[‡]*Calculation: Anion gap: $(Na^+) - (Cl- - HCO_3-)$ (mEq/L)*
[§]*Per Kg of body weight*

FIGURE 3-6. Diagnostic criteria and typical total body deficits of water and electrolytes in diabetic ketoacidosis (DKA) and hyperglycemic hyperosmolar syndrome (HHS). (*Adapted from* Kitabchi, *et al.* [4]; with permission.)

LABORATORY EVALUATION OF METABOLIC CAUSES OF ACIDOSIS AND COMA

Factor Studied	Starvation of high fat intake	DKA	Lactic acidosis	Uremic acidosis	Alcoholic ketosis (starvation)	Salicylate intoxication	Methanol or ethylene glycol intoxication	Hyper-osmolar coma	Hypo-glycemic coma	Rhabdo-myolysis
pH	Normal	↓	↓	Mild ↓	↓ ↑	↓ ↑*	↓	Normal	Normal	Mild ↓ may be ↓ ↓
Plasma glucose	Normal	↑	Normal	Normal	↓ or normal	Normal of ↓	Normal	↑ ↑ >500 mg/dL	↓ ↓<30 mg/dL	Normal
Glycosuria	Negative	++	Negative	Negative	Negative	Negative†	Negative	++	Negative	Negative
Total plasma ketones†	Slight ↑	↑ ↑	Normal	Normal	Slight to moderate ↑	Normal	Normal	Normal or slight ↑	Normal	Normal
Anion gap	Slight ↑	↑	↑	Slight ↑	↑	↑	↑	Normal	Normal	↑ ↑
Osmolality	Normal	↑	Normal	↑ or	Normal	Normal	↑ ↑	↑ ↑>330 mOsm/kg	Normal	Normal or slight ↑
Uric acid	Mild (starvation)	↑	Normal	Normal ↑	↑	Normal	Normal	Normal	Normal	↑
Miscellaneous		May give false positive for ethylene glycol§	Serum lactate >7 mM	BUN > 200 mg/dL		Serum salicylate +	Serum levels positive			Myoglob-inuria, hemo-globinuria

*Acetest and Ketostix measure acetoacetic acid only. Thus, misleading low values may be obtained because the majority of "ketone bodies" are (beta**)-bydroxybutyrate.
†Respiratory alkalosis/metabolic acidosis.
‡May get false-positive or false-negative urinary glucose caused by the presence of salicylate or its metabolites.
§Bjellerup P, et al. Clin Toxicology 1994; 32:85–86.

FIGURE 3-7. Laboratory evaluation of metabolic causes of acidosis and coma. (*Adapted from* Morris and Kitabchi [14]; with permission.)

Pathophysiology of Insulin-Deficient State

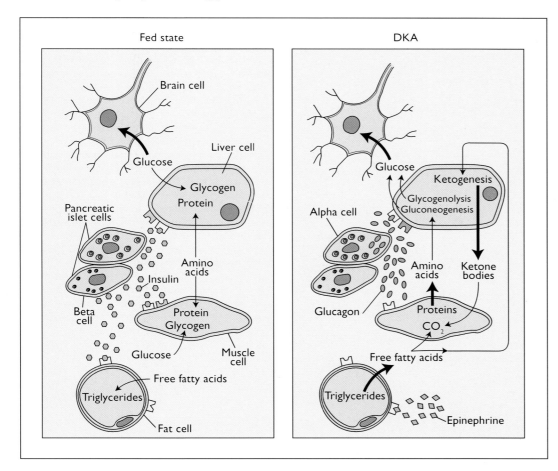

FIGURE 3-8. Normal mechanisms of glucose regulation can maintain supply to the brain when the body has been deprived of caloric intake for days, even weeks. In the fed state (left), assimilation of metabolic fuels and substrates is promoted by insulin in tissues sensitive to the hormone. In the DKA state (right), counterregulatory hormones (notably glucagon and epinephrine) reverse these processes, promoting glycogenolysis and creating substrates for ketogenesis and gluconeogenesis [15–18]. Denial of glucose to insulin-sensitive tissues preserves it for the brain. (*From* Kitabchi and Rumbak [18]; with permission.)

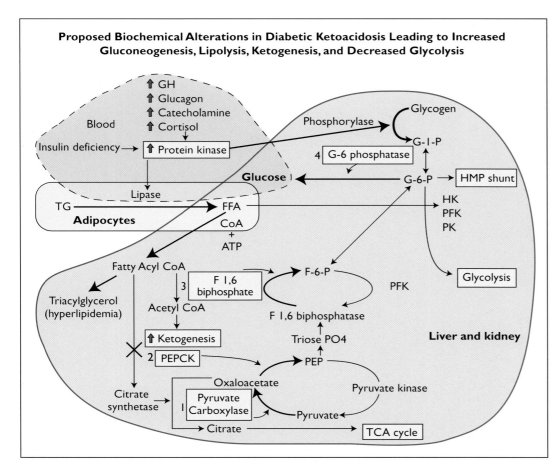

FIGURE 3-9. Proposed biochemical changes that occur during diabetic ketoacidosis. These alterations lead to increased gluconeogenesis and lipolysis and decreased glycolysis. *Note*: Lipolysis occurs mainly in adipose tissue. Other events occur primarily in the liver (except some gluconeogenesis in the kidney) [19]. *Thick arrows* indicate stimulated pathway in DKA which consists of rate limiting enzymes of gluconeogenesis, whereas *thin arrows* indicate inhibitory pathway in glycolysis. The TCA cycle is inhibited by fatty and acyl CoA-induced inhibition of citrate synthesis, a rate-limiting enzyme in the TCA cycle. ATP—adenosine triphosphate; CoA—coenzyme A; FFA—free fatty acids; F-6-P—fructose-6-phosphate; G-(X)-P—glucose-(X)-phosphate; HK—hexokinase; HMP—hexose monophosphate; PC—pyruvate carboxylase; PFK—phosphofructokinase; PEP—phosphoenolpyruvate; PEPCK—PEP carboxykinase; PK—pyruvate kinase; TCA—tricarboxylic acid; TG—triglycerides. (*From* Kitabchi, *et al.* [8]; with permission.)

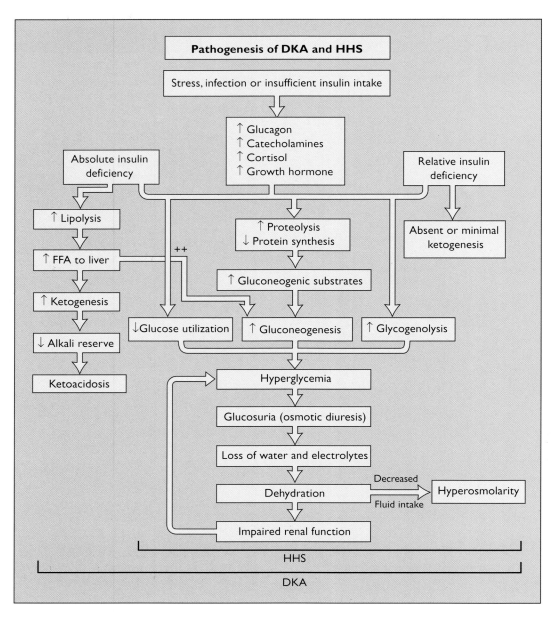

Pathogenesis of DKA and HHS

Stress, infection or insufficient insulin intake

↑ Glucagon
↑ Catecholamines
↑ Cortisol
↑ Growth hormone

Absolute insulin deficiency

Relative insulin deficiency

↑ Lipolysis

↑ Proteolysis
↓ Protein synthesis

Absent or minimal ketogenesis

↑ FFA to liver

++

↑ Ketogenesis

↑ Gluconeogenic substrates

↓ Alkali reserve

↓ Glucose utilization   ↑ Gluconeogenesis   ↑ Glycogenolysis

Ketoacidosis

Hyperglycemia

Glucosuria (osmotic diuresis)

Loss of water and electrolytes

Dehydration   Decreased   Hyperosmolarity
Fluid intake

Impaired renal function

HHS

DKA

FIGURE 3-10. Pathogenesis of DKA and HHS. Alteration of fat, protein and carbohydrate metabolism leads to metabolic changes toward catabolic states and symptoms of polyuria, polydipsia, polyphagia, osmotic diuresis, severe hydration and, if not treated, coma and death. The hallmark of these events is the insulin deficient state and increased counterregulatory hormones. In HHS, in addition to the relative insulin deficiency and greater dehydration, there is also greater amount of hyperglycemia (secondary to lower intake of fluid) than in DKA. Although the mechanism for the lack of a significant amount of ketosis and acidemia in HHS (as compared with DKA) is not entirely clear, in one study the level of C-peptide (as an indication of pancreatic insulin reserve) was shown to be five- to ten-fold lower in DKA than in HHS [20]. This has been offered as a part of the explanation for the lack of ketonemia in HHS. Since the required amount of insulin for its antilipolytic action is about five- to ten-fold lower than for the glucose transport action [21], it follows that the larger amount of residual insulin (C-peptide) in HHS is sufficient to prevent lipolysis (thus no ketogenesis in HHS), but this amount of insulin is not enough to promote glucose transport and its metabolism, thus resulting in the hyperglycemia that one notes in HHS without severe ketonemia.(*From* Kitabchi, *et al.* [4]; with permission.)

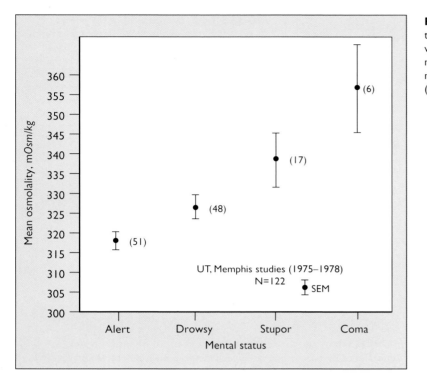

FIGURE 3-11. Calculated serum osmolality in 122 DKA patients with relation to mental status. About 1/3 of patients with hyperglycemic crises may present with altered mental status [6]. This can be correlated to serum osmolality but needs to be differentiated from various clinical conditions associated with altered mental status or coma (see Fig 3-7), which may be present in diabetic patients. (*From* Kitabchi and Fisher [6]; with permission.)

Treatment of Acute Diabetic Complications

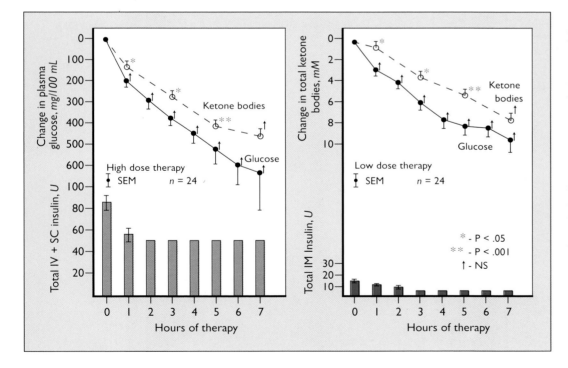

FIGURE 3-12. The efficacy of low dose versus conventional therapy of insulin for treatment of DKA. Treatment of hyperglycemic crises has undergone numerous modifications since the discovery of insulin. In the early decades of insulin discovery, and partially due to limited availability of insulin, low-dose therapy was the norm, but in subsequent decades, doses of insulin were modified from physiologic to pharmacologic and even suprapharmacologic doses of insulin until the mid-1970s. The initial observation of Alberti, *et al* [22] showed the effectiveness of low-dose insulin and gave impetus to the first prospective randomized study, which is summarized here [22]. This study confirms the similarity of the responses to low-dose and high-dose insulin in DKA without the disadvantages of greater hypoglycemia and hypokalemia associated with high-dose insulin therapy. (*From* Kitabchi, *et al.* [23]; with permission.)

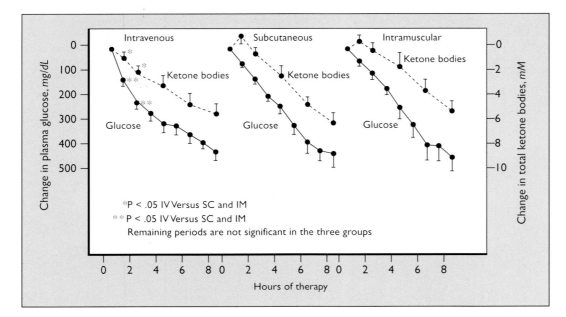

FIGURE 3-13. Comparison of the effects of randomized intravenous, subcutaneous, and intramuscular low-dose insulin regimens on changes in plasma glucose and total ketone bodies in patients with DKA (15 patients in each group). The low-dose insulin therapy was effective in lowering blood glucose in DKA therapy by any route of administration. (*From* Fisher, *et al.* [24]; with permission.)

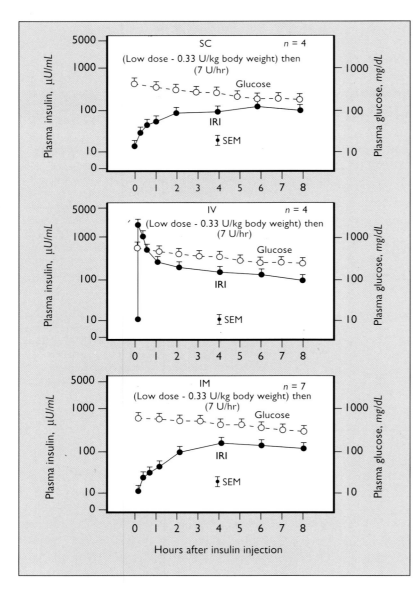

FIGURE 3-14. Comparison of the effect of low-dose insulin regimen (7 U/h) administered by subcutaneous (SC), intravenous (IV), and intramuscular (IM) injections on plasma immunoreactive insulin levels and plasma glucose decrements in three groups of DKA patients who had not previously been treated with insulin. However, IV insulin in these patients caused serum insulin to rise immediately to supraphysiologic levels, whereas SC and IM injections of the same amount of insulin provided low serum insulin concentrations, which reached near physiologic concentrations (postprandially) only after two to three hours. This low level of insulin may be the reason for the slow clearance of ketone bodies noted in Figure 3-13 for the IM and SC routes as compared to the IV route of the same amount of insulin injection (7 U/h). (*From* Kitabchi, *et al.* [25]; with permission.)

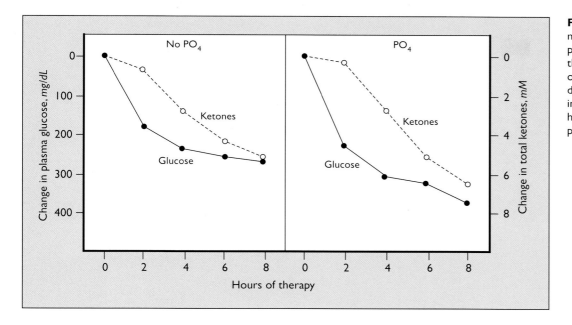

FIGURE 3-15. Another controversial issue in management of DKA prompted study on the use of phosphate in DKA. This study shows that phosphate therapy does not effect the clinical and biochemical outcomes (plasma glucose and ketone bodies) of low dose insulin therapy. However, the use of phosphate in DKA was associated with a certain degree of hypocalcemia. (*From* Fisher and Kitabchi [26]; with permission.)

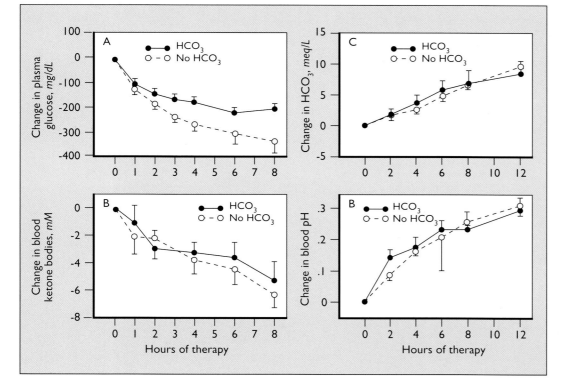

FIGURE 3-16. Another controversial issue in therapy of DKA has been the role of bicarbonate [27]. This prospective randomized study shows the effect of bicarbonate therapy on various recovery parameters of DKA indicating that bicarbonate did not alter outcomes of DKA therapy on hours of recovery from hyperglycemia, acidosis or hypocapnia [28]. There is therefore very little reason for the use of HCO_3 in DKA, particularly for a PH level that is ≥ 7 [27]. (*From* Fisher and Kitabchi [26]; with permission.)

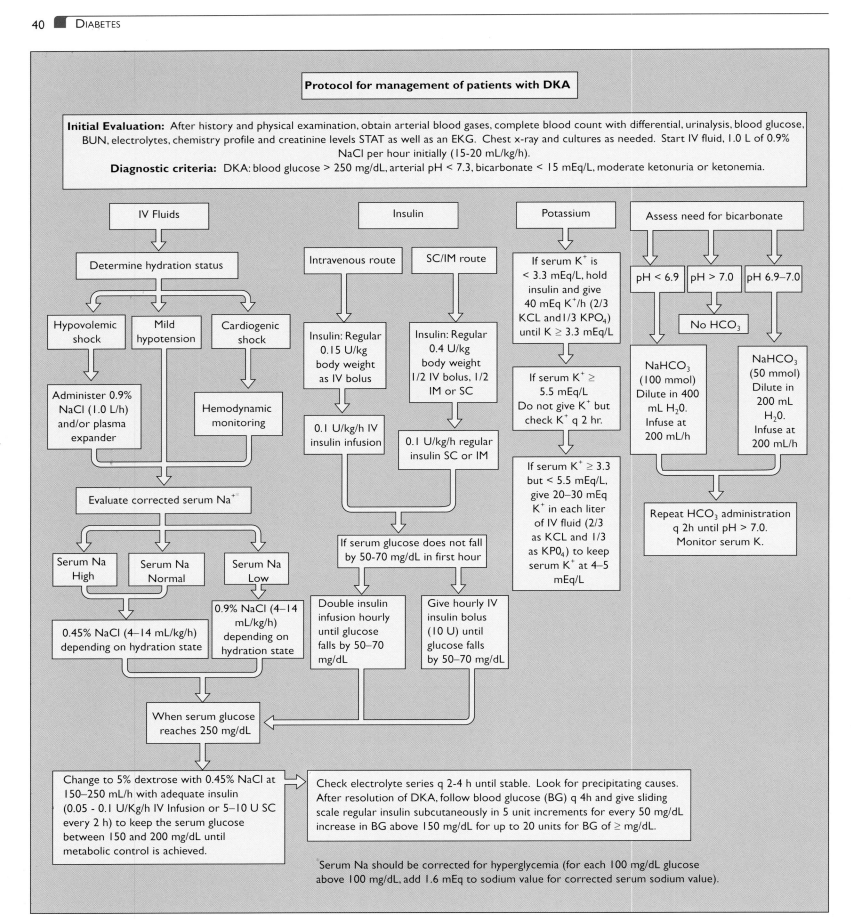

Protocol for management of patients with DKA

Initial Evaluation: After history and physical examination, obtain arterial blood gases, complete blood count with differential, urinalysis, blood glucose, BUN, electrolytes, chemistry profile and creatinine levels STAT as well as an EKG. Chest x-ray and cultures as needed. Start IV fluid, 1.0 L of 0.9% NaCl per hour initially (15-20 mL/kg/h).
Diagnostic criteria: DKA: blood glucose > 250 mg/dL, arterial pH < 7.3, bicarbonate < 15 mEq/L, moderate ketonuria or ketonemia.

IV Fluids

Determine hydration status

Hypovolemic shock | Mild hypotension | Cardiogenic shock

Administer 0.9% NaCl (1.0 L/h) and/or plasma expander

Hemodynamic monitoring

Evaluate corrected serum Na^{+*}

Serum Na High | Serum Na Normal | Serum Na Low

0.45% NaCl (4–14 mL/kg/h) depending on hydration state

0.9% NaCl (4–14 mL/kg/h) depending on hydration state

Insulin

Intravenous route | SC/IM route

Insulin: Regular 0.15 U/kg body weight as IV bolus

Insulin: Regular 0.4 U/kg body weight 1/2 IV bolus, 1/2 IM or SC

0.1 U/kg/h IV insulin infusion

0.1 U/kg/h regular insulin SC or IM

If serum glucose does not fall by 50-70 mg/dL in first hour

Double insulin infusion hourly until glucose falls by 50–70 mg/dL

Give hourly IV insulin bolus (10 U) until glucose falls by 50–70 mg/dL

Potassium

If serum K$^+$ is < 3.3 mEq/L, hold insulin and give 40 mEq K$^+$/h (2/3 KCL and 1/3 KPO$_4$) until K ≥ 3.3 mEq/L

If serum K$^+$ ≥ 5.5 mEq/L Do not give K$^+$ but check K$^+$ q 2 hr.

If serum K$^+$ ≥ 3.3 but < 5.5 mEq/L, give 20–30 mEq K$^+$ in each liter of IV fluid (2/3 as KCL and 1/3 as KPO$_4$) to keep serum K$^+$ at 4–5 mEq/L

Assess need for bicarbonate

pH < 6.9 | pH > 7.0 | pH 6.9–7.0

No HCO$_3$

NaHCO$_3$ (100 mmol) Dilute in 400 mL H$_2$O. Infuse at 200 mL/h

NaHCO$_3$ (50 mmol) Dilute in 200 mL H$_2$O. Infuse at 200 mL/h

Repeat HCO$_3$ administration q 2h until pH > 7.0. Monitor serum K.

When serum glucose reaches 250 mg/dL

Change to 5% dextrose with 0.45% NaCl at 150–250 mL/h with adequate insulin (0.05 - 0.1 U/Kg/h IV Infusion or 5–10 U SC every 2 h) to keep the serum glucose between 150 and 200 mg/dL until metabolic control is achieved.

Check electrolyte series q 2-4 h until stable. Look for precipitating causes. After resolution of DKA, follow blood glucose (BG) q 4h and give sliding scale regular insulin subcutaneously in 5 unit increments for every 50 mg/dL increase in BG above 150 mg/dL for up to 20 units for BG of ≥ mg/dL.

*Serum Na should be corrected for hyperglycemia (for each 100 mg/dL glucose above 100 mg/dL, add 1.6 mEq to sodium value for corrected serum sodium value).

FIGURE 3-17. This figure provides step by step methods for therapeutic management of patients with DKA. Important steps besides use of insulin is hydration and frequent monitoring of such patients [4,6,13]. (*From* Kitabchi, *et al.* [8]; with permission.)

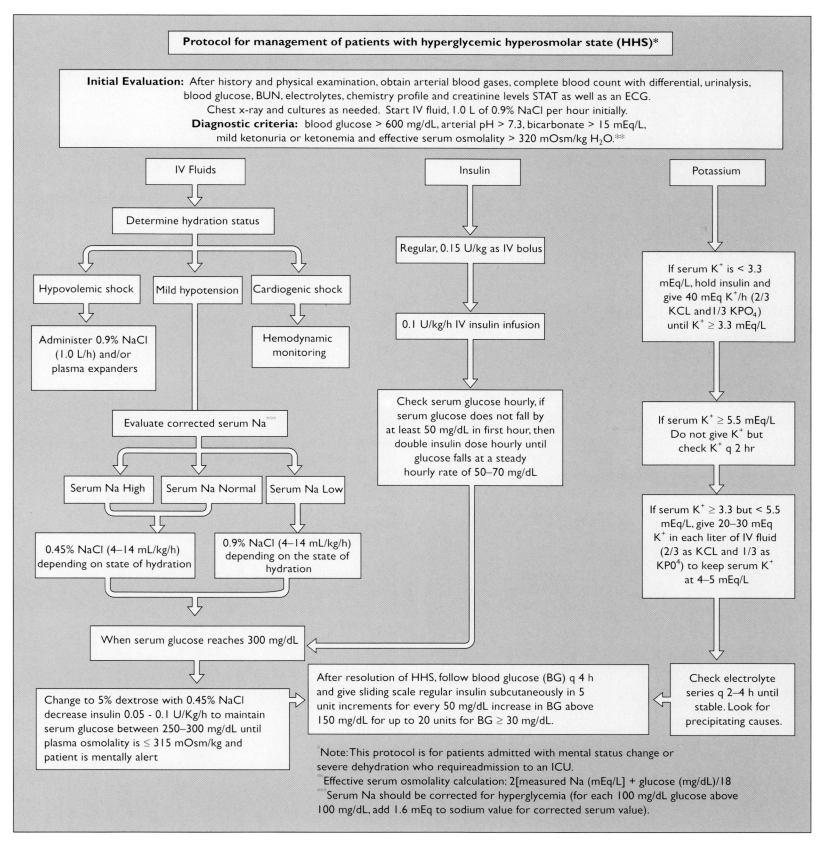

Protocol for management of patients with hyperglycemic hyperosmolar state (HHS)*

Initial Evaluation: After history and physical examination, obtain arterial blood gases, complete blood count with differential, urinalysis, blood glucose, BUN, electrolytes, chemistry profile and creatinine levels STAT as well as an ECG. Chest x-ray and cultures as needed. Start IV fluid, 1.0 L of 0.9% NaCl per hour initially.
Diagnostic criteria: blood glucose > 600 mg/dL, arterial pH > 7.3, bicarbonate > 15 mEq/L, mild ketonuria or ketonemia and effective serum osmolality > 320 mOsm/kg H_2O.**

IV Fluids

Insulin

Potassium

Determine hydration status

Regular, 0.15 U/kg as IV bolus

If serum K^+ is < 3.3 mEq/L, hold insulin and give 40 mEq K^+/h (2/3 KCL and 1/3 KPO_4) until K^+ ≥ 3.3 mEq/L

Hypovolemic shock

Mild hypotension

Cardiogenic shock

Administer 0.9% NaCl (1.0 L/h) and/or plasma expanders

Hemodynamic monitoring

0.1 U/kg/h IV insulin infusion

Evaluate corrected serum Na⁺

Serum Na High

Serum Na Normal

Serum Na Low

Check serum glucose hourly, if serum glucose does not fall by at least 50 mg/dL in first hour, then double insulin dose hourly until glucose falls at a steady hourly rate of 50–70 mg/dL

If serum K^+ ≥ 5.5 mEq/L Do not give K^+ but check K^+ q 2 hr

0.45% NaCl (4–14 mL/kg/h) depending on state of hydration

0.9% NaCl (4–14 mL/kg/h) depending on the state of hydration

If serum K^+ ≥ 3.3 but < 5.5 mEq/L, give 20–30 mEq K^+ in each liter of IV fluid (2/3 as KCL and 1/3 as KPO_4) to keep serum K^+ at 4–5 mEq/L

When serum glucose reaches 300 mg/dL

Change to 5% dextrose with 0.45% NaCl decrease insulin 0.05 - 0.1 U/Kg/h to maintain serum glucose between 250–300 mg/dL until plasma osmolality is ≤ 315 mOsm/kg and patient is mentally alert

After resolution of HHS, follow blood glucose (BG) q 4 h and give sliding scale regular insulin subcutaneously in 5 unit increments for every 50 mg/dL increase in BG above 150 mg/dL for up to 20 units for BG ≥ 30 mg/dL.

Check electrolyte series q 2–4 h until stable. Look for precipitating causes.

Note: This protocol is for patients admitted with mental status change or severe dehydration who require admission to an ICU.
*Effective serum osmolality calculation: 2[measured Na (mEq/L) + glucose (mg/dL)/18
**Serum Na should be corrected for hyperglycemia (for each 100 mg/dL glucose above 100 mg/dL, add 1.6 mEq to sodium value for corrected serum value).

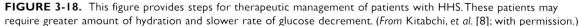

FIGURE 3-18. This figure provides steps for therapeutic management of patients with HHS. These patients may require greater amount of hydration and slower rate of glucose decrement. (*From* Kitabchi, *et al.* [8]; with permission.)

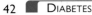

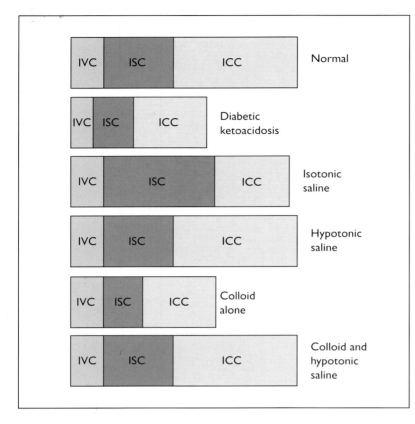

FIGURE 3-19. The use of hypotonic versus isotonic saline and plasma expanders has been the subject of controversy. This figure demonstrates the effect of these solutions in various cellular compartments. The diagram depicts the decreased intravascular (IVC), interstitial (ISC), and intracellular (ICC) compartments present in patients with diabetic ketoacidosis, as compared with normal subjects. Subsequent panels show the effects of fluid resuscitation of DKA with different solutions. Isotonic solutions replete only IVC and ISC compartments, whereas hypotonic solutions replete all compartments. However, larger volumes of hypotonic solutions are required to produce equivalent increases in IVC. Colloid alone is restricted to the IVC; therefore, combined use of colloid plus hypotonic solution can lead to a rapid increase in IVC, followed by more gradual replacement of the other compartments. It is also important to remember that hydration in DKA and HHS dilutes concentrations of the stress hormones and thus make peripheral tissues more sensitive to lower doses of insulin [31]. (*From* Hillman [30]; with permission.)

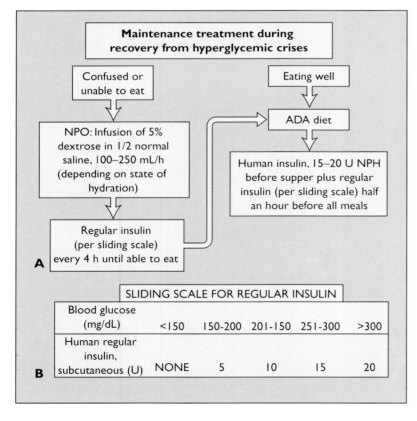

FIGURE 3-20. This figure depicts the procedure proposed for the use of insulin after remission of hyperglycemic crises (**A**). The use of sliding scale regular insulin based on blood glucose is recommended every four hours for those patients who are on IV therapy and are not eating (**B**). This is to prevent relapse of the DKA state, as circulating level of insulin in low dose insulin protocol is very low and decreases precipitously with cessation of insulin injection.

Suggested DKA/HHS Flowsheet											
Date											
Mental Status*											
Temperature											
Pulse											
Respiration/Depth**											
Blood Pressure											
Serum Glucose mg/dL											
Serum "ketones"											
Urine "ketones"											
Serum Na+ mEq/L											
Serum K+ mEq/L											
Serum Cl- mEq/L											
Serum HCO3- mEq/L											
Serum BUN mg/dL											
Effective Osmolality 2 [measured Na mEq/L]+ glucose mg/dL/18											
Anion gap											
pH venous (V) arterial (A)											
pO2											
pCO2											
O2 SAT											
Units past hour											
Route											
0.45% NaCl (mL) past hour											
0.9% NaCl (mL) past hour											
5% Dextrose (mL) past hour											
KCL (mEq) past hour											
PO4 (mmol) past hour											
Other											
Urine (mL)											
Other											

Weight: 0° ___ 24° ___

*A - Alert D-Drowsy S-Stuporous C-Comatose
**D-Deep S-Shallow N-Normal

FIGURE 3-21. Flow sheet to document serial changes in laboratory/clinical values and supplementary measures during recovery from DKA. (*From* Kitabchi, et al. [8].)

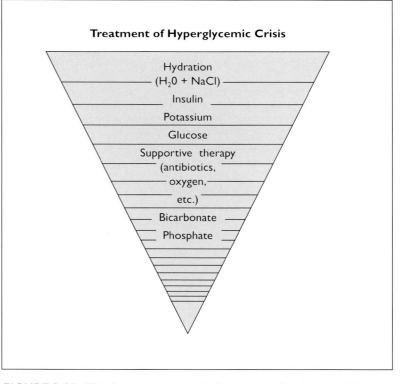

FIGURE 3-22. This figure summarizes the importance of various modalities of therapy and their treatment of hyperglycemic crises. The additional caveat on importance and frequent monitoring of patients by health care providers cannot by over emphasized. It is also important to mention that precipitating causes of these crises must be sought while patient is being managed and that inquiry into educational program, as discussed earlier, be initiated for prevention of future recurrence of such events. (*From* Kitabchi, et al. [32]).

References

1. Turnebum A: Of the causes and signs of acute and chronic disease, 1554. Reynolds TF, translator. London: William Pickering, 1837.
2. Faich GA, Fishbein HA, Ellis SE. The epidemiology of diabetic acidosis: a population-based study. .Am J Epidemiol 1983, 117:551.
3. Fishbein HA, Palumbo PJ: Acute metabolic complications in diabetes. Diabetes in America (National Diabetes Data Group). National Institute of Health, (NIH Publication No. 95-1468), 1995, pp 283–291.
4. Kitabchi AE, Umpierrez GE, Murphy MB, Barrett EJ, Kreisberg RA, Malone JI, Wall BM: Management of hyperglycemic crises in patients with diabetes mellitus. Diabetes Care. (In Press)
5. Umpierrez GE, Kelly JP, Navarrete JE, Casals MMC, Kitabchi AE: Hyperglycemic crises in urban blacks. Arch Int Med 1997, 157:669–675.
6. Kitabchi AE, Fisher JN: Insulin therapy of diabetic ketoacidosis: Physiologic versus pharmacologic doses of insulin and their routes of administration. In (Brownlee M, ed). Handbook of Diabetes Mellitus, vol 5, New York: Garland ATPM Press, 1981, 95–149.
7. Carroll P, Matz R: Uncontrolled diabetes mellitus in adults: experience in treating diabetic ketoacidosis and hyperosmolar coma with low-dose insulin and uniform treatment regimen. Diabetes Care 1983, 6:579–585.
8. Kitabchi AE, Fisher JN, Murphy MB, Rumbak MJ: Diabetic ketoacidosis and the hyperglycemic hyperosmolar nonketotic state. In: Joslin's Diabetes Mellitus. 13th ed. Kahn CR, Weir GC, eds. Lea & Febiger, Philadelphia, 1994, pp 738–770.
9. Javor KA, Kotsanos JG, McDonald RC, Baron AD, Kesterson JG, Tierney WM: Diabetic ketoacidosis charges relative to medical charges of adult patients with type 1 diabetes. Diabetes Care 1997, 20:349–354.
10. Orci L: A fresh look at the interrelationships within the islets of langerhans. In: Diabetes Research Today. Meeting of the Minkowski prize-Winners. Symposium Capri. FK Schattauer Verlag. Stuttgart. 1976, 135–151.
11. Orci L, Baetens D, Rufener C, et al.: Hypertrophy and hyperplasia of somatostatin-containing D-cells in diabetes. Proc Nat Acad Sci 1976, 73:1338–1342.
12. Yoon JW, Austin M, Onodera T, Notkins AI: Isolation of a virus from the pancreas of a child with diabetic ketoacidosis. N Engl J Med 1979, 300:1173–1179.
13. Kitabchi AE, Wall BM: Diabetic ketoacidosis. In: Medical Clinics of North America 1995, 79:9–37.

14. Morris LE, Kitabchi AE: Coma in the diabetic. In: Schnatz JD, ed. Diabetes mellitus: problems in management. Menlo Park, CA: Addison-Wesley Publishing. 1982, 234–251.

15. DeFronzo RA, Matsuda M, Barrett E: Diabetic ketoacidosis. A combined metabolic-nephrologic approach to therapy. *Diabetes Review* 1994, 2:209–238.

16. Miles JM, Rizza RA, Haymond MW, Gerich JE: Effects of acute insulin deficiency on glucose and ketone body turnover in man: evidence for the primacy overproduction of glucose and ketone bodies in the genesis of diabetic ketoacidosis. *Diabetes* 1980, 29:926–930.

17. McGarry JD, Woeltje KF, Kuwajima M, Foster DW: Regulation of keto-genesis and the renaissance of carnitine palmitoyl transferase. *Diab Metab Rev* 1989, 5:271–284.

18. Kitabchi AE, Rumbak MJ: Management of diabetic emergencies. *Hosp Pract* 1989, 24:129–160.

19. Myer C, Stumvolle M, Nadkarni V, et al.: Abnormal renal and hepatic glucose metabolism in type 2 dibetes mellitus. *J Clin Invest* 1998, 102:619–624.

20. Chupin M, Charbonnel B, Chupin F: C-peptide levels in ketoacidosis and in hyperosmolar non-ketotic diabetic coma. *Acta Diabet* 1981, 18:123–128.

21. Schade DS, Eaton RP: Dose response to insulin in man: Differential effects on glucose and ketone body regulation. *J Clin Endocrinol Metab* 1977, 44:1038–1053.

22. Alberti KGMM, Hockaday TDR, Turner RC: Small doses of intramuscular insulin in the treatment of diabetic "coma." *Lancet* 1973, 5:515–522.

23. Kitabchi AE, Ayyagari V, Guerra SMO, Medical House Staff: The efficacy of low dose versus conventional therapy of insulin for treatment of diabetic ketoacidosis. *Ann Intern Med* 1976, 84:633–638.

24. Fisher JN, Shahshahani MN, Kitabchi AE: Diabetic ketoacidosis: low-dose insulin therapy by various routes. *N Engl J Med* 1977, 297:238–247.

25. Kitabchi AE, Young RT, Sacks HS, Morris L: Diabetic ketoacidosis: reappraisal of therapeutic approach. *Ann Rev Med* 1979, 30:339–357.

26. Fisher JN, Kitabchi AE: A randomized study of phosphate therapy in the treatment of diabetic ketoacidosis. *J Clin Endocrinol Metab* 1983, 57:177–180.

27. Matz R: Diabetic acidosis: rationale for not using bicarbonate. *NY State J Med* 1977, 76:1299–1303.

28. Morris LR, Murphy MB, Kitabchi AE: Bicarbonate therapy in severe diabetic ketoacidosis. *Ann Intern Med* 1986, 105:836–840.

29. Barnes HV, Cohen RD, Kitabchi AE, Murphy MB: When is Bicarbinate Appropriate in Treating Metabolic Acidosis, Including Diabetic Acidosis? In *Debates in Medicine.* Gitnick G, et al. eds.. Chicago: YearBook Medical Publishers; 1990:200–233.

30. Hillman K: Fluid resuscitation in diabetic emergencies: a reappraisal. *Intensive Care Med* 1987, 13:4–8.

31. Waldhausl W, Kleinberger G, Korn A, et al.: Severe hyperglycemia: effects of hydration on endocrine derangements and blood glucose concentration. *Diabetes* 1979, 28:577–584

32. Kitabchi AE, Matteri R, Murphy MB: Optimum insulin delivery in diabetic ketoacidosis (DKA) and hyperglycemic hyperosmolar nonketotic coma (HHNC) *Diabetes Care* 1982, 5:78–87.

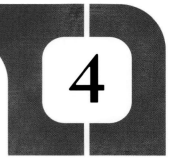

Type 1 Diabetes

Mark A. Atkinson

Type 1 diabetes is a chronic disorder resulting from autoimmune destruction of the insulin-producing pancreatic β cells. The epidemiologic features of type 1 diabetes are described, and the possible contributions of genetics and environment to its development are illustrated. In addition, based on improved knowledge of the immunopathogenesis of this disorder, we report on work that holds promise for future interventions aimed at prevention.

The exact cause or causes of type 1 diabetes remain unclear [1]. It occurs most frequently in whites of Northern European descent, with more than a fortyfold difference observed in disease incidence rates based on geographic location. Environmental factors such as diet, stress, and viruses have been proposed to play a modifying and perhaps even a primary role in the development of type 1 diabetes. Thus, these factors may contribute to its varying prevalence. The disorder was once termed *juvenile diabetes* and thought to occur predominantly in persons under 18 years of age. However, more recent evidence suggests that the number of new cases may be equal in those over and under 30 years of age.

Susceptibility to type 1 diabetes is inherited and increased risk is associated with being a first-degree relative to a person with a diabetic proband. However, approximately 85% of new cases show no such familial lineage. The major genetic region associated with predisposition to the disease is that encoding genes for the highly polymorphic human leukocyte antigens (HLAs). However, nearly 20 other loci have been proposed as contributing from 50% to 70% of the total genetic susceptibility.

Multiple lines of evidence support the theory that type 1 diabetes has an autoimmune nature. The evidence includes the aforementioned association with HLA, presence of a lymphocytic infiltrate within the pancreatic islet cells (*ie,* insulitis), and expression of islet reactive autoantibodies. Although once viewed as an acutely developing illness, today it is known that the natural history of type 1 diabetes is that of a chronic autoimmune process. In most patients the disease exists for months to years in a preclinical asymptomatic phase. Many improvements in our knowledge of the pathogenesis of type 1 diabetes derive from investigations of two spontaneous animal models for the disease (*ie,* BioBreeding rats and nonobese diabetic mice).

Although it remains unclear which immune system component or mechanism plays the major role in β-cell destruction, most studies point toward the cellular immune system as providing a key role. Furthermore, multiple interrelated flaws in immunoregulation may underlie the failure to form a tolerance to self-antigens that results in type 1 diabetes. A large number of islet cell antigens have been associated with type 1 diabetes. Their biochemical identification has led to improved markers for predicting future cases and provided the potential to design antigen-specific therapies aimed at prevention. Numerous intervention studies have been directed toward patients with new-onset type 1 diabetes (predominantly involving immunosuppression), with disappointing degrees of success in terms of disease reversal. Improvements have been made in the ability to predict future cases of type 1 diabetes and assess metabolic activity. Therefore, the more recent clinical trials have sought to use alternatives such as nicotinomide and insulin that are much less likely to have such serious side effects as do immunosuppresive agents, thus providing a safe and effective means of disease prevention.

Clinical Description

COMPARISON OF CLINICAL, GENETIC, AND IMMUNOLOGIC FEATURES OF TYPE I AND TYPE II DIABETES

Characteristic	Type I	Type II
Onset	Abrupt	Progressive
Endogenous insulin	Low to absent	Normal, elevated, or depressed
Ketosis	Common	Rare
Age at onset	Any age	Vast majority in adults
Body mass	Usually nonobese	Obese or nonobese
Treatment	Insulin	Diet, oral hypoglycemics, insulin
Family history	10–15%	30%
Twin concordance	30–50%	70–90%
Human leukocyte antigen (HLA) association	HLA-DR, HLA-DQ	Unrelated
Autoantibodies	Present in most (>85%)	Absent, except in patients with coincident Type I disease

FIGURE 4-1. The terms applied to the subgroup of disorders known collectively as diabetes mellitus are useful. However, they often break down in practice owing to confusion regarding the age at diagnosis or to an overlap or absence of the indicated features normally associated with the specific disorder. In many instances, the terms *type I diabetes* and *insulin-dependent diabetes* are used interchangeably, as are the terms *type 2 diabetes* and *non–insulin-dependent diabetes*. However, enthusiasm has grown for the terms *type I diabetes* or *immune-mediated diabetes* (IMD) to identify the forms of diabetes involving an autoimmune destruction of the insulin-producing pancreatic β cells.

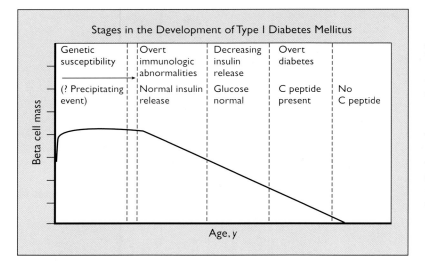

FIGURE 4-2. Five stages of type 1 diabetes mellitus. The natural history of type 1 diabetes has been modeled into a disease comprised of five stages. Stage 1 includes genetic susceptibility (major histocompatibility complex [MHC] and non-MHC) with intact β-cell mass. It is thought that stage 2 follows an environmental insult in the first months to years of life. At that time, insulitis is initiated and, owing to a genetic predisposition that does not properly regulate immune responses, the process of β-cell destruction begins. Autoantibodies to islet cell antigens develop, marking the autoimmune disease process; however, no measurable β-cell dysfunction occurs at this stage. In stage 3, a gradual decline in β-cell mass occurs, with the slope being highly variable between persons (ie, months to years). Incipient β cell damage is first detectable as an abnormal intravenous glucose tolerance test with a deficient first-phase insulin response. In stage 4, an advanced degree of β-cell damage, hyperglycemia symptomatic of type 1 diabetes onset (with minimal C peptide), and exogenous insulin dependence occur. With complete β-cell destruction in stage 5, the C peptide becomes undetectable and autoantibody markers of disease disappear. (*Adapted from* Eisenbarth [2].)

Epidemiology

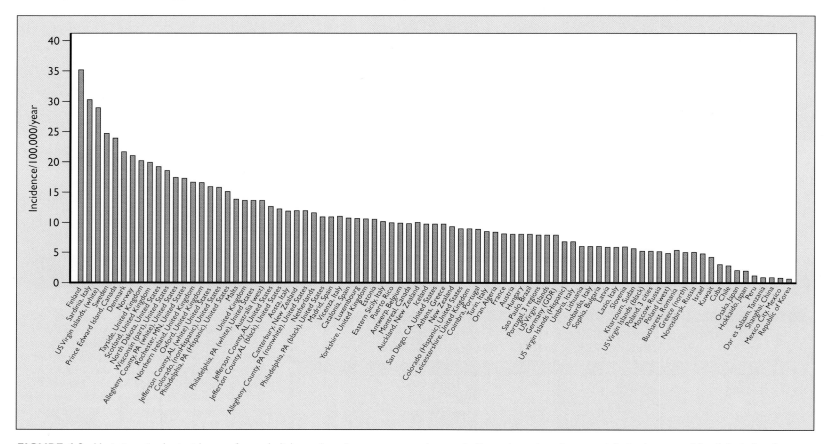

FIGURE 4-3. Variations in the incidence of type 1 diabetes based on geographic location. This disease predominantly affects populations with a substantial white genetic admixture. In Finland the incidence rate approaches 40 cases per 100,000 persons per year, whereas in Korea and Mexico the rate approximates 0.6 per 100,000 per year. In Europe the incidence is highest in the northern-most regions and generally declines in countries that lie in the south. Exceptions do exist, especially in the case of Sardinia, Italy, where the incidence rate approximates that of Finland. Furthermore, the disease incidence in Iceland is only one third that of Finland. Multiple studies suggest a continuing increase in the incidence of the disease, reporting regional increases of 6% to 20% per decade. (*Adapted from* Karvonen *et al.* [3]; with permission.)

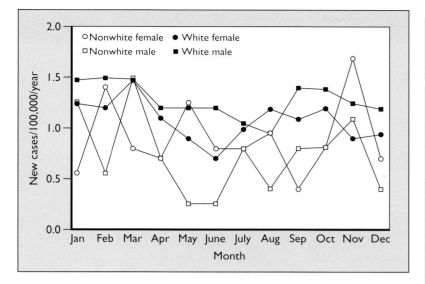

FIGURE 4-4. Variations in the frequency of diagnosing type I diabetes as a function of season. Data from Allegheny County, Pennsylvania, show a decline in newly diagnosed cases in the summer months. Additional studies confirm and expand on this finding, with reports of bimodal peaks in the late Winter and early Spring. Historically, such findings often have been considered as supporting an environmental agent in the pathogenesis of this disease. (*From* Laporte *et al.* [4]; with permission.)

ENVIRONMENTAL AGENTS AND LIFE-STYLE PRACTICES PROPORTED TO INFLUENCE THE INCIDENCE OF HUMAN TYPE I DIABETES

Class	Specific Agent
Viruses	Coxsackie B
	Cytomegalovirus
	Echo
	Encephalomyocarditis
	Epstein-Barr
	Mumps
	Rotoviruses
	Rubella (congenital)
Diet	Cow's milk and cow's milk–based infant formulas
	Caffeine
	Nitrates (*N*-nitroso compounds)
	Duration of breast-feeding
Life-style	Exposure to β-cell toxins (eg, vacor)
	Stress
	Quantitative or qualitative exposure to viral and bacterial agents

FIGURE 4-5. Numerous epidemiologic studies and case reports have associated viral infections or local epidemics with type I diabetes. Likewise, epidemiologists have provided conflicting reports associating specific dietary practices with the disorder. However, when these practices are identified, their association (in terms of relative risk) usually is modest. Indeed, the collective literature to date has not demonstrated a diabetogenic agent that would represent a single major agent responsible for type I diabetes.

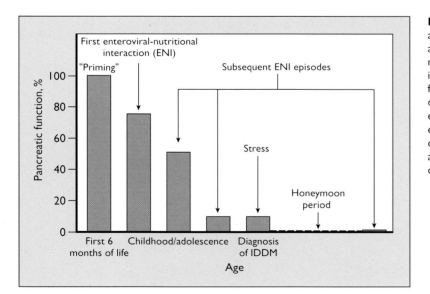

FIGURE 4-6. Multihit nature of action in type I diabetes. Thus far, no single agent has been associated exclusively with the disorder. Therefore, recent models associating environmental agents with type I diabetes have proposed a multihit nature of action. The primary "triggers" for type I diabetes could be those involving a yet to be identified interaction between an enterovirus and a nutritional factor. Subsequent enteroviral-nutritional interactions could lead to further destruction of the pancreas. This situation would go unnoticed until there is not enough insulin-producing capability to respond to stress. Indeed, a stressful life event (*eg,* trauma, other infection, pubescent growth spurt, and pregnancy) could cause a person to exceed the insulin-producing capacity of the pancreas and lead to the clinical diagnosis of type I diabetes. IDDM—insulin-dependent diabetes mellitus. (*Adapted from* Hawkins [5].)

Genetics

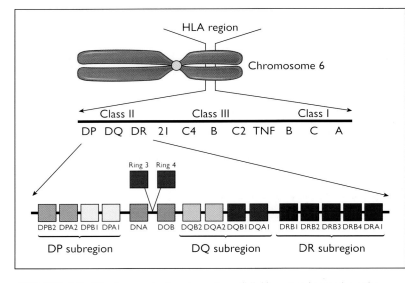

FIGURE 4-7. The human leukocyte antigen (HLA) region located on the short arm of chromosome 6. This region is approximately 3.5 centimorgans long and includes classes I, II, and III loci. Class I gene products (ie, HLA-A, HLA-B, and HLA-C) are expressed on all nucleated cells and serve as the classic transplantation antigens. These proteins present antigenic peptides to CD8+ T cells. Class II gene products are restricted in expression to antigen-presenting cells (eg, macrophages, dendritic cells, and B cells) and function to present peptides to CD4+ T cells. Class III gene products include complement proteins (eg, B, C2, and C4) and tumor necrosis factor.

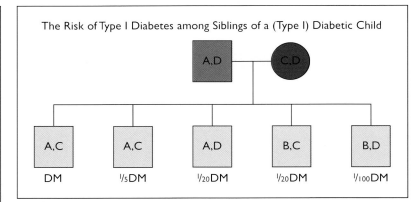

FIGURE 4-8. Familial risk of developing Type I diabetes as a function of the relationship to the disease proband. The prevalence of disease (DM) is 30% to 50% in twins (not shown), 20% in human leukocyte antigen (HLA–) identical siblings (patient A,C), 5% in haploidentical siblings (A,D; B,C), and 1% in non-identical siblings (B,D). The mode of inheritance remains an enigma. Both dominant and recessive patterns of inheritance have been proposed; however, neither model adequately addresses Type I diabetes. This line of investigation is further complicated by the potential interactions between genes and environmental factors, as well as evidence of the polygenic nature (ie, currently 20 additional loci) of the disorder. Furthermore, the risk of developing diabetes is higher in offspring of a father with Type I diabetes than in offspring of a mother with the disorder. The life-time risk for first-degree relatives is 5% to 8%. The probability is shown relative to inheritance of HLA haplotypes, which is indicated as A, B, C, D.

FIGURE 4-9. Note that these associations are representative of those most often observed in whites with a strong Northern European genetic influence. Interestingly, variance in susceptibility and resistance of human leukocyte antigen (HLA) types have been noted with Type I diabetes in patients of different ethnic admixtures, especially those of Asian descent. Approximately 95% of whites with Type I diabetes have either HLA-DR3 or HLA-DR4. However, susceptibility appears to reside predominantly in the HLA-DQ alleles under influence of HLA-DR. Furthermore, depending on the specific haplotype inherited, risk can be modified by the presence of a strong susceptibility or resistance allele, eg, DQB1*0602.

HLA-DR AND HLA-DQ TYPES AND THE RISK FOR TYPE I DIABETES

Risk	Genotype
Susceptible	DR3
	DR4
	DR1 (<DR3 or DR4)
	DQA1*0301
	DQA1*0501
	DQB1*0201
	DQB1*0302
Resistant	DR2
	DR5 (< DR2)
	DQB1*0602
	DQB1*0301

LOCATION AND MAXIMUM LOD SCORE FOR REPORTED SUSCEPTIBILITY INTERVALS FOR HUMAN TYPE I DIABETES

Loci	Region	Maximum LOD Score
IDDM1	6p21	34.0
IDDM2	11p15	2.8
IDDM3	15q26	2.5
IDDM4	11q13	3.9
IDDM5	6q25	4.5
IDDM6	18q	2.8
IDDM7	2q33	1.0
IDDM8	6q27	3.6
IDDM9	3q	1.1
IDDM10	10p13-q11	4.7
IDDM11	14q24-q31	4.0
IDDM12	2q33	0.9
IDDM13	2q33	3.3
IDDM15	6q21	4.2
D14s70-D14s276	14q12-q21	2.0
D16s515-D16S520	16q22-q24	3.4
D19S247-D19S226	19p13	1.7
D19S225	19q13	1.6
D1S1644-AGT	1q	2.8

FIGURE 4-10. Studies over the past 2 decades have suggested a large number of genes or genetic intervals may be implicated in the pathogenesis of insulin-dependent diabetes mellitus (IDDM) [6,7]. These genes are referred to as *susceptibility genes* that, by definition, increase or modify disease risk. Susceptibility genes are neither necessary nor sufficient for disease development. Therefore, some gene carriers may never develop the disease, whereas some noncarriers may develop IDDM. The IDDM1 loci (containing the HLA-DR and HLA-DQ regions) is the only major susceptibility interval, accounting for 30% to 50% of the total aggregated risk for IDDM.

Pathology

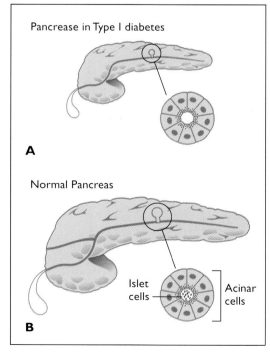

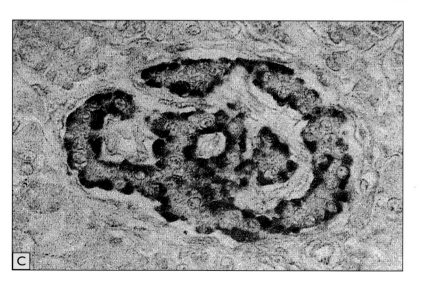

FIGURE 4-11. (see Color Plate) The pancreas of a person with type 1 diabetes (**A**) is often smaller and weighs less (ie, approximately 50% of total organ weight and 30% of endocrine weight) than its healthy counterpart (**B**). This difference is a consequence of the progressive atrophy of exocrine tissue that comprises about 98% of the total pancreatic volume. **C** and **D** demonstrate the pathology of pancreatic specimens from a patient with recent-onset type 1 diabetes. *Panel C,* Insulin-deficient islet stained for glucagon, somatostatin, and pancreatic polypeptide. All endocrine cells appear to have been stained, confirming the lack of β cells.

(*Continued on next page*)

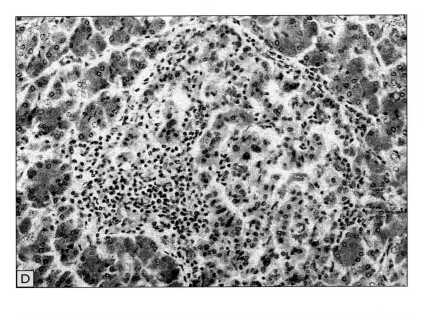

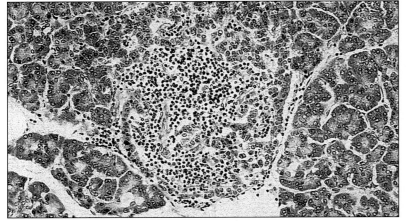

FIGURE 4-11. *(Continued) Panel D,* Insulitis. A chronic inflammatory cell infiltrate is centered on the islet. Insulitis is an elusive lesion to detect in the human pancreas, with only rare detection after 1 year of overt type 1 diabetes. With prolonged duration of disease, a progressive distortion of islet architecture develops with a tendency for α and δ cells to leave the islet and spread as single cells into the exocrine parenchyma. (Part *C,* immuno-alkaline phosphatase stain, ×1150.) (Part *D,* hematoxylin-eosin stain, ×300.) (Parts C and D *from* Foulis [8]; with permission.)

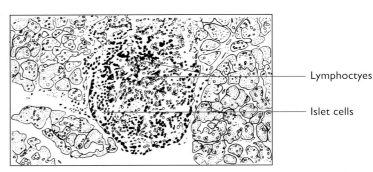

FIGURE 4-12. *(see* Color Plate) Islet of a patient recently diagnosed with type 1 diabetes demonstrating a diffuse lymphocytic infiltration (insulitis) with onset of atrophy of the islet cords. (Hematoxylin-eosin stain, ×300.) *(From* Foulis [8]; with permission.)

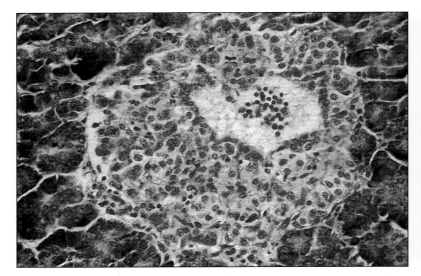

FIGURE 4-13. *(see* Color Plate) Pathology of a regenerating islet in the pancreas of a patient recently diagnosed with type 1 diabetes. Newly formed islet cells are derived from the epithelium of a duct. Lymphocytes are present in the lumen of the duct and in some places at the periphery. Evidence of such regeneration is rare in the pancreatic organs of patients with type 1 diabetes and usually limited to those who die shortly after disease onset. (Hematoxylin-eosin stain, × 400.) *(From* Foulis [8]; with permission.)

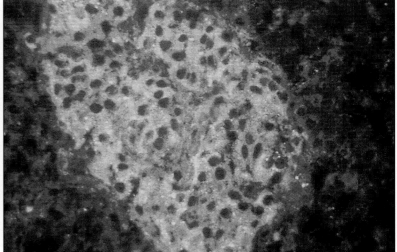

FIGURE 4-14. *(see* Color Plate) Islet cell autoantibodies (ICA). ICAs are present in the serum of approximately 75% of persons at the onset of type 1 diabetes versus 0.4% of healthy persons. The first autoantibody ascribed to type 1 diabetes, the presence of ICAs is identified by indirect immunofluorescence assay using human blood group O pancreas. ICAs specific for β cells have been identified. However, the autoantibodies react with all cells within the islet, including those that secrete insulin (β cells), glucagon (α cells), somatostatin cells (δ cells), and pancreatic polypeptide (PP cells). Autoantigens thus far ascribed to be responsible for the ICA reaction include sialoglycolipids, glutamic acid decarboxylase, and ICA512/IA-2.

AUTOANTIBODY MARKERS OF ISLET IMMUNITY IN HUMAN TYPE I DIABETES

Described in the 1970s
  Islet cell cytoplasmic autoantibodies
  Islet cell surface autoantibodies
Described in the 1980s
  64kD autoantibodies
  Carboxypeptidase-H autoantibodies
  Heat shock protein autoantibodies
  Insulin autoantibodies (IAA)
  Insulin receptor autoantibodies
  Proinsulin autoantibodies
Described in the 1990s
  37kd/40kD tryptic fragment autoantibodies
  52kD rat insulinoma (RIN) autoantibodies
  51kD aromatic-L-amino-acid decarboxylase autoantibodies
  128kD autoantibodies
  152kD autoantibodies
  Chymotrypsinogen-related 30 kD pancreatic autoantibodies
  DNA topoisomerase II autoantibodies
  Glucose transporter 2 autoantibodies
  Glutamic acid decarboxylase 65 autoantibodies
  Glutamic acid decarboxylase 67 autoantibodies
  Glima 38 autoantibodies
  Glycolipid autoantibodies
  GM2-1 islet ganglioside autoantibodies
  ICA512/IA-2 autoantibodies
  IA-2 autoantibodies
  Phogrin autoantibodies

FIGURE 4-15. Since the first description of islet cell autoantibodies (ICAs) in 1974 (see Fig. 4-14), many new autoantibody markers of anti-islet immunity have been identified in persons with type I diabetes. In addition to their presence at disease onset, many of these markers have proved useful in identifying persons in the presymptomatic period, months to years before the clinical onset of type I diabetes. Of these, four markers have gained the most acceptance owing to scientific confirmation, high frequency of expression, and superior disease sensitivity and specificity: ICA, insulin autoantibodies (IAA), glutamic acid decarboxylase, and IA-2 autoantibodies. (Information courtesy of W. Winter, University of Florida)

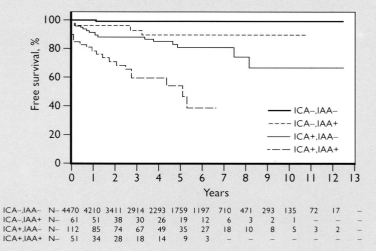

	N–												
ICA–,IAA–	N– 4470	4210	3411	2914	2293	1759	1197	710	471	293	135	72	17	–
ICA–,IAA+	N– 61	51	38	30	26	19	12	6	3	2	1	–	–	–
ICA+,IAA–	N– 112	85	74	67	49	35	27	18	10	8	5	3	2	–
ICA+,IAA+	N– 51	34	28	18	14	9	3	–	–	–	–	–	–	–

FIGURE 4-16. Using autoantibodies to islet cell autoantigens to predict future cases of type I diabetes. A life-table analysis is shown. This analysis indicates the probability of remaining disease-free stratified by the appearance of islet cell cytoplasmic autoantibodies (ICA) and insulin autoantibodies (IAA) in relatives of probands with the disease. The number of relatives followed since identification of the autoantibody is displayed at the bottom for each group. As can be observed, the probability of developing type I diabetes is highest in those persons with two autoantibodies, with approximately half of these persons developing the disease within 4 years. IDDM—insulin-dependent diabetes. (*From* Krischer *et al.* [9]; with permission.)

PREVALENCE OF GLUTAMIC ACID DECARBOXYLASE AUTOANTIBODIES AND THEIR POTENTIAL USE IN IDENTIFYING AUTOIMMUNE ACTIVITY

Subject Group	Autoantibody Frequency, %
Healthy control group	0.3–0.6
First-degree relatives of patients with type I diabetes	3–4
Patients with other autoimmune endocrine disorders	1–2
Patients with newly diagnosed type I diabetes	55–85
Patients with type 2 diabetes	10–15
Patients with gestational diabetes	10

FIGURE 4-17. Glutamic acid decarboxylase (GAD) autoantibodies serve as a marker for predicting future cases and diagnosing new cases of Type I diabetes. Recent investigations summarized in representative form here indicate that GAD autoantibodies may also be useful in identifying autoimmunity in persons diagnosed with other forms of diabetes. These identifications may be useful in terms of imparting appropriate diabetes management and clinical care.

A. THE NONOBESE DIABETIC MOUSE MODEL OF TYPE I DIABETES

Characteristic	Nonobese Diabetic Mice
Disease onset	Spontaneous, 13–30+ weeks of age
Gender bias	Female predominance
Disease frequency	Strong intercolony variation, 50%–80% female, 20%–50% male, typical rates at 26 weeks of age
Clinical presentation	Hyperglycemia, mild ketosis, polydipsia, polyuria, weight loss, insulin dependency
Additional disease model	Thyroiditis, sialoadenitis (Sjögren syndrome), deafness
Insulitis	Appears in nondestructive (5–12 wk) and destructive (13+ wk) phases; macrophages, dendritic cells, T and B lymphocytes, NK cells
Genetic susceptibility	Major histocompatibility complex (MHC) plus >15 non-MHC loci
Immune markers	Autoantibodies, autoreactive T cells

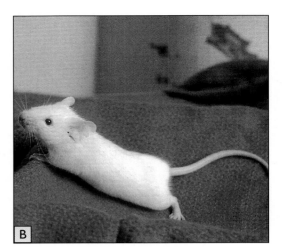

FIGURE 4-18. The nonobese diabetic mouse model of Type I diabetes. **A,** Characteristics. **B,** Photograph of nonobese diabetic mouse.

FIGURE 4-19. The BioBreeding rat model of type I diabetes.

THE BIOBREEDING RAT MODEL OF TYPE I DIABETES

Characteristic	BioBreeding Rats
Disease onset	Spontaneous, 8–14 weeks of age
Gender bias	None
Disease frequency	Minor intercolony variation, 40%–70% at 12 weeks of age
Clinical presentation	Hyperglycemia, mild ketosis, polydipsia, polyuria, weight loss, insulin dependency
Additional disease model	Thyroiditis, T-cell lymphopenia
Insulitis	Rapidly progressive; appears near time of disease onset; macrophages, dendritic cells, T and B lymphocytes, NK cells
Genetic susceptibility	Major histocompatibility complex (MHC) plus *Lyp* (T-lymphopenia) locus (chromosome 4)
Immune markers	Autoantibodies, autoreactive T cells

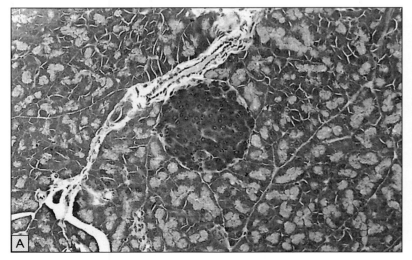
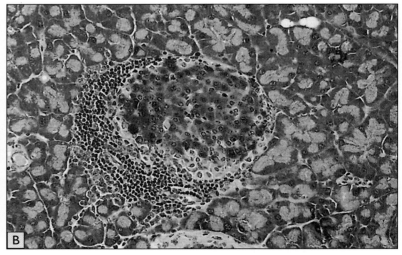

FIGURE 4-20. (*see* Color Plate) Developmental stages of the insulitis lesion in nonobese diabetic mice. Pathology of pancreatic specimens from a normal islet cell devoid of leukocytic infiltrate (**A**) and at various stages of infiltration (**B** *to* **H**).

(Continued on next page)

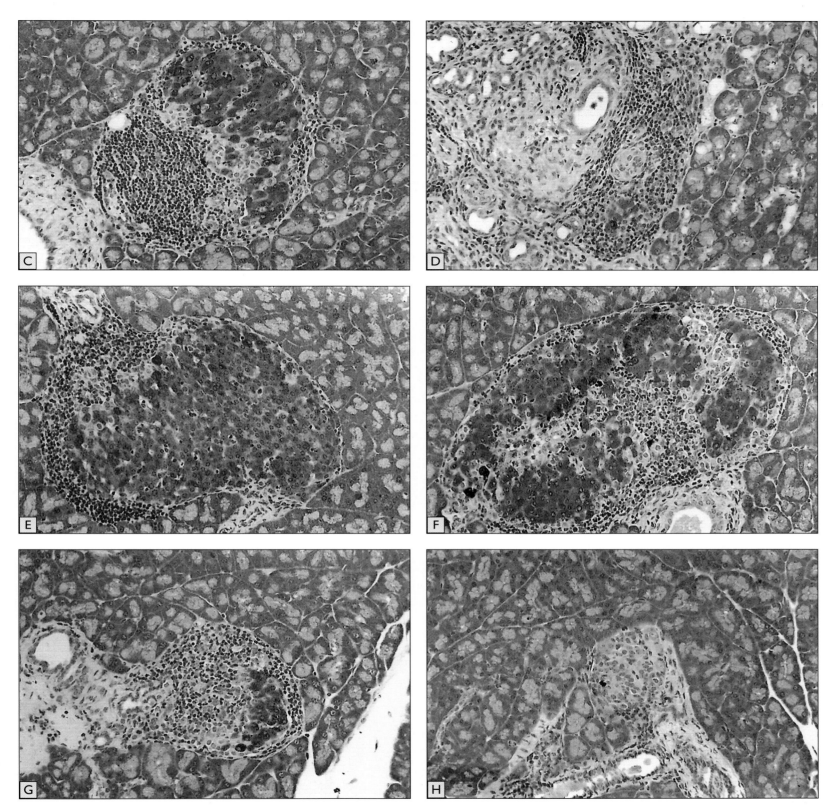

FIGURE 4-20. (*Continued*) Beginning at 5 to 7 weeks of age, leukocytes surround and eventually infiltrate the islets in increasing numbers. Beginning at 12 to 14 weeks, this early insulitis (often termed *non-destructive*) is replaced with an insulitis that destroys the insulin-producing β cells. When the islet is devoid of β cells the leukocytic infiltrate disappears, leaving only α, τ, and δ cells (*panel H*). (Hematoxylin-eosin stain followed by counterstaining with anti-insulin antibody and avidin-biotin, × 300.) (Photomicrographs *courtesy of* A. Peck, University of Florida.)

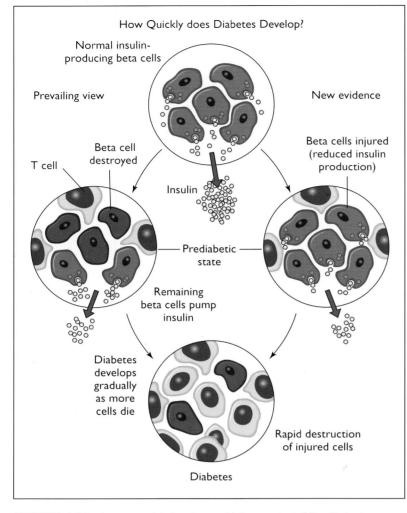

How Quickly does Diabetes Develop?

Normal insulin-producing beta cells

Prevailing view

New evidence

Beta cell destroyed

T cell

Beta cells injured (reduced insulin production)

Insulin

Prediabetic state

Remaining beta cells pump insulin

Diabetes develops gradually as more cells die

Rapid destruction of injured cells

Diabetes

FIGURE 4-21. A new model showing rapid destruction of β cells in the pathogenesis of type 1 diabetes. Until recently, most models assessing the rate of β-cell destruction have presumed a gradual (ie, modified linear; see Fig. 4-1) endocrine cell loss characterized by small periods of "waxing and waning" in the immune response. However, recent investigations of nonobese diabetic mice have suggested that actual β-cell destruction occurs in a very limited time period immediately before symptomatic onset. The composition of the insulitic lesion, destructive activity, or both before this event would be of nondestructive or limited destructive capacity. Although limited evidence exists for this model in terms of human type 1 diabetes, it is the subject of ongoing investigation.

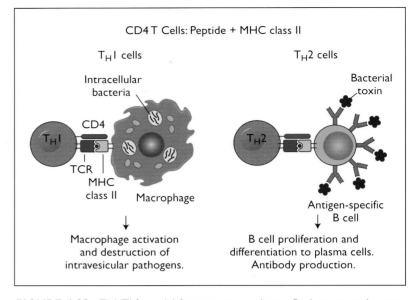

CD4 T Cells: Peptide + MHC class II

T$_H$1 cells

T$_H$2 cells

Intracellular bacteria

Bacterial toxin

CD4

TCR

MHC class II

Macrophage

Antigen-specific B cell

Macrophage activation and destruction of intravesicular pathogens.

B cell proliferation and differentiation to plasma cells. Antibody production.

FIGURE 4-22. Th1/Th2 model for immune regulation. Both *in vivo* and *in vitro* studies have supported the notion that activities of CD4+ "helper-T" cells may directly or indirectly relate to the production of specific cytokines. Evolutionary immunologists indicate that the compartmentalization of such responses provides for a more efficient development of an immune response against pathogens of divergent origins and modes of evasion. Although somewhat of an overgeneralization, Th1 cytokines are viewed as enhancing cellular immune activities, whereas Th2 cytokines support those of humoral immunity. Specifically, Th1 activity appears to be enhanced by production of the lymphokines interferon γ (IFN-γ), interleukin 2 (IL-2), and IL-12. Conversely, Th2 augmentation of humoral immunity occurs through the release of IL-4 and IL-10. Note that IL-4 appears to be a strong inhibitor of Th1 immunity. The production of specific cytokines, both systemic and at the site of pancreatic inflammation, may have important implications for the pathogenesis of diabetes as well as the potential for developing methods aimed at disease prevention (*see* Fig. 4-29). MHC—major histocompatibility complex; TCR—T-cell receptor.

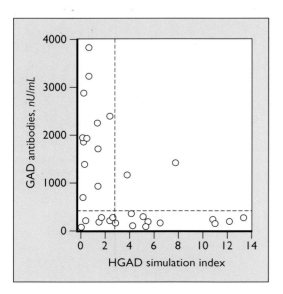

FIGURE 4-23. Evidence supporting an inverse relationship (ie, the Th1/Th2 model) for type 1 diabetes in humans. Persons having high levels of autoantibodies against glutamic acid decarboxylase (GAD) demonstrate minimal T-cell reactivity to the same antigen. Conversely, persons with high anti-GAD T-cell response present with low levels of GAD autoantibody. In terms of disease prediction, persons with the latter phenotype exhibit a higher rate of developing Type 1 diabetes (*From* Harrison *et al.* [10]; with permission.)

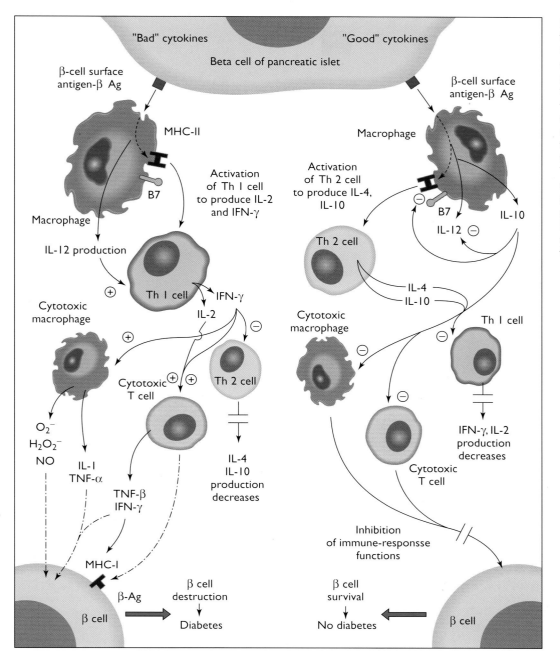

FIGURE 4-24. The "good and bad" cytokine model for the pathogenesis of type 1 diabetes. As modeled in accordance with Figures 4-22 and 4-23, production of Th2 cytokines would be viewed as providing a pathway of avoidance of β-cell destruction (hence the label "good" cytokine). Production of interleukin 4 (IL-4) and IL-10 would block the destructive actions of the cellular immune response. By contrast, immune responses characterized by "bad" Th1 cytokines would be considered as promoting β-cell destruction through enhancement of actions ascribed to cytotoxic T cells or macrophages (through oxygen radical–mediated damage). Ag—antigen; H_2O_2—hydrogen peroxide; IFN—interferon; MHC—major histocompatibility complex; minus sign—inhibitory pathway; NO—nitric oxide; O_2^-—oxygen free radical; plus sign—promoting pathway; TNF-α—tumor necrosis factor α.

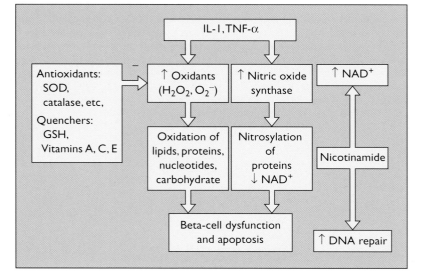

FIGURE 4-25. The lymphokine model for β-cell destruction in type 1 diabetes. Under this scenario, lymphokines produced in response to a nonspecific infection would, by their mode of action, impart a limited degree of initial β-cell destruction owing to an usual susceptibility of β cells to such agents. The predominant lymphokines cited in this model are those produced by macrophages and include tumor necrosis factor α (TNF-α) and interleukin 1 (IL-1). Despite the benefits of recovery from infection, this process of anti-β cell immunity would result in those genetically susceptible to the disease. The continuing process of β-cell destruction would occur through the action of various cytotoxic agents (eg, oxidants and nitric oxide) as well as a lack in activity of numerous compounds associated with cellular or DNA repair mechanisms (eg, anti-oxidants). GSH—glomerulus-stimulating hormone; H_2O_2—hydrogen peroxide; NAD^+—oxidized nicotinamide adenine dinucleotide; O_2^-—oxygen free radical; SOD—superoxide dismutase. (Adapted from Kolb and Kolb-Bachofen [11].)

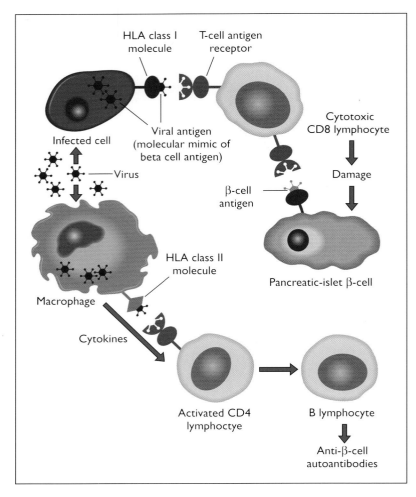

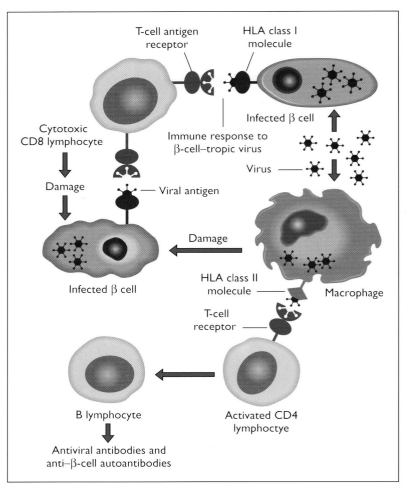

FIGURE 4-26. Potential role for viruses in the pathogenesis of Type I diabetes: the molecular mimicry model. In this model, the autoimmune process begins after a "normal" immune response to a cell infected with a virus whose proteins share a similar sequence to that of a β-cell protein. The infected cells display processed viral antigens (by way of Class I molecules) to CD8+ T cells. Macrophages having phagocytosed and processed virus present the viral peptides to CD4+ T cells through Class II molecules. The CD4+ T cells amplify the actions of the CD8+ T cells to become cytotoxic effector cells that can kill β cells that express a peptide common to the viral protein. Despite exhaustive research efforts to demonstrate molecular mimicry as an underlying cause of Type I diabetes, it remains an unproved model. Contemporary support predominantly derives from studies demonstrating amino acid sequence similarity between β-cell proteins (eg, glutamic acid decarboxylase and IA-2) with those of viruses (eg, Coxsackie and Rotavirus) and the ability of human lymphocyte antigen (HLA) molecules with susceptibility and resistance for Type I disease to bind these regions of mimicry. Studies, in particular those of cellular immunity, of the natural history of diabetes in humans and nonobese diabetic mice have failed to elevate this model beyond the hypothetical stage. (*Adapted from* Atkinson and Maclaren [1].)

FIGURE 4-27. Potential role for viruses in the pathogenesis of type I diabetes: β tropic virus–viral superantigen models. In these models, initiation of the autoimmune process follows direct viral infection of β cells or the expression in β cells of a virus acting as a superantigen. In both situations, leukocytes are recruited to pancreatic islets. Recruitment increases the release of cytokines (eg, interferon α) and adhesion of leukocytes within the pancreatic islets. In the β-cell tropic model, the infected β cell is susceptible to direct attack by antiviral cytotoxic lymphocytes. In both models, cytokines and free radicals produced by macrophages activated within the islet cells may augment the cytotoxic response to the β cells; the cytokines also recruit CD4+ T cells to the lesion. Macrophages present autoantigens derived from virus-damaged β cells, thus leading to the development of lymphocytes and autoantibodies that react with β-cell proteins. Support for both of these models exists, yet they remain hypothetical. Whereas viruses capable of β-cell destruction have been isolated from an extremely limited number of human pancreatic organs, examination of a large number of these tissues from patients with Type I diabetes has failed to reveal the presence of such viruses. Support for the superantigen model exists through the identification of T cells characteristic of superantigen activation in the pancreatic organs of a limited number of patients with new-onset Type I diabetes. To date, however, no such viral superantigen has been unequivocally identified. HLA—human leukocyte antigen. (*Adapted from* Atkinson and Maclaren [1].)

Future Directions

THERAPIES DELAYING OR PREVENTING THE ONSET OF TYPE I DIABETES IN THE NONOBESE DIABETIC MOUSE MODEL

Androgens
Anesthesia
Azathioprine
Anti–B7-I
Bacillus Calmette-Guérin
Baculofin
Anti-beta 7 integrin
Blocking peptide of major histocompatibility complex class II
Bone marrow transplantation
Castration
Anti-CD3
Anti-CD4
Anti-CD8
Anti-CD28
Cholera toxin-B subunit
Clip peptide
Cold exposure
Anti-complement receptor
Complete Freund adjuvant
Anti–CTLA4
Cyclosporin
Cyclosporin A
Deflazacort
Dendritic cells from pancreatic lymph node
Deoxyspergualin
Diazoxide
1,25-dihydroxylvitamin D_3
Elevated temperature
Escherichia coli extract
Encephalomyocarditis virus
Essential fatty acid deficient diets
FK506
Gallium nitrate

Glucose (neonatal)
Glutamic acid decarboxylase: intraperitoneal, intrathymic, intravenous, oral
Glutamic acid decarboxylase peptides: intraperitoneal, intrathymic, intravenous, oral
Gonadectomy
Heat shock protein 65
Heat shock protein peptide (p277)
Anti–intracellular adhesion molecule I
Immobilization
Immunoglobulin
Anti–integrin α 4
Inomide
Insulin: intraperitoneal, oral, subcutaneous, nasal
Insulin B chain, B chain amino acids 9-23: intraperitoneal, oral, subcutaneous, nasal
Interferon γ
Anti–interferon γ
Interleukin I
Interleukin-I receptor
Interleukin 2
Interleukin-2 fusion toxin
Interleukin 3
Interleukin 4
Interleukin 10
Interleukin 12 antagonist
Islet cells: intrathymic
Lactate dehydrogenase virus
Lazaroid
Linomide
Anti–lymphocyte function–associated antigen I
Anti-*L*-selectin
Lymphocyte choriomeningitis virus
Anti–lymphocyte serum

LZ8
MDL 29311
Anti–MHC class I
Anti–MHC class II
Mixed allogeneic chimerism
Monosodium glutamate
Murine hepatitis virus
Mycobacterium
Natural antibodies
Nicotinamide
OK432
Overcrowding
Pancreatectomy
Pertussigen
Poly [I:C]
Pregestimil diet
Probucol
Prolactin (Abbott Diagnostics; Abbott Park, IL)
Rampamycin
Saline (repeated injection)
Semipurified diet (*eg*, AIN-76)
Silica
Sodium fusidate
Somatostatin
Nonspecific pathogen-free conditions
Streptococcal enterotoxins
Superantigens
Superoxide dismutase–desferrioxamine
Anti–T-cell receptor
Anti–-thy-I
Thymectomy (neonatal)
Tolbutamide
Tumor necrosis factor α
Vitamin E
Anti–VLA 4

FIGURE 4-28. Therapies delaying or preventing the onset of Type I diabetes in the nonobese diabetic mouse model.

TREATMENTS AIMED AT INDUCING CLINICAL REMISSION OR PREVENTING HUMAN TYPE I DIABETES

Group Studied	Agent or Treatment
Patients with new-onset Type I disease	Cyclosporine
	Azathioprine
	Anti-CD5 antibodies (CD5 plus)
	Intensive insulin therapy
	High-dose insulin therapy
	Antibody against interleukin 2 receptor
	Nicotinamide
	Intravenous immune globulin
	Plasmapheresis
	Anti–lymphocyte globulin
	Prednisone
	Bacillus Calmette-Guérin
Persons at high risk for Type I disease	Intensive therapy with intravenous insulin
	Prophylactic insulin therapy
	Nicotinamide
	Oral insulin
	Avoidance of cow's milk–based infant formulas

FIGURE 4-29. Since the first description of islet cell autoantibodies (ICAs) in 1974 (see Fig. 4-4), many new autoantibody markers of anti-islet immunity have been identified in persons with Type I diabetes. In addition to their presence at disease onset, many of these markers have proved useful in identifying persons in the presymptomatic period, months to years before the clinical onset of Type I diabetes. Of these, four markers have gained the most acceptance owing to scientific confirmation, high frequency of expression, and superior disease sensitivity and specificity: ICA, insulin autoantibodies, glutamic acid decarboxylase, and insulin antibody-2 autoantibodies.

References

1. Atkinson MA, Maclaren NK: The pathogenesis of insulin-dependent diabetes mellitus. *N Engl J Med* 1994, 331:1428–1436.

2. Eisenbarth GS: Type I diabetes mellitus. A chronic autoimmune disease. *N Engl J Med* 1986, 314:1360–1368.

3. Karvonen M, Tuomilehto J, Libman I, LaPorte R: WHO Diamond Project Group: a review of the recent epidemiological data on incidence of Type I (insulin-dependent) diabetes mellitus worldwide. *Diabetologia* 36:883–892.

4. LaPorte RE, Matsushima M, Chang Y-F: Prevalence and incidence of insulin dependent diabetes. In *Diabetes in America*. Edited by Harris M. NIH publications, Bethesda, MD; 1995:37–46.

5. Hawkins HW: Could the aetiology of IDDM be multifactorial? *Diabetologia* 1997, 40:1235–1240.

6. She JX: Susceptibility to Type I diabetes: HLA-DQ and DR revisited. *Immunol Today* 1996, 17:323–329.

7. Lernmark A, Ott J: Sometimes it's hot, sometimes it's not. *Nat Genetics* 1998, 19:213–214.

8. Foulis AK: In *Textbook of Diabetes*. Vol. 1. edited by Pickup J, Williams G.. Oxford, England: Blackwell Scientific; 1991.

9. Krischer JP, Schatz D, Riley WJ, et al.: Insulin and islet cell autoantibodies as time-dependent covariates in the development of insulin-dependent diabetes. *J Clin Endocrinol Metab* 1993, 77:743–749.

10. Harrison LC, Honeymoon MC, De Aizpurua HJ, et al.: Inverse relation between humoral and cellular immunity to glutamic acid decarboxylase in subjects at risk of insulin-dependent diabetes. *Lancet* 1993, 341:1365–1369.

11. Kolb H, Kolb-Bachofen V: Nitric oxide in autoimmune disease: cytotoxic or regulatory mediator? *Immunol Today* 1998, 19:556-561.

MANAGEMENT AND PREVENTION OF COMPLICATIONS IN TYPE 1 DIABETES MELLITUS

David M. Nathan

Therapy for type 1 diabetes mellitus has a relatively short history that can be divided conveniently into three eras: pre-insulin, insulin, and the era after the Diabetes Control and Complications Trial (DCCT). Before the introduction of insulin therapy, persons with the form of diabetes we currently call type 1 had a uniform mortality rate approaching 100% within the first 2 years of diagnosis. The existence of a distinct form of diabetes, now designated as type 2, was not well recognized until the mid-1930s. Considering the short life span of patients with type 1 diabetes, it is not surprising that the long-term complications of diabetes were virtually unknown. Two dramatic events accompanied the introduction of insulin therapy in 1922. First, type 1 diabetes was no longer an acutely fatal disease. Second, with longer survival, previously unheard of complications began to occur, including retinopathy, nephropathy, and neuropathy [1]. The consequences of these complications and the desire to prevent or delay them have been the focus of clinical care and research, culminating in the DCCT [2].

The DCCT and a series of smaller clinical studies, including the Kroc [3], Steno [4], Oslo [5], and Stockholm Diabetes [6] studies, examined whether the long-term complications of diabetes could be prevented or delayed by implementing therapies aimed at achieving blood glucose levels as close as possible to the normal range. These so-called intensive therapies were made possible by the development of self-glucose monitoring techniques and insights into the physiologic pattern of delivery of insulin necessary to achieve and maintain glucose levels in the near normal range [7]. Insulin therapy with long-acting and short-acting insulins was adjusted based on glucose self-monitoring results, meal content, and anticipated exercise. Short-acting insulins were given at least two to three times per day with multiple daily injection (MDI) therapy or with continuous subcutaneous insulin infusion (CSII) provided by an external pump. The development of an objective accurate index of long-term glycemia, the *glycohemoglobin assay*, complemented these other developments and facilitated the performance of the clinical trials [8].

The DCCT was initiated in 1982 and completed in 1993. Patients with type 1 diabetes with either no retinopathy (primary prevention) or minimal to moderate nonproliferative retinopathy (secondary intervention) were randomly assigned to conventional or intensive therapy [2]. In conventional therapy, patients used one to two daily insulin injections and daily glucose monitoring. Conventional therapy was designed to avoid symptoms of hyperglycemia and hypoglycemia but had no specific blood glucose level goals. In contrast, intensive therapy was aimed at achieving blood glucose levels between 70 and 120 mg/dL before meals, under 180 mg/dL at 90 to 120 minutes after meals, and over 65 mg/dL at a weekly test performed at 3 AM to monitor and decrease the occurrence of nocturnal hypoglycemia. In addition, intensive therapy was aimed at achieving hemoglobin A_{1c} (HbA$_{1c}$) levels in the normal range (<6.05%).

A total of 1441 patients with type 1 diabetes aged 13 to 40 were recruited between 1983 and 1990, and follow-up examinations were performed for a mean of 6.5 years. Intensive therapy resulted in a decrease in mean HbA$_{1c}$ levels of 1.8% to 2.0% and a consistent and impressive reduction in the occurrence and progression of retinopathy, nephropathy, and neuropathy. When compared with conventional therapy, intensive therapy reduced the development of both early and later manifestations of retinopathy (three-step change, severe nonproliferative retinopathy, and the need for laser therapy), nephropathy (microalbuminuria and clinical grade albuminuria), and peripheral and autonomic neuropathy [2]. Included in the costs of intensive therapy were frequent supervision by a highly trained and expert staff and increased monitoring compared with conventional therapy. In addition, intensive therapy was accompanied by a threefold increased risk for severe hypoglycemia, including episodes that resulted in coma or seizure, and an increased risk for weight gain. No significant cognitive impairment occurred in the intensive treatment group, even in those patients who experienced repeated episodes of severe hypoglycemia.

The DCCT and other studies, especially the Stockholm Diabetes Study [6], have established intensive therapy as the standard of therapy for type 1 diabetes. Until new and improved therapies that are safer and more user-friendly supplant MDI and CSII, they will remain the staples for patients with type 1 diabetes. For those patients who cannot perform all of the myriad of tasks intensive therapy requires or who cannot achieve and maintain near-normal glycemia, any lowering of HbA$_{1c}$ is likely to decrease the rate of development and slow the progression of long-term complications [9]. Note that intensive therapy has not been demonstrated to decrease the excessive cardiovascular disease (CVD) that affects patients with type 1 diabetes; however, longer-term studies may be expected to demonstrate a decrease in CVD owing to the decrease in renal failure, a major contributor to accelerated atherosclerosis.

Improvements in intensive therapy have been made in the relatively brief period of time since the completion of the DCCT. Improved glucose self-monitoring devices are now available. A new understanding of the pathogenesis of hypoglycemia and hypoglycemia unawareness exists that promises to decrease the risk of hypoglycemia accompanying intensive therapy [10–12]. The development of new insulin analogues, such as lispro, is now making physiologic replacement easier [13]. In addition, advances in whole-organ pancreas transplantation have made it an increasingly appropriate and acceptable procedure in the setting of kidney transplantation and, arguably, even as a solitary transplantation. Finally, progress in islet transplantation and the development of continuous and less invasive, or even noninvasive, monitoring technology may make these therapies a reality in the next decade.

For those patients who do not or cannot take advantage of the improvement in long-term outcome provided by intensive therapy, laser therapy, vitrectomy, renal replacement therapy, and treatments for painful neuropathy and the manifestations of autonomic neuropathy remain [14].

Herein, the seminal insights and developments that allowed physiologic replacement of insulin in type 1 diabetes, consequences of such therapy on long-term complications, and several new treatments are reviewed.

History of Type 1 Diabetes and Its Treatment

Pre-insulin		Insulin	Post-DCCT
1500 BC　　　1889	1922	1930-	1993

Pre-insulin / Insulin / Post-DCCT

1500 BC　　1889　　1922　　1930-　　1993

Diabetes described as a wasting illness in Ebers papyrus	von Mering and Minkowski discover importance of pancreas in diabetes	Banting and Best first give insulin to human diabetic	Retinopathy, nephropathy and neuropathy diagnosed in increasing numbers of diabetic patients who survive more than 10 years	DCCT establishes means of delaying onset and slowing progression of all diabetic complications

FIGURE 5-1. The history of type 1 diabetes can be divided conveniently into three eras. In the pre-insulin era, diabetes was usually fatal within 1 to 2 years of its development. In the insulin era, acute mortality was eliminated but chronic complications were first noted. The Diabetes Control and Complications Trial (DCCT) [2] proved that intensive therapy would decrease the development and progression of long-term complications.

Therapy for Type 1 Diabetes

FORMS OF MODIFIED INSULIN

Insulin form	Modification	Onset of Action	Duration of Activity
Very rapid acting			
Lispro*	B-chain proline (amino acid 28) and lysine (amino acid 29) reversed	10–15 min	2–3 h
Rapid-acting			
Crystalline zinc insulin (CZI)†	Zinc	30–45 min	4–6 h
Intermediate-acting			
Neutral protamine Hagedorn (NPH)†	Protamine	1–2 h	6–12 h
Lente†	Zinc	1–2 h	6–12 h
Long-acting			
Ultralente*	Zinc	6–8 h	18 h
Premixed combinations:			
70/30*	70% NPH and 30% CZI	30–45 min	6–12 h
50/50*	50% NPH and 50% CZI	30–45 min	6–12 h

*Available only as recombinant human insulin.
†Available as human, beef and pork, and pure pork. Effective January 1999, animal species insulin to be eliminated.

FIGURE 5-2. The available forms of modified insulin provide a spectrum of action that facilitates near normalization of glucose levels when used in conjunction with frequent monitoring of glucose levels. Selection of dose size and timing of administration are dependent on an understanding of the impact of exercise and meal size and composition on glucose fluctuations. Even with these tools, intensive therapy is imperfect. True normalization of glucose levels rarely, if ever, is achieved. Realistically, hemoglobin A_{1c} levels can be maintained at 4 to 5 standard deviations above the mean nondiabetic level, and then only with a substantial frequency of hypoglycemic reactions.

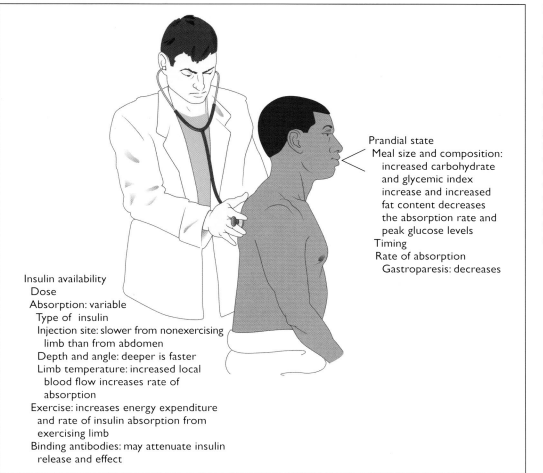

Prandial state
Meal size and composition:
    increased carbohydrate
    and glycemic index
    increase and increased
    fat content decreases
    the absorption rate and
    peak glucose levels
Timing
Rate of absorption
    Gastroparesis: decreases

Insulin availability
Dose
Absorption: variable
    Type of insulin
    Injection site: slower from nonexercising
        limb than from abdomen
    Depth and angle: deeper is faster
    Limb temperature: increased local
        blood flow increases rate of
        absorption
Exercise: increases energy expenditure
    and rate of insulin absorption from
    exercising limb
Binding antibodies: may attenuate insulin
    release and effect

FIGURE 5-3. Causes of lability of glycemia in type I diabetes. After a variable but usually brief period of preserved insulin secretion, often called a honeymoon period, type I diabetes is characterized by a complete deficiency of endogenous insulin production. Whereas glucose levels in the nondiabetic state are maintained in a very limited range owing to the exquisite and coordinated responsiveness of the β cells (insulin) and α cells (glucagon) to ambient glucose levels and gut peptides, glucose levels are extremely labile once type I diabetes has been established. The patient with type I diabetes is entirely dependent on exogenous insulin delivery, which can be affected by many variables. In addition, the rate of increase in glucose levels is dictated by meal size and composition. Finally, a host of other factors, including exercise timing and intensity, can affect energy use and glucose levels.

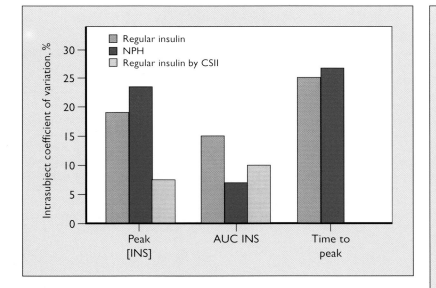

FIGURE 5-4. Variability (coefficients of variation) for insulin absorption. The absorption of insulin from the subcutaneous depot determines its delivery to its target tissues. Absorption is influenced by many factors (see Fig. 5-3), and it is highly variable. In the study results shown here, the same dose of subcutaneous insulin was administered repeatedly by nurses using the same anatomic site and standardized injection techniques. Alternatively, insulin was administered by continuous subcutaneous insulin infusion (CSII) with an external pump. The coeffficients of variation within individuals for peak insulin level (Peak[INS]), area under the curve (AUC) for insulin levels, and time to peak level after a subcutaneous injection were as high as 25% to 30%. Variabilities in peak insulin level and area under the curve were somewhat less with CSII, suggesting that external pump therapy may provide more consistent insulin delivery than conventional subcutaneous insulin delivery therapy. (*From* Galloway [15].)

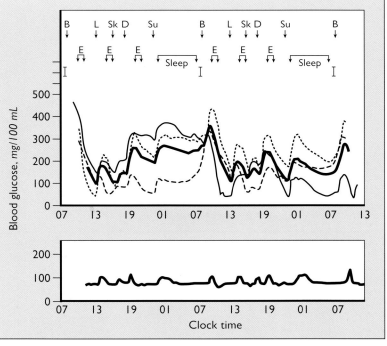

FIGURE 5-5. Daily blood glucose profiles in persons without diabetes and in patients with type I diabetes treated with nonphysiologic insulin replacement. Studies were performed in the highly regimented environment of an inpatient clinical research center, with standardized uniform meals and exercise. These studies demonstrate the relatively constant blood glucose levels maintained by persons without diabetes. In contrast, even in a highly regimented setting, patients with type I diabetes who are treated with a single dose of intermediate-acting insulin (I) have gross and seemingly unpredictable fluctuations in blood glucose levels. (*From* Molnar *et al.* [16]; with permission.)

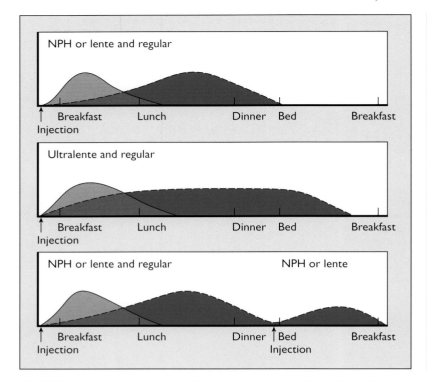

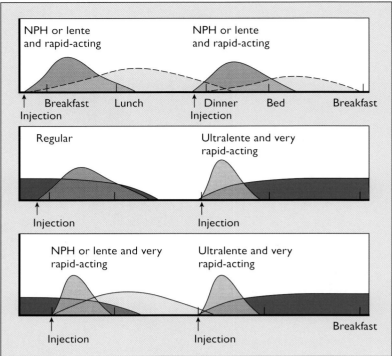

FIGURE 5-6. Insulin activity profiles and algorithms. Insulin profiles achieved with different injection regimens are shown. Minimal regimens are likely to be associated with intermittent symptoms of hyperglycemia and hemoglobin A_{1c} levels exceeding 10% (nondiabetic range, 4% to 6.1%). These relatively nondemanding insulin regimens will prevent ketosis most of the time. In addition to once or twice daily insulin injections, self-glucose monitoring should be performed daily. Patients should perform monitoring more often before traveling, with changes in schedule or regimen, and during illness. Urine ketone testing should be performed in the setting of unusually elevated glucose levels (>300 mg/dL) or in the presence of illness, especially when gastrointestinal symptoms are present.

FIGURE 5-7. Moderate intensity regimens. These regimens include twice daily insulin injections coupled with glucose self-monitoring. Insulin doses are adjusted based on glucose levels and meal size. Such regimens are associated with hemoglobin A_{1c} levels of 8% to 9%. In general, patients should be asymptomatic, with infrequent symptoms of hyperglycemia.

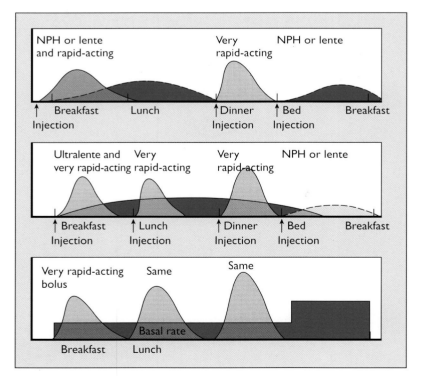

FIGURE 5-8. Intensive treatment regimens. These regimens include at least three injections of insulin daily or administration of insulin by an external pump. Self-monitoring of blood glucose levels is performed 4 times per day and at 3 AM once per week to detect and prevent episodes of otherwise unrecognized nocturnal hypoglycemia. Insulin doses, and especially the rapid or very rapid-acting insulins, are adjusted for each meal based on glucose level, meal size and composition, and anticipated exercise and activity. Intensive regimens can achieve a hemoglobin A_{1c} of 7% or less but at a cost of a threefold increase in episodes of severe hypoglycemia. An episode of severe hypoglycemia is defined as requiring help for treatment. An expert team including a diabetologist, diabetes educator, and dietitian is helpful in implementing and supervising such regimens. Intensive regimens have been recommended as the standard of therapy since the Diabetes Control and Complications Trial (DCCT) demonstrated their efficacy in preventing the development and slowing the progression of diabetic complications.

Results of Therapy: Glycemia

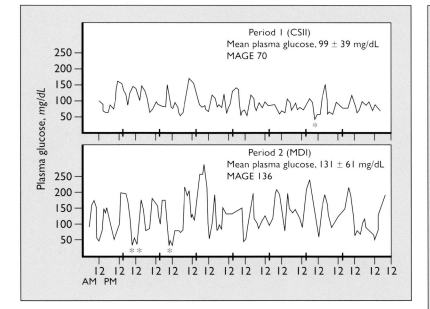

FIGURE 5-9. Glycemia in type 1 diabetes treated with physiologic insulin replacement using a multiple daily injection (MDI) regimen or continuous subcutaneous insulin infusion (CSII) with an external pump. In this study, a patient with type 1 diabetes performed multiple (15) self-glucose monitoring tests in a single day as an outpatient. Other than the frequent glucose checks, the accuracy of which were confirmed by simultaneous laboratory assay, the patient maintained a normal outpatient schedule, including self-selected meals and sedentary office work. During one 24-hour period (*see* bottom section of Fig. 5-8), the patient used a continuous subcutaneous insulin infusion with an external insulin pump and gave himself multiple daily injections with insulin placebo. During a second 24-hour period (*see* middle section of Fig. 5-8), the patient reversed therapy, using insulin placebo in the pump and active insulin in the injections. Although the glucose profile is somewhat less labile with CSII than with MDI, both therapies achieved blood glucose levels that are close to or within the normal range for much of the day. (*From* Nathan *et al.* [17]; with permission.)

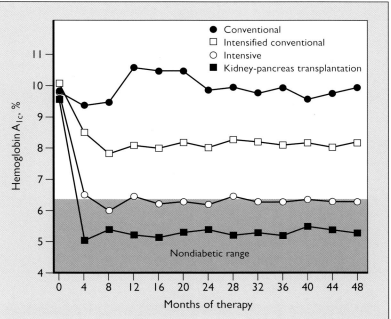

FIGURE 5-10. Comparison of long-term glycemia, as measured by hemoglobin A_{1c} (HbA$_{1c}$), for different treatments of type 1 diabetes. Patients were nonrandomly assigned to one of three groups: conventional therapy, intensified conventional therapy, or intensive therapy with continuous subcutaneous insulin infusion (CSII) or multiple daily injection (MDI) (n = 18, 22, and 21, respectively). *Conventional therapy* was defined in 1980 to 1984 as 1 or 2 daily insulin injections without frequent self-monitoring of glucose levels or dose adjustment. The injections usually consisted of a combination of intermediate-acting and rapid-acting insulin before breakfast and dinner. *Intensified conventional therapy* is similar to conventional therapy but with the addition of twice-daily glucose monitoring and adjustment of the pre-breakfast and pre-dinner doses based on monitoring results. The fourth group represents patients with end-stage renal disease after receiving a simultaneous kidney-pancreas transplantation (n = 34). MAGE— mean amplitude of glycemic excursions. *Asterisk* indicates clinical hypoglycemia.

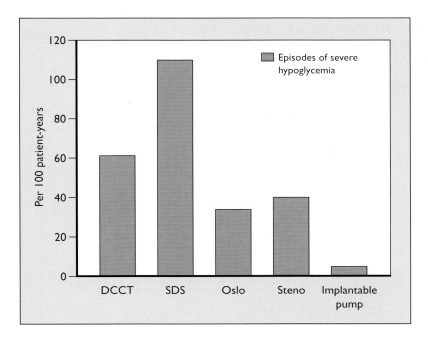

FIGURE 5-11. Frequency of severe hypoglycemia with intensive therapy of diabetes mellitus. As in the Diabetes Control and Complications Trial (DCCT), *Severe hypoglycemia* is defined as any episode of chemical hypoglycemia (usually with plasma glucose <60 mg/dL) requiring help from another person to treat. Severe hypoglycemia includes a spectrum of hypoglycemia, ranging from only minimal confusion to episodes of loss of consciousness or seizures. If the patient is able to swallow, 15 g of a rapidly absorbable simple sugar should be given in the form of 4 oz of orange juice, soda, or sugar candy. If unable to swallow, intramuscular glucagon, usually 1 mg, or intravenous dextrose, 12.5–50 mL of 50% dextrose, is administered. The DCCT [2], SDS (Stockholm Diabetes Study) [18], Oslo Study [5], and Steno Studies [4] studied patients with type 1 diabetes and used either multiple daily injections or external insulin pump therapy. The only intensive therapy for patients with type 1 diabetes with demonstrably lower rates of severe hypoglycemia has used implantable pumps delivering insulin intravenously or intraperitoneally [19].

Long-term Complications: Pathophysiology and Results of Intensive Therapy

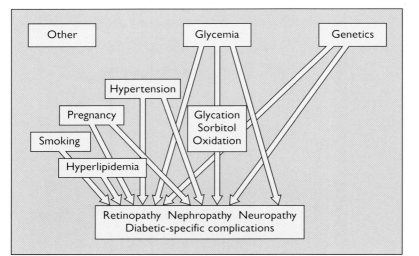

FIGURE 5-12. Pathogenesis of complications. The specific mechanism or mechanisms that cause the microvascular and neurologic complications of diabetes remain unidentified. Several obvious contributing factors, however, have been noted in epidemiologic studies, animal models, and interventional studies. Whereas no single mechanism is likely to explain the myriad of complications, glycemia appears to be an underlying cause for all of them, as demonstrated in interventional studies such as the Diabetes Control and Complications Trial (DCCT) [2]. It is probable that different clinical stages of specific complications, eg, nonproliferative and proliferative retinopathy, have different causes. Genetic susceptibility to retinopathy and neuropathy is suggested by familial clustering [20]. Hypertension and pregnancy are well known to accelerate the development of retinopathy and nephropathy. In addition, interventional studies using anti-hypertensive agents, and especially angiotensin-converting enzyme inhibitors, have demonstrated attenuation of the otherwise inexorable progression of nephropathy [21–23].

LONG-TERM COMPLICATIONS OF TYPE 1 DIABETES AND THE RISK OF DEVELOPING CLINICAL MANIFESTATIONS OF SPECIFIED COMPLICATIONS

Cataract: 25% to 30% lifetime risk with 3% to 5% requiring cataract extraction

Glaucoma (open angle): 10% risk after 30 years

Retinopathy: 90% develop some degree over lifetime; 40% to 50% require laser and 3% to 5% blind after 30 years' duration

Adhesive capsulitis: frozen shoulder, prevalence 10%

CAD: major cause of mortality

Gastroparesis: 1% to 5% develop symptoms - lifetime risk

Carpal tunnel syndrome: 30% with electrophysiologic evidence, 9% with symptoms (prevalence)

Nephropathy: 35% develop end-stage renal disease over lifetime

Trigger finger, DuPuytren's contractures: 10% prevalence

Autonomic neuropathy (prevalence): bladder, 1% to 5% with dysfunction; impotence, 10% to 40%; diarrhea, 1%

Peripheral vascular disease

Peripheral neuropathy: 54% lifetime risk; 2% to 3% foot ulcers/y

FIGURE 5-13. Long-term complications of type 1 diabetes and the risks of developing clinical manifestations of specified complications. Data for some complications are sparse. The estimates provided reflect the era before the –Diabetes Control and Complications Trial (DCCT). Intensive therapy of type 2 diabetes is anticipated to reduce the lifelong development of retinopathy, nephropathy, and neuropathy by 50% to 80%. The overall effect of diabetic complications results in a substantial 15-year reduction in life span, predominantly owing to the development of nephropathy and cardiovascular disease.

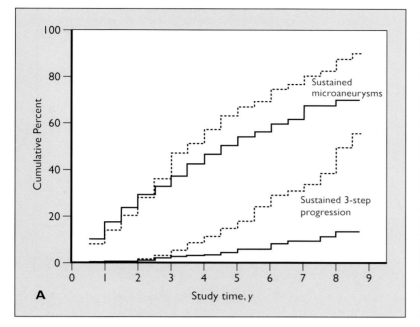

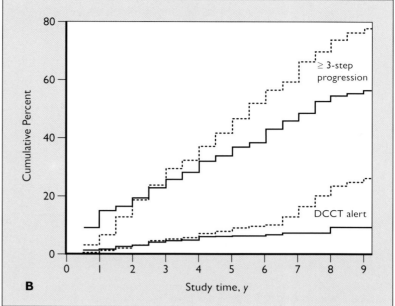

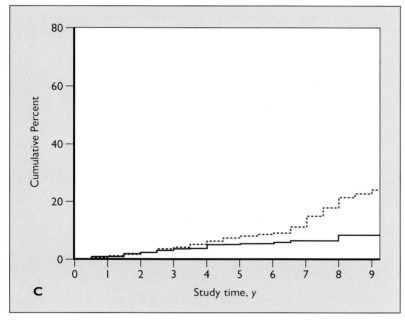

FIGURE 5-14. In the Diabetes Control and Complications Trial (DCCT), retinopathy measured in 18,000 sets of photographs with seven-field stereoscopic fundus photography performed every 6 months. The development and progression of retinopathy at virtually every stage were decreased by intensive therapy. The primary prevention cohort had 1 to 5 years' duration of diabetes and no retinopathy at baseline. In the primary cohort, the development of *sustained microaneurysms*, defined as one or more microaneurysms detected at two consecutive 6-month examinations, and of sustained three-step or greater progression according to the Early Treatment of Diabetic Retinopathy Study (ETDRS) scale, were decreased by 27% and 76% ($P < 0.002$), respectively (**A**). The secondary intervention cohort was defined as having 1 to 15 years' duration of diabetes and at least one microaneurysm in either eye at baseline. In the secondary intervention cohort, intensive therapy was highly effective at reducing the progression to more severe levels of retinopathy, including a 34% reduction in three-step or greater progression ($P < 0.001$) and a 47% reduction ($P < 0.02$) in severe nonproliferative retinopathy (DCCT alert) (**B**). The development of even more severe retinopathy, defined as neovascularization either on the disc or elsewhere, was reduced by 48% ($P < 0.02$) (**C**). (*From* DCCT Research Group [24]; with permission.)

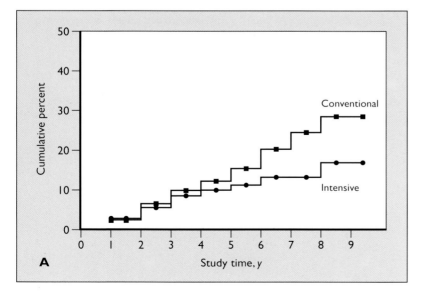

FIGURE 5-15. Nephropathy. Nephropathy in patients with type 1 diabetes progresses through several stages, usually over 15 to 25 years. The development of microalbuminuria, defined as between 20 and 40 mg of albumin excretion per 24 hours, is the first detectable stage, progressing to clinical albuminuria (> 300 mg albumin excretion per 24 h), usually over more than a decade. Albumin excretion progresses to the level consistent with nephrotic syndrome followed by decreasing glomerular filtration rate and culminating in end-stage renal disease (ESRD). Hypertension uniformly accompanies the development of nephropathy. Treatment of hypertension, especially with angiotensin-converting enzyme (ACE) inhibitors, and use of ACE inhibitors during the microalbuminuric stage, even in the absence of hypertension, have been shown to attenuate the progression rate of nephropathy.

The Diabetes Control and Complications Trial (DCCT) demonstrated a uniformly beneficial effect of intensive therapy on the development of microalbuminuria (40 mg/24 h). **A,** In patients with primary prevention, 34% risk reduction ($P = 0.04$).

Continued on next page)

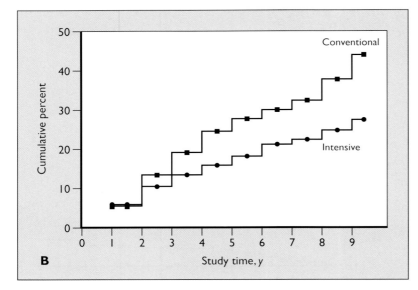

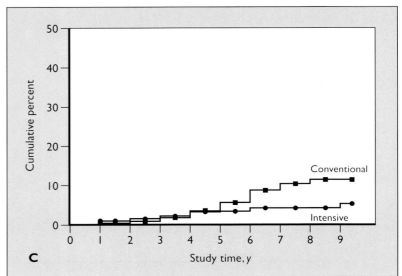

FIGURE 5-15. (*Continued*) **B,** In patients with secondary intervention, a 43% reduction (*P* < 0.0001). **C,** A 56% reduction in the development of more

advanced stages of nephropathy, such as clinical albuminuria (*P* < 0.01). (*From* DCCT Research Group [25]; with permission.)

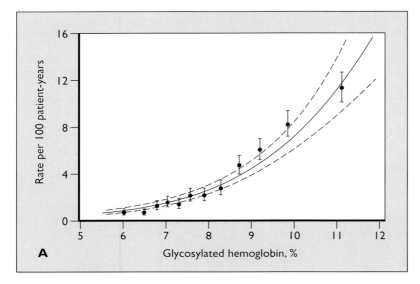

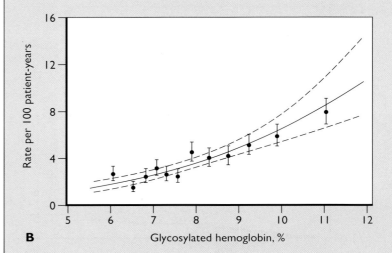

FIGURE 5-16. Glycemia and complications. The Diabetes Control and Complications Trial (DCCT) performed primary analyses comparing the effects of intensive and conventional therapy on long-term complications. In addition, the DCCT performed secondary analyses examining the relationship of glycemia (mean of all hemoglobin A_{1c} [HbA_{1c}] values for each subject during the trial) and the development or progression of complications, independent of treatment assignment. These analyses provide an assessment of the expected risk for different complications based on HbA_{1c} achieved. **A,** Rate of retinopathy progression in combined treatment groups. **B,** Rate of development of microalbuminuria (>40 mg/24h) in combined treatment groups. In addition, the risk reduction for a specified decrease in HbA_{1c} can be calculated (**C**). (*From* DCCT Research Group [9]; with permission.)

C. CALCULATED RELATIVE RISK REDUCTIONS ASSOCIATED WITH 10% LOWER MEAN HEMOGLOBIN A_{1c}

Complication	Risk Reduction, %*
Retinopathy:	
Onset	35
Sustained progression	39
Severe nonproliferative	37
Nephropathy:	
Microalbuminuria ($\geq$ 40 mg/24 h)	25
Microalbuminuria ($\geq$ 100 mg/24 h)	39
Albuminuria ($\geq$ 300 mg/24 h)	34
Neuropathy	30

*Calculated reduction in risk for every 10% lowering of hemoglobin A_{1c}.

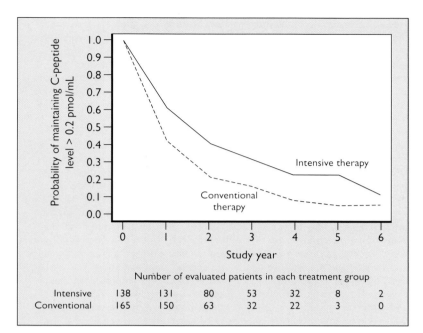

FIGURE 5-17. Preservation of endogenous insulin secretion with intensive therapy. In the Diabetes Control and Complications Trial (DCCT), patients with less than 5 years' duration of diabetes could have a modest degree of residual insulin secretion (C-peptide level 0.2–0.5 pmol/mL 90 min after a standardized meal). Of the patients, 303 fulfilled this criteria; 138 were randomly assigned to intensive therapy and 165 to conventional therapy. During the DCCT, repeated tests of endogenous insulin secretion were performed. As shown, intensive therapy was more likely to preserve endogenous secretion of insulin than was conventional therapy, extending the residual secretion by at least 2 years. Compared with patients having intensive treatment without residual insulin secretion, those having intensive treatment with residual insulin secretion maintained lower HbA$_{1c}$ levels with less exogenous insulin and had less frequent severe hypoglycemia and a lower risk of retinopathy progression. Thus, preservation of endogenous insulin secretion is clinically important, facilitating the safe implementation of intensive therapy. Intensive therapy should be initiated as early as possible in the course of type 1 diabetes. (*From* DCCT Research Group [26].)

New Approaches to Therapy

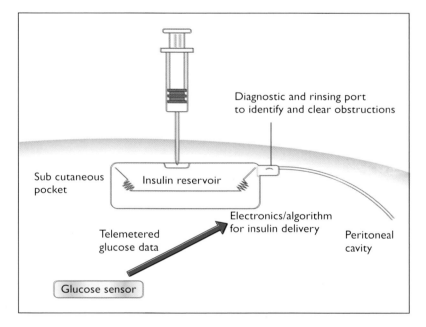

FIGURE 5-18. Implantable pump. The first step in creating an artificial pancreas was the development of a totally enclosed implantable pump. Ideally, the pump should deliver insulin reliably and in physiologic patterns to achieve normoglycemia. In addition, the requirement for rapid changes in insulin levels precludes subcutaneous delivery. Either intravenous or intraperitoneal delivery can achieve rapid changes and avoid peripheral hyperinsulinemia. Intraperitoneal delivery has a slight advantage in delivering insulin directly to the liver.

Several implantable pumps have been developed and tested extensively. The pumps share many characteristics. They hold enough insulin for 4 to 8 weeks and are filled subcutaneously through a port. The pumps are implanted in either a subclavian pocket or in the lower abdomen, with a catheter tunneled either into the subclavian vein or peritoneal cavity. The catheters become obstructed, on average, every 4 to 9 months and usually can be cleared through a flushing procedure, although occasionally catheter replacement is necessary. All pumps operate by telemetry and can be programmed to provide many different insulin profiles. The pumps are capable of achieving glycemic control similar to conventional intensive therapy but with a lower risk of severe hypoglycemia. A functional and practical glucose sensor has yet to be developed.

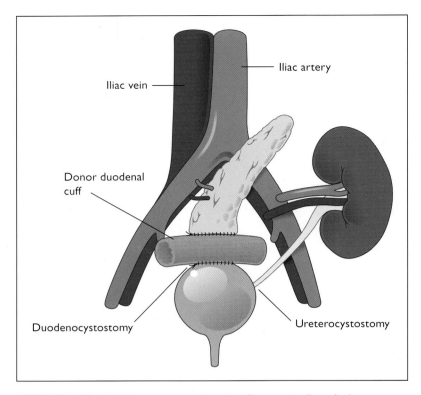

FIGURE 5-19. Whole-organ transplantation. Pancreatic allografts have become increasingly successful as a form of hormone replacement therapy. When successful, they obviate the need for exogenous insulin, "diabetes diets,"

frequent self-monitoring, and the panoply of other day-to-day chores and life-style adjustments that are a part of the management of type 1 diabetes. Whereas most pancreas transplantations are performed in type 1 diabetes with cadaveric organs and simultaneously with kidney transplantation (to treat end-stage renal disease), some centers perform isolated pancreas transplantations, partial pancreatic transplantations from living donors, and, rarely, transplantation in type 2 diabetes. The current consensus is that simultaneous kidney-pancreas transplantation is most acceptable because the risks of immunosuppression and surgery are subsumed by renal transplantation. Moreover, pancreas transplantation survival is superior in the setting of a combined kidney-pancreas transplantation compared with an isolated pancreas transplantation. However, patients who come to kidney transplantation always have a high burden of well-established, long-term complications, including decreased vision from retinopathy and peripheral and cardiovascular disease, and neuropathy. As such, these patients are less likely to benefit from the putative improvement in long-term complications that might be expected from transplantation at an earlier stage of the disease. The balance, therefore, is between the acute risk of surgery and recognized complications of long-term immunosuppression and the putative benefit of pancreas transplantation at an earlier age, before the development of complications. Current recommendations suggest that patients with type 1 diabetes undergoing kidney transplantation, and those rare patients with very brittle diabetes that interferes substantially with their day-to-day existence because of repeated hypoglycemia and ketoacidosis, be considered as candidates for pancreas transplantation.

The most common procedure is shown below. It includes anastomosis of the pancreas attached to the duodenal cuff to the bladder for exocrine drainage, and anastomosis of the pancreatic blood supply into the iliac vessels, resulting in systemic rather than mesenteric insulin delivery. More physiologic approaches also are being used, including enteric drainage of the exocrine pancreas and mesenteric vessel anastomoses to provide more direct insulin delivery to the liver.

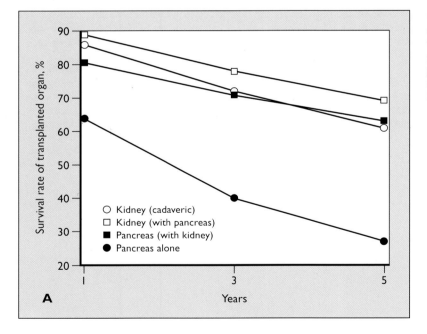

A

FIGURE 5-20. Transplantation results. Increasingly successful technical results of pancreas transplantation have made it a viable choice of therapy, especially in the setting of a kidney transplantation (*see* Fig. 5-19). The metabolic results of pancreas transplantation, *ie,* pancreas transplantation "survival" defined as normal glycemia (fasting glucose or hemoglobin A_{1c} results) without any exogenous insulin or other hypoglycemic agents, are beginning to parallel the results of kidney transplantation (**A**).

(Continued on next page)

B. OUTCOMES OF WHOLE-ORGAN PANCREATIC TRANSPLANTATION

	Simultaneous with Kidney	After Kidney	Solitary
Patient survival, %:			
1 y	93	97	90
3 y	86	88	85
5 y	82	83	77
Pancreas graft survival, %:			
1 y	81	73	64
3 y	71	42	40
5 y	63	34	27
Kidney graft survival, %	86		
Effect on diabetic complications:			
Retinopathy	None		
Neuropathy	Reduces peripheral and autonomic		
Nephropathy:			
Native kidney			Reverses lesions after >5 y
Transplanted kidney	May prevent development	Prevents progression	
Quality of life	Improves (compared with solitary kidney transplantation)		

FIGURE 5-20. (*Continued*) The complications of pancreas transplantation are relatively frequent and must be considered before recommending the procedure to patients. No controlled clinical trials have been performed. However, studies of retinopathy, nephropathy, and neuropathy have been performed that compare patients who have had kidney transplantation alone or failed pancreas transplantation with patients who have had successful pancreas transplantations. These studies have demonstrated improvements in outcome that generally support the role of pancreas transplantation in ameliorating long-term complications (**B**). All data based on published or registry data for 1988 to 1996 [27–39]. Of all pancreas transplantations in patients with diabetes, 87% have been performed as simultaneous kidney-pancreas procedures. Approximately 8% have been done as pancreas after kidney transplantation and 5% as solitary pancreas transplantations. Results from pancreas transplantation performed before 1986 generally were less successful, whereas results from the most recently performed pancreas transplantations reveal better short-term pancreas survival. (*From* UNOS [27]; with permission.)

POTENTIAL ADVANTAGES AND DISADVANTAGES OF WHOLE-ORGAN VERSUS ISLET TRANSPLANTATION

	Whole Organ	Isolated Islets
Surgery	Major surgery required; must drain exocrine secretions	Can be infused in minor procedure
Postoperative complications	Frequent	None
Transplantation tissue:		
Source	Human allograft	Human or other species
Number	Single donor	Islets harvested from multiple donors
Immunosuppression	Major	May be minimal for immunoprotected (encapsulated or masked antigenic sites)
Current efficacy (restoration of normoglycemia at 1 y with no exogenous insulin)	80%–90% success rate	<10%

FIGURE 5-21. Islet transplantation. Many of the drawbacks of whole-organ transplantation, including major abdominal surgery, requirement for long-term immunosuppression, and postoperative complications are potentially eliminated with the use of isolated islets,. Masking of antigenic sites or immunoprotection with encapsulation may not only reduce the need for immunosuppression but may allow the use of islets from other species.

References

1. Dolger H: Clinical evaluation of vascular damage in diabetes mellitus. *JAMA* 1947, 134:1289–1291.

2. DCCT Research Group: The effect of intensive diabetes treatment on the development and progression of long-term complications in insulin-dependent diabetes mellitus: The Diabetes Control and Complications Trial. *N Engl J Med* 1993, 329:978–986.

3. The Kroc Collaborative Study Group: Blood glucose control and the evolution of diabetic retinopathy and albuminuria. *N Engl J Med* 1994, 311:365–372.

4. Feldt-Rasmussen B, Mathiesen ER, Deckert T: Effect of two years of strict metabolic control on progression of incipient nephropathy in insulin-dependent diabetes. *Lancet* December 6, 1986, 1300–1304.

5. Binchmann-Hansen O, Dahl-Jorgensen K, Hanssen KR, Sandvik L: The response of diabetic retinopathy to 41 months of multiple insulin injections, insulin pumps, and conventional insulin therapy. *Arch Ophthalmol* 1988, 106:1242–1246.

6. Reichard P, Nilsson B-Y, Rosenqvist U: The effect of long-term insulin treatment on the development of microvascular complications of diabetes mellitus. *N Engl J Med* 1993, 329:304–309.

7. Nathan DM: The modern management of insulin-dependent diabetes mellitus. *Med Clin NA* 1988, 72:1365–1378.

8. Nathan DM, Singer DE, Hurxthal K, Goodson JD: The clinical information value of the glycosylated hemoglobin assay. *N Engl J Med* 1984, 310:341–346.

9. DCCT Research Group: The absence of a glycemic threshold for the development of long-term complications. *Diabetes* 1996, 45:1289–1298.

10. Cryer PE, Fisher JN, Shamoon H: Hypoglycemia. *Diabetes Care* 1994, 17:734–751.

11. Fanelli C, Epifano L, Rambotti AM, *et al.*: Meticulous prevention of hypoglycemia normalizes the glycemic thresholds and magnitude of most of neuroendocrine responses to, symptoms of, and cognitive function during hypoglycemia in intensively treated patients with short-term IDDM. *Diabetes* 1993, 42:1683–1689.

12. Saleh TY, Cryer PE: Alanine and terbutaline in the prevention of nocturnal hypoglycemia in IDDM. *Diabetes Care* 1997, 20:1231–1236.

13. Zinman B, Tildesley H, Chiasson J-L, *et al.*: Insulin Lispro in CSII. *Diabetes* 1997, 46:440–443.

14. Nathan DM: Long-term complications of diabetes mellitus. *N Engl J Med* 1993, 328:676–685.

15. Galloway JA, *et al.*: Intrasubject differences in pharmacokinetic and pharmacodynamic responses: the immutable problem of present-day treatment? In *Diabetes*. Edited by Serrano-Rios M, Lefebvre PJ. New York: Elsevier Science: 1985.

16. Molnar GD *et al.*: Plasma immunoreactive insulin patterns in insulin-treated diabetics. Studies during continuous blood glucose monitoring *Mayo Clin Proc* 1972, 47:709–719.

17. Nathan DM, Lou P, Avruch J: Intensive conventional and insulin pump therapies in type 1 diabetes. A crossover study. *Ann Intern Med* 1982, 97:31–36.

18. Reichard P, Pihl M: Mortality and treatment side effects during long-term intensified conventional insulin treatment in the Stockholm Diabetes Intervention Study. *Diabetes* 1994, 43:313–317.

19. Dunn FL, Nathan DM, Scavini M, Selam J-L: Long-term therapy of IDDM with an implantable insulin pump. *Diabetes Care* 1997, 20:59–63.

20. DCCT Research Group: Clustering of long-term complications in families with diabetes in the Diabetes Control and Complications Trial. *Diabetes* 1997, 46:1829–1839.

21. Parving HH, Smidt UM, Friisberg B, *et al.*: A prospective study of glomerular filtration rate and arterial blood pressure in insulin-dependent diabetics with nephropathy. *Diabetologia* 1981, 20:457–461.

22. Klein BEK, Moss SE, Klein R: Effect of pregnancy on progression of diabetic retinopathy. *Diabetes Care* 1990, 13:34–40.

23. Lewis EJ: The effect of angiotensin-converting-enzyme inhibition on diabetic nephropathy. *N Engl J Med* 1993, 329:1456–1462.

24. Progression of retinopathy with intensive versus conventional treatment in the Diabetes Control and Complications Trial. Diabetes Control and Compications Trial Research Group. *Opthamology* 1995, 102:647–661.

25. Effect of intensive therapy on the development and progression of diabetic nephropathy in the Diabetes Control and Complications (DCCT) Research Group. *Kidney Int* 1995, 47:1703–1720.

26. DCCT Research Group. Effect of intensive therapy on residual β cell function in patients with type 1 diabetes in the Diabetes Control and Complications Trial. *Ann Int Med* 1998, 128:517–523.

27. UNOS. 1997 Annual Report: U.S. Scientific Registry of Transplant Recipients and The Organ Procurement and Transplantation Network. Bethesda, MD: Department of Health and Human Services, ISBN 1-886651-25-6.

28. Gruessner RW, Sutherland DER: Simultaneous kidney and segmental pancreas transplants from living related donors: the first two successful cases. *Transplantation* 1996, 61:1265–1268.

29. Stegall M, Wachs M, Kam I: Successful pancreas transplantation in adult-onset diabetes mellitus. *Diabetes* 1997, 46(Suppl 1):64A.

30. American Diabetes Association: Pancreas transplantation for patients with diabetes mellitus. *Diabetes Care* 1998, 21(Suppl 1):S79.

31. Sutherland DER, Gruessner RWG: Current status of pancreas transplantation for the treatment of type 1 diabetes mellitus. *Clin Diabetes* 1997, 15:152–156.

32. Ramsay RC, Goetz FC, Sutherland DER, *et al.*: Progression of diabetic retinopathy after pancreas transplantation for insulin-dependent diabetes mellitus. *N Engl J Med* 1988, 318:208–214.

33. Navarro X, Sutherland DER, Kennedy WR: Long-term effects of pancreatic transplantation on diabetic neuropathy. *Ann Neurol* 1997, 42:727–736.

34. Navarro X, Kennedy WR, Sutherland DER: Autonomic neuropathy and survival in diabetes mellitus: effects of pancreas transplantation. *Diabetologia* 1991, 34(Suppl 1): S108–S112.

35. Fioretto P, Steffes MW, Sutherland DER, *et al.*: Reversal of lesions of diabetic nephropathy after pancreas transplantation. *N Engl J Med* 1998, 339:69–75.

36. Bohman SO, Tyden G, Wilczek, *et al.*: Prevention of kidney graft diabetic nephropathy by pancreas transplantation in man. *Diabetes* 1985, 34:306–308.

37. Bilous RW, Mauer SM, Sutherland DER, *et al.*: The effects of pancreas transplantation on the glomerular structure of renal allografts in patients with insulin-dependent diabetes. *N Engl J Med* 1989, 321:80–85.

38. Nathan DM Fogel HA, Norman D, *et al.*: Long-term metabolic and quality of life results with pancreatic/renal transplantation in IDDM. *Transplantation* 1991, 52:85–91.

39. Milde FK, Hart LK, Zehr PS: Quality of life of pancreatic transplant recipients. *Diabetes Care* 1992, 15:1459–1463.

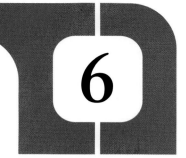

THE PATHOGENESIS OF TYPE 2 NON–INSULIN-DEPENDENT DIABETES

C. Ronald Kahn

Non–insulin-dependent diabetes mellitus, or type 2 diabetes (the currently preferred nomenclature), is among the most common chronic diseases, affecting about 6% of the U.S. population (approximately 15 million people) [1]. The prevalence of this disease in the United States has increased rapidly over the past 50 years (Fig. 6-1). It has been estimated that the number of people affected with non–insulin-dependent diabetes worldwide will increase from 135 million to over 300 million by 2025, with most of this increase occurring in developing countries. The prevalence of non–insulin-dependent diabetes in the United States is highest in minority populations, including African Americans, Mexican Americans, and especially Native Americans. In the Pima Indians of Arizona, 50% of adults older than age 35 years have the disease [2]. In all populations, the prevalence increases with age; in white persons, the prevalence reaches 17% by the age of 80 years [1]. Non–insulin-dependent diabetes is frequently associated with other metabolic abnormalities, sometimes called the "metabolic syndrome" or syndrome X, which includes central obesity, hyperlipidemia, hypertension, and accelerated atherosclerosis [3].

Glucose homeostasis in the fasting state is the balance between glucose production by the liver and glucose utilization by muscle and fat (Fig. 6-2). Although the fine-tuning of glucose metabolism may be influenced by many hormones and metabolic intermediates, normal glucose disposal depends primarily on only four factors: 1) the ability of the body to secrete insulin both acutely and in a sustained fashion; 2) the ability of insulin to inhibit hepatic glucose output; 3) the ability of glucose to promote glucose disposal, ie, insulin sensitivity; and 4) the ability of glucose to enter the cells in the absence of insulin, sometimes called glucose sensitivity or glucose effectiveness [4] (Fig. 6-3).

The pathogenesis of type 2 diabetes appears to involve at least two defects in this system of regulation (Figs. 6-2 and 6-4). The earliest detectable lesion is insulin resistance in peripheral tissues [2,5,6]. The beta cells of the pancreas detect the insulin resistance and respond by increasing insulin secretion, as measured by an elevation in the fasting insulin level. As the prediabetic state progresses, insulin resistance increases and insulin levels gradually rise [7]. Eventually, the pancreas appears to lose its ability to meet this demand, insulin levels begin to decrease, and non–insulin-dependent diabetes develops (Fig. 6-5). At this point, the beta cell is desensitized to glucose stimulation but still responds to other insulin secretagogues (Fig. 6-6).

Considerable evidence indicates that both type 2 diabetes and the accompanying fundamental defects are the result of an interaction between genes and the environment [6,8] (Fig. 6-7). Studies in populations at high risk for developing non–insulin-dependent diabetes, such as offspring of diabetic parents and Pima Indians, have demonstrated that insulin resistance both precedes and predicts the development of non–insulin-dependent diabetes [2,5]. In these populations, low insulin sensitivity can be detected in normoglycemic persons in their teens or early twenties. There is also familial clustering of insulin sensitivity [2,9] (Fig. 6-8). Longitudinal studies have shown that offspring with a low insulin sensitivity are much more likely to develop type 2 diabetes than offspring with normal or high insulin sensitivity (Fig. 6-9). Type 2 diabetes is both polygenic and heterogeneous (Fig. 6-10). In general, the monogenic forms of diabetes develop in younger patients, whereas the polygenic forms occur later in life. The best characterized of these are the forms called maturity-onset diabetes of the young (MODY) [10,11] (Figs. 6-11 to 6-13). The role of the environment is multifaceted. The major predisposing factors to non–insulin-dependent diabetes are obesity, decreased activity, and increasing age [6] (Fig. 6-14).

Because insulin resistance is the earliest defect in most patients with non–insulin-dependent diabetes, understanding the molecular mechanism of insulin action and its alterations in insulin resistance is essential to understanding the disease. Over the past 20 years, tremendous progress has been made in understanding insulin action at a molecular level [12–15] (Figs. 6-15 to 6-19). In type 2 diabetes, a combination of genetic, physiologic, environmental, and disease factor changes occur (Figs. 6-20 to 6-24). Although there has been a long debate about the value of treatment of non–insulin-dependent diabetes, the recently completely United Kingdom Prospective Diabetes Study [UKPDS] has conclusively demonstrated that improved glucose control of non–insulin-dependent diabetes significantly reduces the incidence of long-term complications and prolongs life [16,17] (Fig. 6-25). Understanding the physiologic basis for non–insulin-dependent diabetes also allows us to understand the basis for treatment of the disease [18] (Fig. 6-26).

Pathogenesis of Type 2 Non–Insulin-Dependent Diabetes

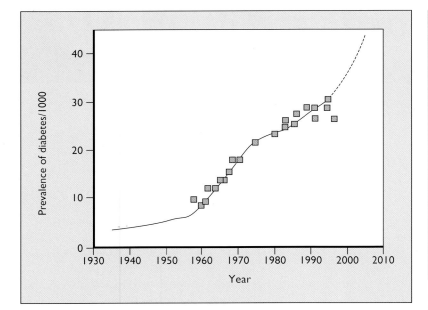

FIGURE 6-1. Increasing prevalence of diabetes in the United States. The prevalence of diagnosed diabetes in the United States has risen steadily since 1930 and is expected to continue to increase rapidly in the early part of the 21st century. About 90% of cases of diagnosed diabetes are of non–insulin-dependent diabetes. It is estimated that at any given time, at least one-third of persons with non–insulin-dependent diabetes are undiagnosed. (*Adapted from Harris et al.* [1]; *with permission.*)

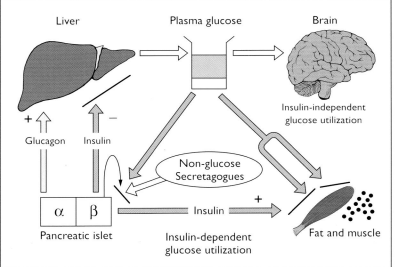

FIGURE 6-2. Regulation of glucose homeostasis. The blood glucose level is a balance between glucose production by the liver and glucose utilization by insulin-independent tissues (such as the brain, kidney, and erythrocytes) and insulin-dependent tissues (such as fat and muscle). This balance is orchestrated by hormones of the endocrine pancreas: insulin from the beta cell and glucagon from the alpha cell. In non–insulin-dependent diabetes, there is insulin resistance in the liver, muscle, and fat and a decrease in the ability of the beta cell to sense glucose and increase insulin levels appropriately. This figure also shows the defects in insulin action on the liver, muscle, and fat and defects in glucose sensing by the beta cell in non–insulin-dependent diabetes. Recent evidence suggests that insulin action at the beta cell may be important in glucose sensing and that this is another site of insulin resistance in non–insulin-dependent diabetes [19].

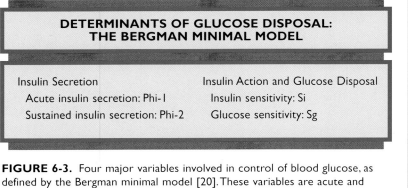

FIGURE 6-3. Four major variables involved in control of blood glucose, as defined by the Bergman minimal model [20]. These variables are acute and sustained insulin secretion (sometimes called first- and second-phase secretion), the ability of insulin to act on peripheral tissues (insulin sensitivity), and the ability of glucose to enter cells in the absence of insulin or in the presence of basal insulin only (glucose sensitivity).

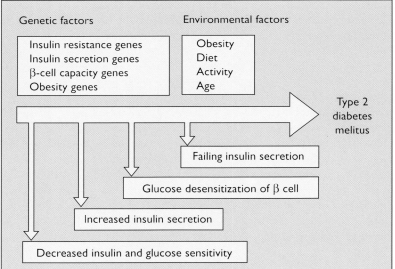

FIGURE 6-4. The progressive pathogenesis of type 2 diabetes. The pathogenesis of the disease develops over many years. The earliest detectable lesion is insulin resistance. Initially, increased insulin secretion compensates for this defect. Eventually, the beta cell becomes desensitized to the glucose stimulus and insulin levels decrease, leading to clinically overt diabetes. Both the insulin resistance and beta-cell failure are genetically programmed and influenced by environmental factors, such as diet, activity, and aging.

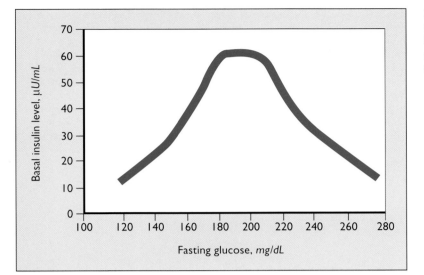

FIGURE 6-5. The "Starling curve" of the pancreas. In early non–insulin-dependent diabetes, insulin levels increase as glucose levels increase. Eventually, however, the beta cell loses its glucose-sensing ability and insulin levels begin to decrease. This creates a bell-shaped curve, reminiscent of Starling's curve for cardiac contractility.

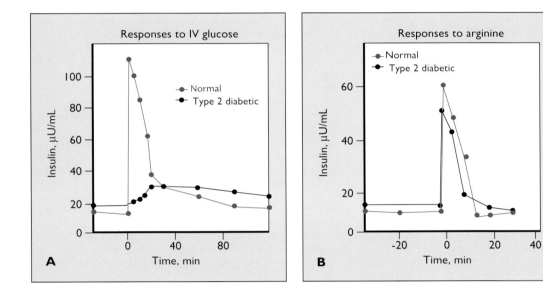

FIGURE 6-6. Typical insulin secretory defect in patients with non–insulin-dependent diabetes. This consists of a loss of first-phase insulin secretion to an intravenous glucose stimulus (**A**); the responses to intravenous (IV) arginine (**B**) and other secreta-gogues are maintained [21]. This lesion indicates the glucose-specific sensing defect present in this disease. A similar lesion is also seen in early insulin-dependent diabetes. The exact mechanism is unclear but may involve a decrease in GLUT2 glucose transporters in the pancreas.

The Role of Genes and the Environment

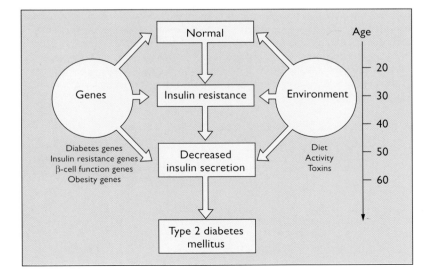

FIGURE 6-7. Genes and the environment in the development of type 2 diabetes. The early prediabetic phase begins in young adulthood and can be identified as insulin resistance in peripheral tissues. Initially, insulin levels are elevated in response to the resistance, but as glucose desensitization develops, insulin secretion decreases. This eventually leads to clinical non–insulin-dependent diabetes. Both the insulin resistance and the decreased insulin secretion are genetically programmed. This program is modified by a variety of environmental factors, especially diet and activity. (*Adapted from* Kahn [6]; with permission.)

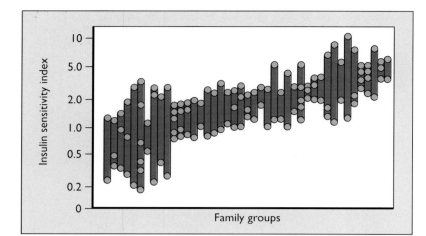

FIGURE 6-8. Familial clustering of insulin sensitivity. Insulin sensitivity is inherited within families. In this figure, each vertical bar represents a family cluster for offspring of diabetic parents, and each dot represents a sibling in this family who has had his or her insulin sensitivity assessed by using the Bergman minimal model of glucose clearance during and intravenous glucose tolerance test [9]. Some families consist primarily of individuals with low insulin sensitivity, whereas other families are composed of individuals with high insulin sensitivity. This clustering suggests some genetic control of insulin sensitivity. Similar results have been observed in family studies of Pima Indian populations [2] and in Mexican Americans [22]. Of note, familial clustering is also observed for measurements of first-phase insulin secretion [23] but not for insulin-independent glucose uptake (*ie*, glucose sensitivity).

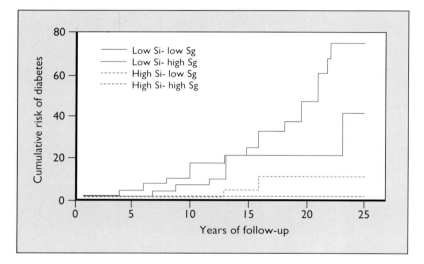

FIGURE 6-9. Cumulative risk for non–insulin-dependent diabetes. Low insulin sensitivity and low glucose effectiveness precede and predict the development of this disease. To determine the effect of low insulin sensitivity and glucose sensitivity on the development of diabetes, a prospective study was performed

among offspring of two parents with non–insulin-dependent diabetes at the Joslin Diabetes Center [5]. The normoglycemic offspring were screened by using an intravenous glucose tolerance test; results were analyzed with the Bergman minimal model [20]. This allowed the participants to be divided into four groups on the basis of their initial insulin sensitivity (Si) and glucose sensitivity (Sg) values: a group with low insulin sensitivity (*ie*, insulin sensitivity below the mean), a group with high insulin sensitivity (insulin sensitivity above the mean), a group with low glucose sensitivity, and a group with high glucose sensitivity. The cumulative risk for developing non–insulin-dependent diabetes over the subsequent 25 years of follow-up in these four groups of offspring was defined by the insulin sensitivity and glucose sensitivity. If an individual had both low insulin sensitivity and low glucose sensitivity (*ie*, values in the lower half of the normal range), he or she had a greater than 80% probability of developing non–insulin-dependent diabetes during follow-up. By contrast, if the offspring had high insulin sensitivity and high glucose sensitivity, none developed diabetes, even though they had two diabetic parents. If one value was high and the other value was low, they had intermediate risk for non–insulin-dependent diabetes, although low insulin sensitivity produced a greater risk than low glucose sensitivity. By contrast, insulin secretory response to the intravenous glucose challenge did not predict development of diabetes; indeed, the "prediabetics" had higher, rather than lower, values of first-phase insulin secretion. This finding suggests that in this phase of the disease, the beta cell was compensating for the insulin resistance of peripheral tissues [24].

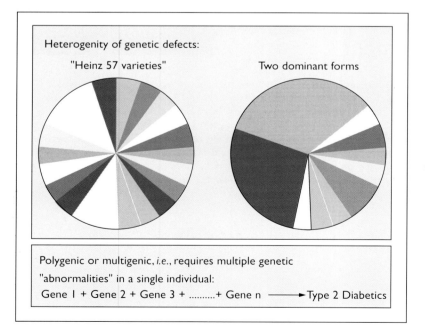

FIGURE 6-10. Two major features of the genetics of non–insulin-dependent diabetes mellitus in the general population. First, this disease is a genetically heterogeneous disorder. At present, however, it is not clear how many forms of diabetes exist, whether there are one or two predominant forms, or whether each form represents only a small percentage of the total population. For most patients, the disease is polygenic: Some abnormality or sequence polymorphism is present in several genes, each contributing a small amount to the overall pathogenesis. Although there is no definitive information on the number of genes involved in each form, most investigators believe that at least three genes, and perhaps as many as 10 or 20, may contribute to the final phenotype. Most likely, these are "normal" genetic variants or sequence polymorphisms, which slightly alter insulin action or insulin secretion [6].

A GENETIC CLASSIFICATION OF HUMAN TYPE 2 DIABETES MELLITUS

Monogenic forms of Type 2 diabetes

Defects in insulin synthesis or secretion

MODY 1: HNF-4α

MODY 2: Glucokinase

MODY 3: HNF-1α

MODY 4: PDX-1 (IPF-1)

MODY 5: HNF-1β

Mutations in mitochondrial DNA tRNA^{leu}

Maternally inherited diabetes associated with nerve deafness

Defects in insulin receptor

Leprechaunism

Type A syndrome of insulin resistance and acanthosis nigricans

Rabson-Mendenhall syndrome

Polygenic forms of diabetes

Type 2 (non–insulin-dependent) diabetes

Epidemiology suggests both genetic heterogeneity and polygenic pathogenesis

No single major locus identified, however, several signaling proteins show sequence polymorphism

FIGURE 6-11. Genetic classification of non–insulin-dependent diabetes. There are several monogenic forms of the disease. The best characterized are the several forms of maturity-onset diabetes of the young (MODY). Mutations in mitochondrial DNA that encode the transfer RNA (t-RNA) for leucine are also associated with a maternally inherited form of non–insulin-dependent diabetes associated with nerve deafness. Defects in the insulin receptor may also cause diabetes. The most common forms of non–insulin-dependent diabetes, however, are polygenic. HNF—hepatic nuclear factor; IPF—insulin promoter factor; PDX—pancreatic development factor.

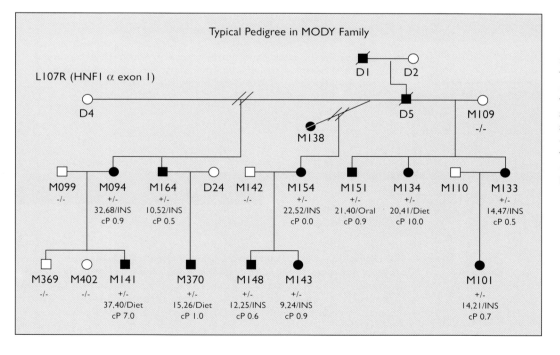

Typical Pedigree in MODY Family

FIGURE 6-12. Typical pedigree of a family with maturity-onset diabetes of the young (MODY). Note that affected individuals occur in three successive generations; the gene can be passed from either parent to children of either sex, a pattern consistent with an autosomal dominant form of transmission. The various forms of MODY are listed in Figure 6-11, and the molecular defects are shown in Figure 6-13. The family shown has a defect in HNF-1alpha and is therefore a MODY3 family. This is the most common form of MODY in the United States. (Family tree kindly provided by A. Doria)

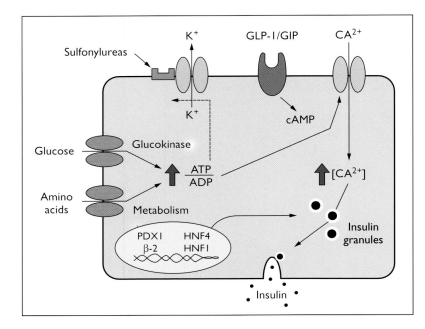

FIGURE 6-13. Nutrient sensing and insulin secretion by the pancreatic beta cell. The beta cell takes up glucose and amino acids via specific transporters on the cell membrane, such as the GLUT2 glucose transporter. This isoform of transporter is expressed only by the beta cell and the liver and has a Km in the physiologic range. Once inside the cell, glucose is phosphorylated by a specialized form of hexokinase called glucokinase. The subsequent metabolism of glucose results in a change in the adenosine triphosphate (ATP):adenosine diphosphate (ADP) ratio in the cell, which in turn causes activation of the ATP-sensitive potassium channel. This results in depolarization of the cell, an influx of calcium, and subsequent release of insulin from secretory granules. The sulfonylurea receptor can also activate the ATP-sensitive potassium channel, mimicking the effect of glucose. Other secretagogues, such as glucagon-like peptide-1 (GLP-1), bypass this system by changing cellular cyclic adenosine monophosphate (cAMP) levels. The level of expression of the several molecules involved in glucose sensing, including the GLUT2 glucose transporter, and the development of the beta cell are controlled by several nuclear transcription factors. The best studied of these are HNF-1alpha, HNF-1beta, HNF-4alpha, and PDX-1 (IPF-1). Maturity-onset diabetes of the young can result from genetic defects in any of these transcription factors or a genetic defect in glucokinase. In non–insulin-dependent diabetes, the exact site of the defect in glucose sensing in unknown, but studies in animal models of disease have suggested that this may be the result of a down-regulation of the GLUT2 glucose transporter [25].

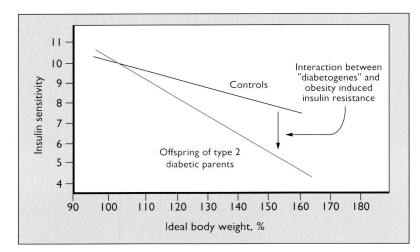

FIGURE 6-14. Interaction between obesity and genetic predisposition to type 2 diabetes. Obesity causes insulin resistance and potentiates the genetic defect in non–insulin-dependent diabetes. More than 70% of diabetic patients and 50% of all Americans are overweight, and almost one third of the latter group are obese. It is well known that obesity itself causes insulin resistance [26]. Thus, in normal individuals, as body weight increases above ideal, insulin sensitivity decreases. In individuals with a family history of non–insulin-dependent diabetes, the decrease in insulin sensitivity is greater for every increment in body weight than in the normal population (*ie*, obesity causes even more insulin resistance). This is bad news for the person who has inherited these diabetogenes. The good news is that for every increment of weight reduction, the genetically susceptible individual has a greater improvement in insulin sensitivity than the control. Thus, weight reduction is still an important component of diabetes management and the prevention of diabetes in susceptible individuals.

Insulin Action and Insulin Resistance at the Molecular Level

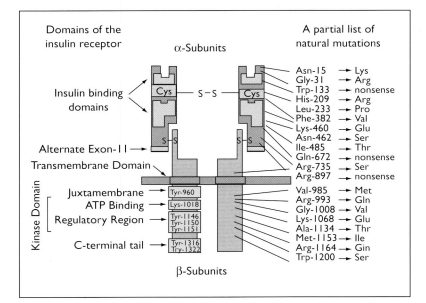

FIGURE 6-15. The structure of the insulin receptor and some typical insulin receptor mutations. The insulin receptor consists of two alpha subunits (which are entirely extracellular and bind the insulin molecule) linked to each other and to two beta subunits by disulfide bonds to form a tetramer. The beta subunits are transmembrane proteins that contain the tyrosine kinase activity in their intracellular domains. This kinase is activated by insulin binding to the alpha subunit and conducts the insulin signal to the intracellular substrates. About 100 different mutations have been identified in the insulin receptor; these mutations occur throughout the length of the receptor [27]. Many are missense mutations causing changes in receptor sequence or premature truncation of the receptor protein. Patients with receptor mutations usually present with a syndrome of severe insulin resistance, such as leprechaunism, the type A syndrome of insulin resistance, and acanthosis nigricans or the Rabson-Mendenhall syndrome. ATP—adenosine triphosphate.

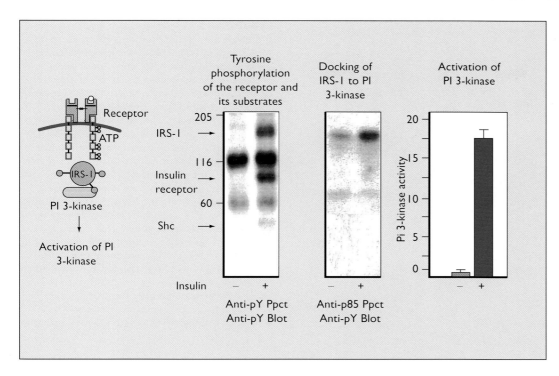

FIGURE 6-16. Three early steps in insulin action depicted schematically (*left panel*) and experimentally (*right three panels*). Insulin binds to the receptor and activates the tyrosine kinase activity present in the receptor. This leads to autophosphorylation of the receptor beta subunit and substrates such as insulin receptor substrate-1 (IRS-1). This can be detected in immunoblots by using antiphosphotyrosine (anti-pY) antibody. The phosphorylated IRS-1 binds to the regulatory (p85) subunit of phosphatidylinositol 3-kinase (PI 3-kinase). This interaction can be detected by immunoprecipitating the cell extract the anti-p85 antibodies, applying this precipitate to sodium dodecyl sulfate (SDS) gels, and immunoblotting the result gel transfer with anti-pY antibody. This results in a 10- to 20-fold activation of PI 3-kinase. Shc—a low molecular weight insulin receptor substrate; Ppct—precipitate.

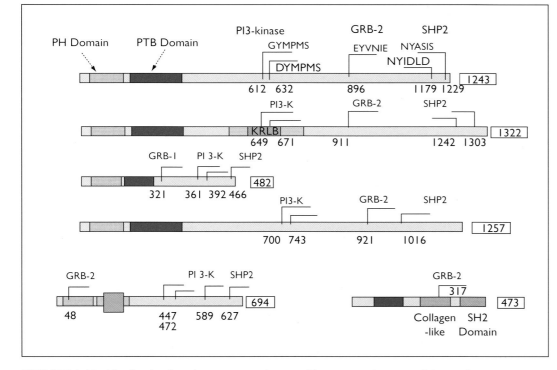

FIGURE 6-17. The family of insulin receptor substrates. The major substrates of the insulin receptor are a group of high-molecular-weight cytosolic proteins termed the insulin receptor substrate (IRS) proteins [28]. Four members of this IRS family have been identified. These IRS proteins vary in molecular weight

between 60,000 and 180,000. All possess many (up to 22) potential sites of tyrosine phosphorylation, each occurring in a specific sequence motif. The IRS proteins serve as intracellular "docking proteins," interacting with other intracellular signaling molecules. The IRS proteins usually bind to other proteins in the cell through the phosphorylation motifs in IRS proteins and specific domains on the target proteins termed SH2 (src homology 2) domains [29]. Over the past few years, many proteins containing SH2 domains (and some that do not contain SH2 domains) have been identified in cells that interact with the IRS proteins. The best studied of these is the lipid-modifying enzyme phosphatidylinositol 3-kinase (PI 3-kinase). When phosphorylated IRS-1 or IRS-2 bind to PI 3-kinase, enzymatic activity is rapidly stimulated. This is critical to many of the metabolic effects of insulin, including stimulation of glucose transport. Docking of IRS to other proteins stimulates other pathways as well, leading to a complex insulin signaling network.

The other insulin receptor substrates shown are GAB1, which is similar in character to the IRS proteins but lacks a phosphotyrosine-binding (PTB) domain and the Shc proteins. The latter are a family of three proteins, about 50 to 60 kDa in size, that have only one tyrosine phosphorylation site and are involved in GRB-2 binding. PH—plextrin homology domain; PTB—phosphotyrosine-binding domain.

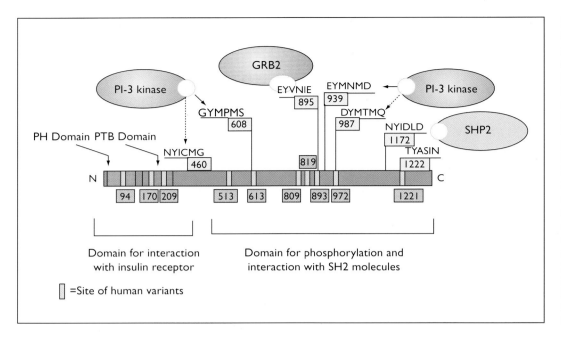

FIGURE 6-18. The structure of insulin receptor substrate type 1 (IRS-1) and sites of human variants. After phosphorylation, IRS-1 and other IRS proteins serve as "docking sites" for other intracellular proteins involved in insulin signaling. The proteins bind to the phosphorylation sites in the IRS proteins through specialized domains called SH2 (src homology 2) domains. The SH2-domain proteins include enzymes such as phosphatidylinositol 3-kinase (PI 3-kinase) and the phosphotyrosine phosphatase SHP2, as well as adaptor proteins such as GRB2. At least 10 sequence polymorphisms have been described in the IRS-1 protein. The most common of these is the change of a glycine residue at position 972 to arginine [30]. In most studies, these polymorphisms occur in about 5% of nondiabetic persons and slightly more than 10% of patients with non–insulin-dependent diabetes. In general, these variant IRS-1 proteins are 30% to 60% as effective as normal IRS-1 proteins in transmitting the insulin signal to PI 3-kinase. In affected individuals, this defect may contribute to the polygenic cause of non–insulin-dependent diabetes. PTB—phosphotyrosine-binding.

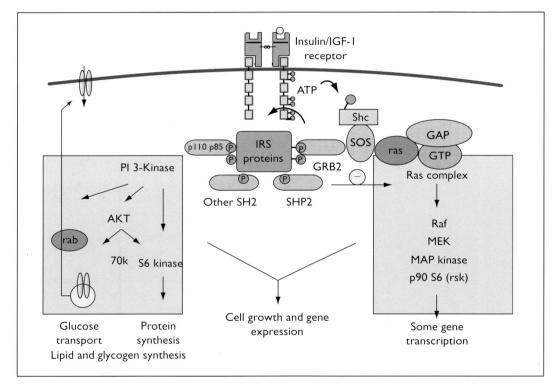

FIGURE 6-19. The insulin signaling network. The full network is complex and can be divided into five levels: 1) activation of the insulin receptor tyrosine kinase and closely linked events; 2) phosphorylation of a family of substrate proteins; 3) interaction of the receptor and its substrates with several intermediate signaling molecules via SH2 (src homology 2) and other recognition domains; 4) activation of serine and lipid kinases, resulting in a broad range of phosphory-lation-dephosphorylation events; and 5) regulation of the final biological effectors of insulin action, such as glucose transport, lipid synthesis, gene expression, and mitogenesis. The SH2 proteins link the insulin receptor substrate (IRS) proteins to a series of cascading reactions involving serine/threonine kinases and phosphatases such as the MAP kinases, S6 kinases, and protein phosphatase-1A. These serine kinases act on enzymes such as glycogen synthase, transcription factors, and other proteins to produce many of the final biological effects of the hormone. In adipose tissue and muscle, insulin stimulation also increases glucose uptake by promoting translocation of an intracellular pool of glucose transporters to the plasma membrane. Exactly how this action is linked to the phosphorylation cascade is unknown, but several studies suggest that this important action of insulin, as well as most metabolic effects, are downstream of the enzyme phosphatidylinositol 3-kinase (PI 3-kinase). Other effects of insulin, such as stimulation of glycogen and lipid synthesis, occur through additional intracellular effects to stimulate the enzymes involved in these reactions. ATP—adenosine triphosphate; GAP—GTPase activating protein; GRB2—growth-factor receptor binding protein 2; GTP—guanosine triphosphate; IGF—insulin-like growth factor; MAP kinase—mitogen activated protein kinase MEK—MAP-Erk kinase; SOS—son-of-seven less protein.

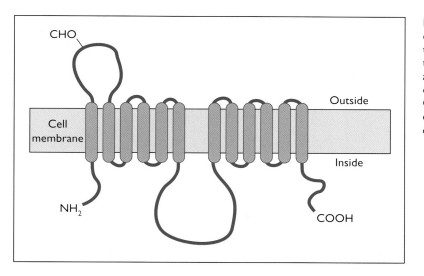

FIGURE 6-20. Schematic structure of a glucose transporter. The most typical effect of insulin in muscle and fat is stimulation of glucose transport. This occurs through a translocation of glucose transporters from an intracellular pool to the plasma membrane. Mammals have six isoforms of glucose transporters. Five are involved in facilitated transport. Each transporter has 12 membrane-spanning domains, which form a channel for glucose to pass through the cell membrane. GLUT4 is the insulin-sensitive glucose transporter. There is also a sodium-dependent glucose transporter (or, more likely, two forms) involved in absorption of glucose from the intestine and reabsorption of glucose in the kidney.

The Molecular Mechanisms of Insulin Resistance

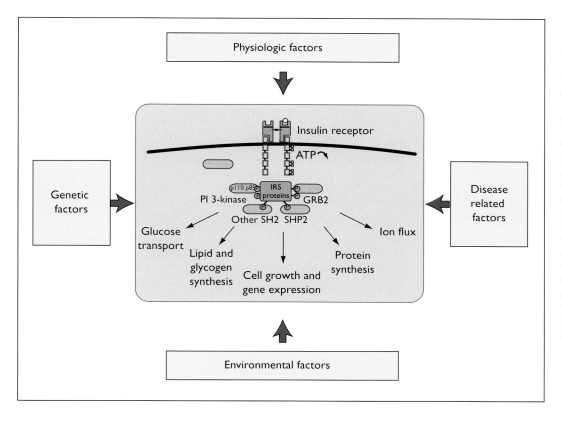

FIGURE 6-21. Range of factors that can regulate insulin action at the cellular level. This regulation often occurs at early steps in insulin action. In animal models of non–insulin-dependent diabetes, such as the ob/ob mouse, considerable evidence suggests alterations in the early steps of insulin action [31]. For example, insulin receptor phosphorylation decreases by 50% and phosphorylation of insulin receptor substrate (IRS) type 1 decreases by 90% in the obese diabetic mouse. Similar alterations occur in tissues of humans with non–insulin-dependent diabetes [32]. These defects appear to be acquired in most patients because patients with non–insulin-dependent diabetes usually do not have mutations in the insulin receptor or IRS-1 itself, and the alteration in receptor function and kinase activity improves with weight reduction. Patients with non–insulin-dependent diabetes also have decreases in many other intracellular steps in insulin action, including stimulation of glycogen synthesis and nonoxidative glucose metabolism [26,33]. ATP—adenosine triphosphate; GRB2—growth-factor receptor-binding protein 2; PI 3-kinase—phosphatidylinositol 3-kinase; SH2—src homology 2.

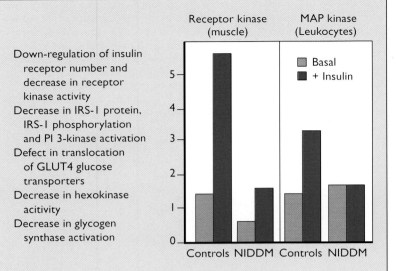

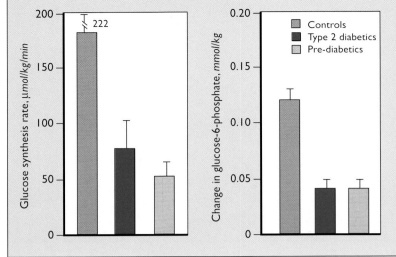

FIGURE 6-22. Development of insulin resistance in humans with non–insulin-dependent diabetes. It is still unclear where, at a molecular level, the genetic defects in this disease are. As noted above, non–insulin-dependent diabetes (NIDDM) is a heterogeneous, polygenic disease. A few genes have proven potential for causing some forms of the disease, but the genes causing the common form remain unknown. At least one contributing factor may be sequence polymorphisms in insulin-signaling proteins, such as insulin resistance substrate type I (IRS-I), which could combine with other genetic or acquired defects to produce severe insulin resistance [30]. **Right,** The decreased insulin stimulation of insulin receptor and the decreased activation of MAP kinase in cells of a patient with non–insulin-dependent diabetes. **Left,** some of the other defects present in this disease. Most of these are aquired.

FIGURE 6-23. Insulin resistance in offspring of diabetic parents. **Right,** Insulin action on glucose transport and phosphorylation was measured in normal individuals, individuals with non–insulin-dependent diabetes, and normoglycemic offspring of patients with non–insulin-dependent diabetes by using 31P-NMR. Both the diabetic patients and the normoglycemic offspring demonstrate insulin resistance at the level of glucose transport. **Left,** Glycogen synthesis was assessed in the same individuals by using 13C-NMR and showed similar levels of insulin resistance. NMR—nuclear magnetic resonance spectroscopy protein. (*Adapted from* Rothman *et al.* [34]; with permission).

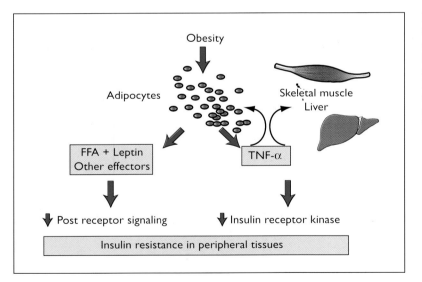

FIGURE 6-24. Mechanisms of insulin resistance in obesity are multiple. Obesity adds to the genetic predisposition of insulin resistance in non–insulin-dependent diabetes. This most likely occurs through the production of some inhibitors of insulin action by the fat cell. These inhibitors might include free fatty acids (FFA), tumor necrosis factor-alpha (TNF-alpha), and the appetite-regulating hormone leptin. Tumor necrosis factor-alpha inhibits the insulin receptor kinase by increasing the serine phosphorylation of insulin receptor substrate type I [35]. Free fatty acids have been postulated to produce insulin resistance by several mechanisms, but, the exact mechanism remains unknown [36].

The Physiologic Basis for Treatment of Type 2 Diabetes

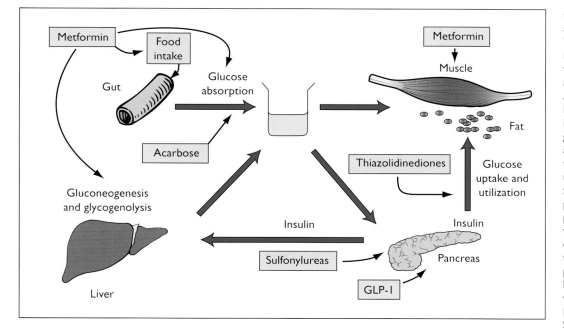

that the major site of action of metformin is the liver and an inhibition of hepatic glucose output [38,39]. The thiazolidinediones improve insulin sensitivity in muscle and fat [39,40]. This occurs via interaction with a nuclear receptor PPARγ2, which also serves as the initial regulator of fat cell differentiation. Activation of this nuclear receptor increases the level of gene expression of many proteins involved in insulin action and insulin sensitivity. An interesting group of obese patients were recently described with activating mutations in PPARγ; the phenotype of these patients includes massive obesity but relatively normal insulin sensitivity [41]. There are several thiazolidinediones, including troglitazone, rosiglitazone, pioglitazone, and englitazone. About one-third of patients with type 2 diabetes cannot be managed with the combination of lifestyle modification and oral agents and must be treated with insulin. Although there has been concern about the use of insulin in patients with type 2 diabetes because hyperinsulinemia has been associated with increased cardiovascular morbidity in several population studies [42], the United Kingdom Prospective Diabetes Study has definitively demonstrated that patients with non–insulin-dependent diabetes receiving insulin have improved outcomes compared with less aggressively treated patients not receiving insulin (see Fig. 6-26).

FIGURE 6-25. Sites of action of drugs used to treat non–insulin-dependent diabetes. Diet and exercise are directed at improving insulin sensitivity by reducing the effects of obesity and sedentary lifestyle. Different oral hypoglycemic agents have different sites of action. Sulfonylureas act on a receptor on the pancreatic beta cell to stimulate insulin secretion, thus bypassing the glucose sensing apparatus [37]. Most studies suggest

FIGURE 6-26. Results of the United Kingdom Prospective Diabetes Study (UKPDS) showed an unequivocal effect of intensive insulin therapy on long-term complications of diabetes and mortality [16,17]. HbA$_{1c}$—glycated hemoglobin; Rx—therapy.

UKPDS: EFFECTS OF INTENSIVE TREATMENT OF TYPE 2 DIABETES

Reduced HbA1c by 11% with intensive Rx (7.9 vs. 7.0%)
This leads to
  12% decrease in any diabetes-related endpoint
  25% decrease in microvascular endpoints
  21% decrease in retinopathy at 12 years
  33% decrease in microalbuminuria at 12 years
  24% decrease in cataract
  16% decrease in myocardial infarction (ns)
  5% decrease in stroke (ns)

References

1. *Diabetes in America*, edn 2. Edited by Harris RA, Cowie CC, Stern MP, *et al.* Bethesda: National Institutes of Health; 1995.

2. Bogardus C, Lillioja S, Bennett PH: Pathogenesis of NIDDM in Pima Indians. *Diabetes Care* 1991, 14:685–690.

3. Reaven GM: Pathophysiology of insulin resistance in human disease. *Physiol Rev* 1995, 75:473–486.

4. Bergman RN, Steil GM, Bradley DC, *et al.*: Modeling of insulin action in vivo. *Annu Rev Physiol* 1992, 54:861–883.

5. Martin BC, Warram JH, Krolewski AS, *et al.*: Role of glucose and insulin resistance in development of Type II diabetes mellitus: results of a 25-year follow-up study. *Lancet* 1992, 340:925–929.

6. Kahn CR: Insulin action, diabetogenes, and the cause of type II diabetes (Banting Lecture). *Diabetes* 1994, 43:1066–1084.

7. Bogardus C, Lillioja S, Howard BV, *et al.*: Relationships between insulin secretion, insulin action, and fasting plasma glucose concentration in nondiabetic and noninsulin-dependent diabetic subjects. *J Clin Invest* 1984, 74:1238–1246.

8. Permutt MA, Chiu K, Ferrer J, *et al.*: Genetics of Type II diabetes. *Recent Prog Horm Res* 1998, 53:216.

9. Martin BC, Warram JH, Rosner B, *et al.*: Familial clustering of insulin sensitivity. *Diabetes* 1992, 41:850–854.

10. Fajans SS, Bell GI, Bowden DW, *et al.*: Maturity-onset diabetes of the young. *Life Sci* 1994, 55:413–422.

11. Zhang Y, Proenca R, Maffei M, *et al.*: Positional cloning of the mouse obese gene and its human homologue. *Nature* 1994, 372:425–432.

12. Cheatham B, Kahn CR: Insulin action and the insulin signaling network. *Endocr Rev* 1995, 16:117–142.

13. White MF, Kahn CR: The insulin signaling system. *J Biol Chem* 1994, 269:1–4.

14. White MF: The insulin signalling system and the IRS proteins. *Diabetologia* 1997, 40:S2-S17.

15. Kahn BB: Glucose transport: pivotal step in insulin action (Lilly Lecture 1995). *Diabetes* 1996, 45:1644–1654.

16. UK Prospective Diabetes Study (UKPDS) Group. Intensive blood-glucose control with sulphonylureas or insulin compared with conventional treatment and risk of complications in patients with type 2 diabetes (UKPDS 33). *Lancet* 1998, 352:837–853.

17. Turner RC: The U.K. Prospective Diabetes Study. A review. *Diabetes Care* 1998, 21:C35–C38.

18. Caligo MA, Cipollini G, Fiore L, *et al.*: NM23 gene expression correlates with cell growth rate and S-phase. *Int J Cancer* 1995, 60:837–842.

19. Kulkarni RN, Bruning JC, Winnay JN, *et al.*: Tissue-specific knockout of the insulin receptor in pancreatic b cells creates an insulin secretory defect similar to that in Type 2 diabetes. *Cell* 1999, 96:329–339.

20. Bergman RN: Toward physiological understanding of glucose tolerance. Minimal model approach (Lilly Lecture 1989). *Diabetes* 1989, 38:1512–1527.

21. Porte D Jr.: BETA cells in type II diabetes mellitus (Banting Lecture 1990). *Diabetes* 1991, 40:166–180.

22. Gulli G, Ferrannini E, Stern M, *et al.*: The metabolic profile of NIDDM is fully established in glucose-tolerant offspring of two Mexican-American NIDDM parents. *Diabetes* 1992, 41:1575–1568.

23. Turner R, Hattersley A, Cook J: Type II diabetes: search for primary defects. *Ann Med* 1992, 24:511–516.

24. Galuska D, Nolte LA, Wahlstrom E, *et al.*: Effects of non-esterified fatty acids on insulin-stimulated glucose transport in isolated skeletal muscle from patients with Type 2 (non-insulin-dependent) diabetes mellitus. *Acta Diabetol* 1994, 31:169–172.

25. Thorens B, Wu YJ, Leahy JL, *et al.*: The loss of GLUT2 expression by glucose-unresponsive beta cells of db/db mice is reversible and is induced by the diabetic environment. *J Clin Invest* 1992, 90:77–85.

26. Felber JP, Haesler E, Jequier E: Metabolic origin of insulin resistance in obesity with and without type 2 (non-insulin-dependent) diabetes mellitus. *Diabetologia* 1993, 36:1221–1229.

27. Taylor SI, Accili D: Mutations in the genes encoding the insulin receptor and insulin receptor substrate-1. In: *Diabetes Mellitus: A Fundamental and Clinical Text*. Edited by LeRoith D, Taylor SI, Olefsky JM. Philadelphia: Lippincott–Raven; 1996: 575.

28. Sun XJ, Rothenberg PL, Kahn CR, *et al.*: The structure of the insulin receptor substrate IRS-1 defines a unique signal transduction protein. *Nature* 1991, 352:73–77.

29. Pawson T: Protein modules and signaling networks. *Nature* 1995, 373:573–580.

30. Almind K, Inoue G, Pedersen O, *et al.*: A common amino acid polymorphism in insulin receptor substrate-1 causes impaired insulin signaling. Evidence from transfection studies. *J Clin Invest* 1996, 97:2569–2575.

31. Kerouz NJ, Horsch D, Pons S, *et al.*: Differential regulation of insulin receptor substrates-1 and -2 (IRS-1 and IRS-2) and phosphatidylinositol 3-kinase isoforms in liver and muscle of the obese diabetic (ob/ob) mouse. *J Clin Invest* 1997, 100:3164–3172.

32. Rondinone CM, Wang LM, Lonnroth P, *et al.*: Insulin receptor substrate (IRS) 1 is reduced and IRS-2 is the main docking protein for phosphatidylinositol 3-kinase in adipocytes from subjects with non-insulin-dependent diabetes mellitus. *Proc Natl Acad Sci U S A* 1997, 94:4171–4175.

33. Roden M, Shulman GI: Applications of NMR spectroscopy to study muscle glycogen metabolism in man. *Annu Rev Med* 1999, 50:277–290.

34. Rothman DL, Magnusson I, Cline G, *et al.*: Decreased muscle glucose transport/phosphorylation is an early defect in the pathogenesis of non-insulin-dependent diabetes mellitus. *Proc Natl Acad Sci U S A* 1995, 92:983–987.

35. Hotamisligil GS, Peraldi P, Budvari A, *et al.*: IRS-1 mediated inhibition of insulin receptor tyrosine kinase activity in TNF-alpha- and obesity-induced insulin resistance. *Science* 1996, 271:665–668.

36. Coffer PJ, Jin J, Woodgett JR: Protein kinase B (c-Akt): a multifunctional mediator of phosphatidylinositol 3-kinase activation. *Biochem J* 1998, 335:1–13.

37. Tobe K, Sabe H, Yamamoto T, *et al.*: Csk enhances insulin-stimulated dephosphorylation of focal adhesion proteins. *Mol Cell Biol* 1996, 16:4765–4772.

38. Stumvoli M, Nurjhan N, Perriello G, *et al.*: Metabolic effects of metformin in non-insulin-dependent diabetes mellitus. *N Engl J Med* 1995, 333:550–554.

39. Inzucchi SE, Maggs DG, Spollett GR, *et al.*: Efficacy and metabolic effects of metformin and troglitazone in type II diabetes mellitus. *N Engl J Med* 1998, 338:867–872.

40. Jackson RS, Creemers JWM, Ohagi S, *et al.*: Obesity and impaired prohormone processing associated with mutations in the human prohormone convertase 1 gene. *Nat Genet* 1997, 16:303–306.

41. Ristow M, Muller-Wieland D, Pfeiffer A, *et al.*: Obesity associated with a mutation in a genetic regulator of adipocyte differentiation. *N Engl J Med* 1998, 339:953–959.

42. Stout RW: Hyperinsulinemia and atherosclerosis. *Diabetes* 1996, 45:S45–S46.

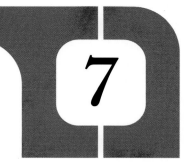

MANAGEMENT AND PREVENTION OF DIABETIC COMPLICATIONS

Sunder R. Mudaliar and Robert R. Henry

Type 2 diabetes is a chronic disease characterized by insulin resistance, impaired insulin secretion, and hyperglycemia. The long-term complications of diabetic retinopathy, nephropathy, neuropathy and accelerated atherosclerosis lead to significant morbidity in the form of preventable blindness, end-stage renal disease, limb amputations, and premature cardiovascular disease [1]. Diabetics suffer from the morbidity of their microvascular complications, and most of them ultimately die from macrovascular coronary artery disease.

A pathophysiologic hallmark of type 2 diabetes is insulin resistance, which has both genetic and acquired components [2]. Glucose intolerance and hyperglycemia supervene only when the pancreatic beta cell is unable to maintain compensatory hyperinsulinemia to overcome tissue resistance to insulin action [3]. In addition to having hyperglycemia and insulin resistance, nearly 80% of diabetics are obese and have a host of other metabolic abnormalities, including dyslipidemia (increased small dense LDL cholesterol, decreased HDL cholesterol, and raised triglyceride levels), hypertension, and abnormalities of coagulation and the fibrinolytic system. This cluster of metabolic abnormalities, which has been termed the *cardiovascular dysmetabolic syndrome*, is associated with a higher incidence of cardiovascular morbidity and mortality [4].

The major cause of tissue damage in diabetes is vascular disease in the micro- and macrovasculature [5]. The molecular and cellular mechanisms by which this damage may occur include increased polyol pathway flux, altered cellular redox state, increased formation of diacyl glycerol (DAG) with subsequent activation of specific protein kinase C isoforms, and accelerated nonenzymatic formation of advanced glycation end products (AGEs). The net result of vascular changes associated with hyperglycemia in diabetes is overproduction of potentially damaging reactive oxygen species and upregulation of cytokines and tissue growth factors. In diabetic macrovascular disease, insulin resistance rather than hyperglycemia may play a role in the selective loss of insulin-dependent vascular homeostasis [5].

The development of diabetic complications is no longer inevitable. Careful glycemic control and modification of major risk factors for micro- and macrovascular disease may prevent or minimize these vascular problems. Recent insights into the pathophysiology of diabetes and its complications make it possible not only to effectively manage diabetic complications, but also possibly to postpone or even prevent them.

Complications of Diabetes

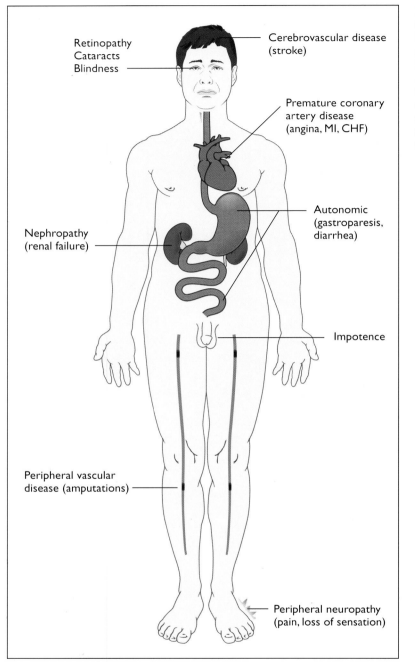

Retinopathy
Cataracts
Blindness

Cerebrovascular disease
(stroke)

Premature coronary
artery disease
(angina, MI, CHF)

Autonomic
(gastroparesis,
diarrhea)

Nephropathy
(renal failure)

Impotence

Peripheral vascular
disease (amputations)

Peripheral neuropathy
(pain, loss of sensation)

FIGURE 7-1. Clinical manifestations of diabetes. The complications of diabetes are protean and encompass nearly all organ systems. Diabetes currently is the leading cause of adult-onset blindness in the United States, and it accounts for more than one third of new cases of end-stage renal disease (ESRD). Accelerated lower extremity arterial disease in diabetics with neuropathy is responsible for 50% of all nontraumatic amputations, and the death rate for cardiovascular disease in diabetics is at least 2.5 times that in nondiabetics [1]. Heart disease appears earlier in type 2 diabetes and is more often fatal. Throughout their lives, diabetics suffer from the microvascular complications of blindness, end-stage renal disease, and neuropathy, and, sooner rather than later, most diabetics ultimately die from the complications of macrovascular cardiovascular disease.

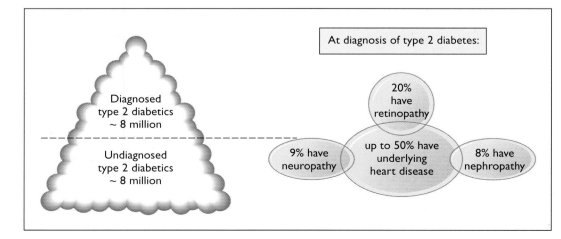

Diagnosed
type 2 diabetics
~ 8 million

Undiagnosed
type 2 diabetics
~ 8 million

At diagnosis of type 2 diabetes:

20%
have
retinopathy

9% have
neuropathy

up to 50% have
underlying
heart disease

8% have
nephropathy

FIGURE 7-2. The epidemiology of diabetes and its complications. Diabetes mellitus is an important clinical and public health problem in the United States. Nearly 8 million adults have been diagnosed with diabetes, 90% to 95% of whom have type 2 diabetes. In addition, it is estimated that a further 8 million persons who meet the diagnostic criteria for diabetes remain undiagnosed. It has been estimated that among patients in the United States, type 2 diabetes may have been present for up to 12 years before clinical diagnosis. During this period of undiagnosed and untreated diabetes, micro- and macrovascular disease progress. By the time of diagnosis, 20% of patients have retinopathy, 8% have nephropathy, 9% have neuropathy, and up to 50% have cardiovascular disease [1,4,18].

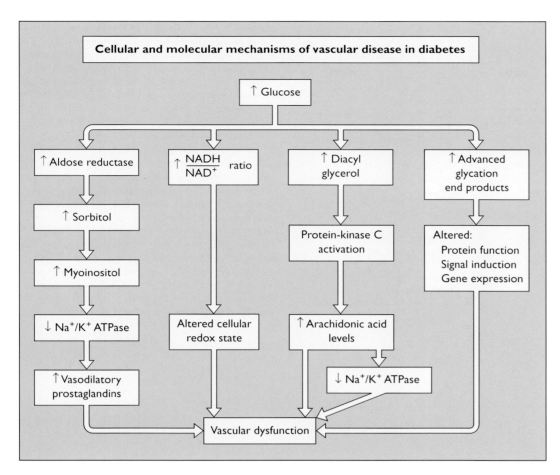

FIGURE 7-3. Possible cellular and molecular mechanisms of vascular disease in diabetes. Hyperglycemia in diabetes causes damage to many tissues, including the retina, the kidney, the nerves, the heart, the brain, and the skin. A major cause of tissue damage is vascular disease affecting both the microvasculature and the macrovasculature. Hyperglycemia-induced mechanisms that induce vascular damage include increased polyol pathway flux, altered cellular redox state, increased formation of diacylglycerol and the subsequent activation of specific protein kinase C isoforms, and accelerated non-enzymatic formation of advanced glycation end products (AGEs). Each of these mechanisms may contribute to vascular dysfunction through a number of mechanisms, including the production of vasodilatory prostaglandins, overproduction of potentially damaging reactive oxygen species, and upregulation of cytokines and growth factors. (*Adapted from King et al.* [5].)

Diabetic Retinopathy

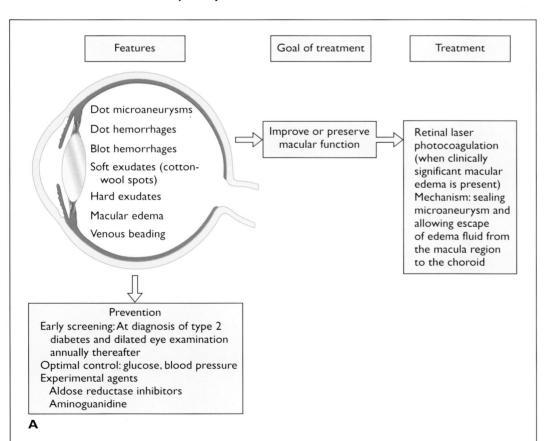

FIGURE 7-4. Clinical features and management. Diabetes is the leading cause of new blindness in adults. Retinopathy is present in a considerable proportion of type 2 diabetics at the time of diagnosis. After 15 or more years of disease, the risk of any retinopathy is about 78%, with about one third of patients having macular edema and about one sixth of patients having proliferative retinopathy [6]. Diabetic retinopathy may be classified as nonproliferative diabetic retinopathy (NPDR) or proliferative diabetic retinopathy (PDR). **A,** Nonproliferative diabetic retinopathy. NPDR is characterized by structural abnormalities of the retinal vessels (primarily capillaries, but also venules and arterioles), varying degrees of retinal nonperfusion, retinal edema, lipid exudates, and intraretinal hemorrhage. NPDR may be mild, moderate, or severe.

(*Continued on next page*)

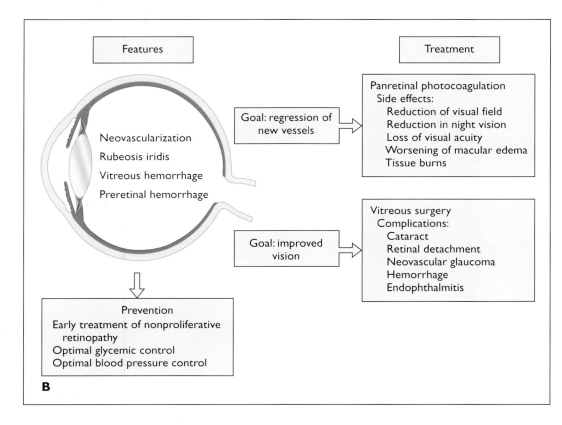

Features

Treatment

Neovascularization
Rubeosis iridis
Vitreous hemorrhage
Preretinal hemorrhage

Goal: regression of
new vessels

Panretinal photocoagulation
Side effects:
    Reduction of visual field
    Reduction in night vision
    Loss of visual acuity
    Worsening of macular edema
    Tissue burns

Goal: improved
vision

Vitreous surgery
Complications:
    Cataract
    Retinal detachment
    Neovascular glaucoma
    Hemorrhage
    Endophthalmitis

Prevention
Early treatment of nonproliferative
retinopathy
Optimal glycemic control
Optimal blood pressure control

B

FIGURE 7-4. (*Continued*) **B**, Proliferative diabetic retinopathy. The presence of extensive areas of hemorrhages, microaneurysms, venous beading, or intraretinal microvascular abnormalities (tortuous dilated vessels adjacent to nonperfused areas of the retina) predicts the progression to proliferative retinopathy. For patients with mild, moderate, or severe NPDR, the risk of developing PDR is 5%, 12% to 24%, and 50%, respectively [6].

All patients with type 2 diabetes should have a dilated eye examination at the time of diagnosis and annually or more often thereafter [7]. Prevention of retinopathy is best accomplished by maintaining near-normal glycemia. Once NPDR develops, intensive attempts should be made to optimize glucose and blood pressure control, and clinically significant macular edema (*ie*, retinal edema that threatens the fovea) should be treated with focal or grid photocoagulation, which reduces the risk of moderate visual loss by about 50%. Panretinal photocoagulation may be beneficial in PDR, along with measures to optimize glucose and blood pressure control [6].

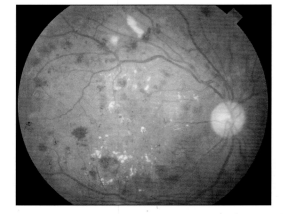

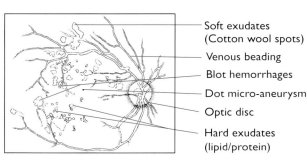

Soft exudates
(Cotton wool spots)
Venous beading
Blot hemorrhages
Dot micro-aneurysm
Optic disc
Hard exudates
(lipid/protein)

FIGURE 7-5. (*see* Color Plate) Nonproliferative diabetic retinopathy (NPDR). The characteristic features of NPDR include dot aneurysms (hypercellular, saccular outpouchings of the capillary wall), blot hemorrhages resulting from vascular occlusion, cotton-wool spots (retinal nerve fiber infarcts due to ischemia), hard exudates (lipid and protein exudates due to excessive vascular permeability), and venous beading (abnormal appearance of retinal veins with localized swellings and constrictions resembling sausage links). (Courtesy of Dr. M. Goldbaum, UCSD/VA San Diego Health Care System, San Diego, CA.)

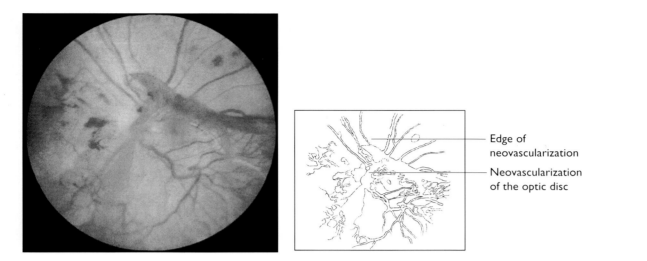

FIGURE 7-6. (see Color Plate) Classical features of proliferative diabetic retinopathy (PDR). The development of neovascularization is pathognomic of this stage. The presence of new vessels on the optic nerve head or on more than one fourth of the disc area, together with preretinal or vitreous hemorrhages, is indicative of high-risk proliferative retinopathy and is an absolute indication for panretinal photocoagulation, if technically possible. (Courtesy of Dr. M. Goldbaum, UCSD/VA San Diego Health Care System, San Diego, CA.)

Diabetic Nephropathy: Clinical Features and Management

URINARY ALBUMIN EXCRETION RATE (AER)

	Urinary AER, 24-h collection	Timed collection, µg/min	Spot collection, µg/mg creatinine
Normal	<30	<20	< 30
Microalbuminuria	30–300	20–200	30–300
Macroalbuminuria (Overt nephropathy)	>300	>200	> 300

FIGURE 7-7. Urinary albumin excretion rate (AER). The incidence of end-stage renal disease (ESRD) in type 2 diabetes ranges from 4% to 20%. Because type 2 diabetes is 10 times or more prevalent than type 1 diabetes, the incidence of ESRD is approximately the same in both types of diabetes [1]. The cost of treatment for ESRD in diabetes exceeds $2 billion annually [8].

A nondiabetic with normal kidneys excretes less than 30 mg of albumin/24 hours (20 µm/min) into the urine, and in a spot urine collection has an albumin:creatinine ratio of less than 30 (µg of albumin/mg of creatinine). Microalbuminuria is present at diagnosis in 3% to 30% of patients with type 2 diabetes. Without specific interventions, 20% to 40% of type 2 diabetes patients with microalbuminuria progress to overt nephropathy. However, 20 years after the onset of overt nephropathy, only about 20% have progressed to ESRD [9]. There is substantial evidence that the onset of microalbuminuria and progression of nephropathy correlate closely with poor glycemic control and, more importantly, that improved glycemic control reduces the onset and progression of microalbuminuria and nephropathy [10]. Screening for microalbuminuria should be performed at the time of diagnosis and annually thereafter by a random/spot urine albumin and creatinine measurement. (This test has good correlation with 24-hour albumin measurements.) Because the urine albumin excretion rate (UAER) is variable, two of three specimens collected within a 3- to 6-month period should be abnormal before a patient is considered to have crossed a diagnostic threshold. Exercise within the preceding 24 hours, fever, heart failure, marked hyperglycemia, and marked hypertension may elevate UAER over borderline values [9].

STAGES OF DIABETIC NEPHROPATHY IN TYPE 2 DIABETES

Asymptomatic	Renal insufficiency	End-stage renal disease
Normal GFR/creatinine	Decreasing GFR	Uremia
Hypertension	Increasing creatinine	Greatly increased creatinine
Microalbuminuria (30–300mg/d)	Proteinuria > 500 mg/day	Greatly decreased GFR (<15 ml/min)

(Data from Friedman [11])

FIGURE 7-8. Stages of diabetic nephropathy in type 2 diabetes. The natural history of nephropathy in type 2 diabetes is not as clear as it is in type 1 diabetes, for which five stages of nephropathy have been described: 1) an early stage of increased glomerular filtration, progressing through 2) a stage of early glomerular lesions with glomerular basement thickening and mesangial matrix expansion, and on to 3) incipient diabetic nephropathy with microalbuminuria (urinary albumin 30 to 300 mg/day). Ultimately, 4) clinical nephropathy with overt proteinuria over 500 mg/day and declining glomerular filtration rate (GFR) develops and culminates in 5) end-stage renal disease (ESRD). The early stages of nephropathy have not yet been well documented in type 2 diabetes. (Data from Friedman [11].)

MEASURES TO PREVENT OR RETARD DIABETIC NEPHROPATHY

Optimal glycemic control: HbA1C < 7% (caution in the elderly)

Adequate blood pressure control: BP < 130/85 (caution in those with autonomic neuropathy)

ACE inhibitors (when microalbuminuria is present with urinary albumin 30–300 mg/day)

Dietary protein restriction (when overt nephropathy is present with urinary protein > 500 mg/day or there is a strong family history of nephropathy)

Experimental: Aminoguanidine (inhibits AGE formation)

FIGURE 7-9. Measures to prevent or retard diabetic nephropathy. The presence of microalbuminuria not only predicts the risk for progression to overt proteinuria and nephropathy, but is also a marker for increased mortality from coronary artery disease (CAD). It should, therefore, serve as an early warning marker to institute aggressive glucose and blood pressure control, among other measures. AGE— advanced glycation end products.

Diabetic Neuropathy

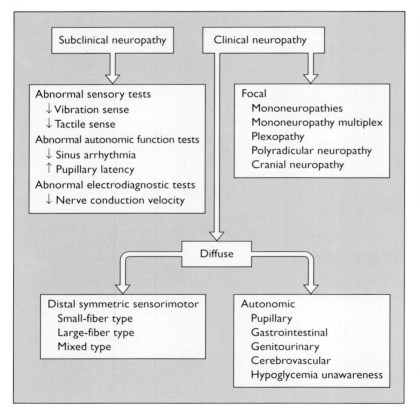

FIGURE 7-10. Clinical features of diabetic neuropathy. Diabetic neuropathy is one of the most common complications of diabetes. Its clinical manifestations cause much suffering among diabetic patients. Acute hyperglycemia decreases nerve function, and chronic hyperglycemia is characterized by progressive loss of nerve fibers, a loss that can be assessed noninvasively by several tests of nerve function, including quantitative sensory tests, autonomic function tests, and electrophysiologic testing [12].

CLINICAL FEATURES OF DISTAL SENSORIMOTOR DIABETIC NEUROPATHY

Large fiber type	Small fiber type
Unsteady gait	Pain predominates
Absent reflexes	Variable reflexes
Decreased vibration/position sense	Variable position/vibration sense
Charcot's joints possible	Variable presence of Charcot's joints
Mimics posterior column lesions	Ultimately leads to sensory loss

FIGURE 7-11. Distal sensorimotor diabetic neuropathy.

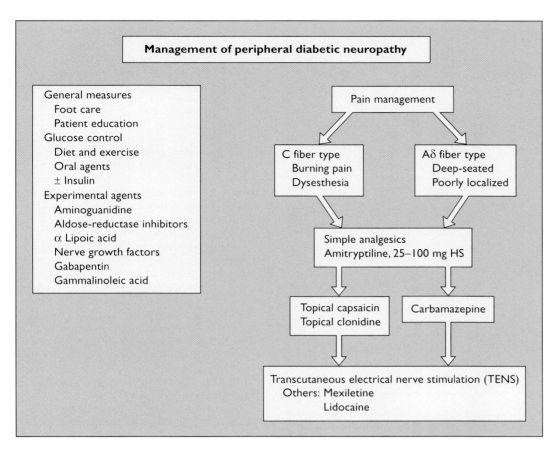

FIGURE 7-12. Management of peripheral diabetic neuropathy. The pathophysiologic mechanisms underlying decreased nerve function and nerve fiber loss in diabetics still are not fully understood but may include formation of sorbitol by aldose reductase and the formation of advanced glycation end products (AGEs) [12]. Like other diabetic complications, the progression of neuropathy is related to glycemic control. Chronic sensory neuropathy with moderate or severe sensory loss involving large-fiber sensation (touch, vibration, and joint position sense) or small-fiber sensation (pain and temperature sense) is associated with a high risk of ulceration.

Current approaches to prevention and treatment of diabetic neuropathy include measures to optimize glucose control, various symptomatic measures for pain control, and use of aldose reductase inhibitors, which appear to slow the progression of neuropathy rather than provide symptomatic relief [13].

Diabetic Foot Disease

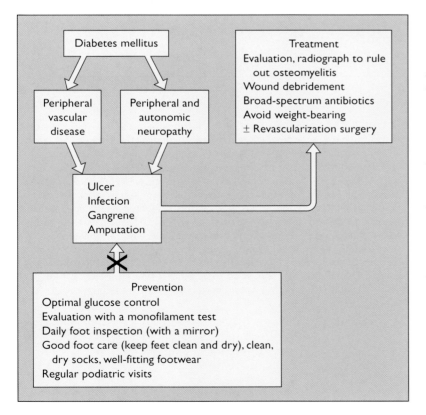

FIGURE 7-13. Clinical features and management of diabetic foot disease. Diabetic foot lesions are a major cause of hospitalization, with approximately 20% of all diabetics entering the hospital because of foot problems. Nearly 55,000 lower extremity amputations are performed each year on diabetics, accounting for 50% of all nontraumatic amputations [14]. Diabetic foot lesions are the result of a combination of peripheral and autonomic neuropathy and peripheral vascular disease (ischemia). The cascade of events begins with foot ulcers, infection, and gangrene, and ultimately results in amputation. Management of diabetic foot ulcers should be aggressive, and should include detailed evaluation of the ulcer and the foot, radiography to exclude osteomyelitis, broad-spectrum antibiotics, wound debridement (if indicated), and avoidance of weight bearing. Topical application of antibacterial agents and platelet-derived growth factors may be useful adjunctive measures. Preventive measures include optimal glycemic control, daily foot inspections (with the aid of a mirror), good foot care (keeping feet clean and dry), wearing clean socks and appropriate, well-fitting shoes, and regular podiatric visits. Good patient education and a team approach are the keys to the prevention and treatment of diabetic foot disease.

Diabetics are particularly prone to foot deformities and the development of cocked-up toes, which results in pressure at the tips of the toes and under the first metatarsal head, leading to ulceration and infection. The ideal treatment is prophylactic surgery to straighten the toes. If this is not feasible, special shoes with a cushioned insole to protect the toes and metatarsal head should be worn.

All diabetics should have the protective sensory function in their feet evaluated with a 10-g Semmestel-Weinstein monofilament. If a patient cannot consistently feel a 10-g monofilament, protective sensory function has been lost, and the patient is at high risk of developing foot ulcers [15].

Diabetic Male Sexual Dysfunction

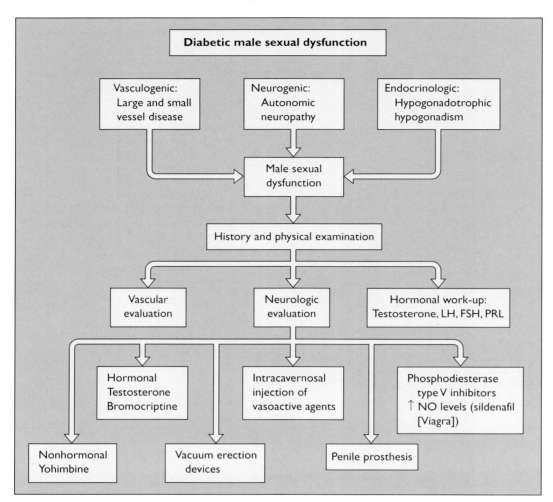

FIGURE 7-14. Evaluation and management of diabetic male sexual dysfunction. The prevalence of erectile dysfunction in diabetic men ranges from 35% to 75%, significantly higher than that in the general population [16]. Its onset is insidious, and it may occur early in the disease. The major underlying abnormalities are vascular (cavernosal artery insufficiency, corporal veno-occlusive dysfunction) and neurologic (autonomic neuropathy). The role of hormonal abnormalities is controversial. All diabetic men with erectile dysfunction require a detailed endocrinologic work-up (luteinizing hormone [LH], follicle-stimulating hormone [FSH], prolactin [PRL], and testosterone levels) and, in select cases, vascular evaluation (intracavernosal injection test, visual sexual stimulation, and penile duplex ultrasonography) and neurologic evaluation (nocturnal penile tumescence test, cavernosal electrical activity potential, somatosensory evoked potentials, and sacral latency test). Treatment options include non-hormonal α-2-adrenergic blocking agents (yohimbine); hormonal therapy, if indicated (testosterone replacement in hypogonadism, bromocriptine/surgery for prolactinomas, discontinuation of medications causing hyperprolactinemia); vacuum erection devices; intracavernosal injection of vasoactive agents; penile prostheses (in selected cases); and the recently introduced phosphodiesterase V inhibitor sildenafil (Viagra), which acts by increasing nitric oxide levels.

Cardiovascular Disease in Diabetes

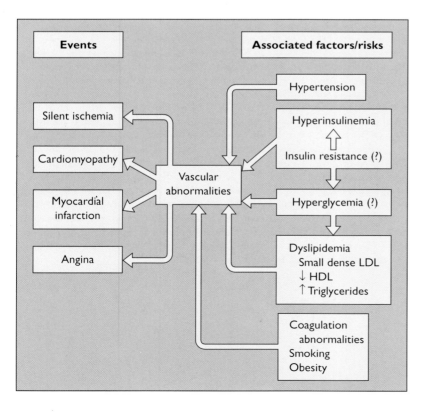

FIGURE 7-15. Pathogenesis and clinical features of heart disease in diabetes. The risk for cardiovascular disease in patients with diabetes is two to five times that in nondiabetic persons [17]. At the time of diagnosis of type 2 diabetes, more than 50% of patients have preexisting coronary artery disease (CAD) [18]. Numerous risk factors contribute to macrovascular dysfunction in type 2 diabetes. Some appear related to the insulin resistance and hyperinsulinemia that is characteristic of the early stages of type 2 diabetes before the onset of pancreatic β-cell exhaustion and overt hyperglycemia. These include the various components of the cardiovascular dysmetabolic syndrome (ie, hypertension, central obesity, dyslipidemia, glucose intolerance, and coagulation abnormalities) [4]. Heart disease in diabetics may result in silent myocardial ischemia, or manifest as angina, myocardial infarction, or congestive heart failure (diabetic cardiomyopathy). HDL—high-density lipoprotein; LDL—low-density lipoprotein.

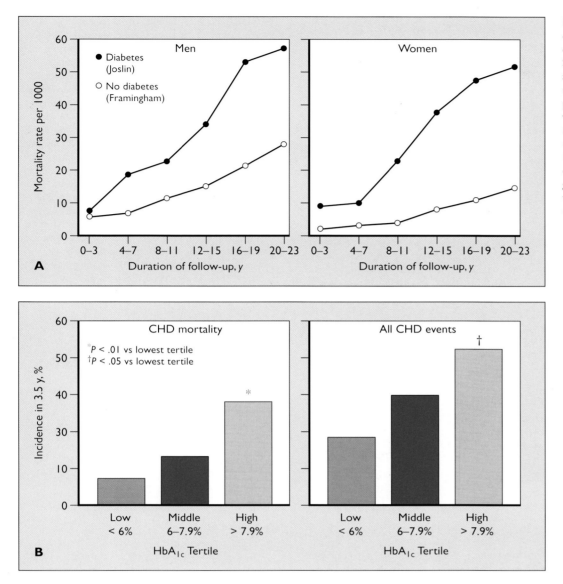

FIGURE 7-16. Cardiovascular disease is the major cause of mortality in type 2 diabetics. **A.** Comparison of data from the Joslin Study and the Framingham Study show that the mortality rate due to coronary artery disease is doubled in men with diabetes and nearly quadrupled in women with diabetes, as compared to the nondiabetic population [19]. Moreover, within the diabetic population, glucose control is an important predictor of coronary artery disease (CAD) mortality and all CAD events. **B.** In the Finnish population, the mortality rate in elderly diabetics (65 to 74 years old at baseline) with poor glycemic control (HbA1C > 7.9%) was more than three times that of those with good glycemic control (HbA1C < 6%) [20]. (Part A *from* Krolewski *et al*, [19]; part B *from* Kuusisto *et al*. [20].)

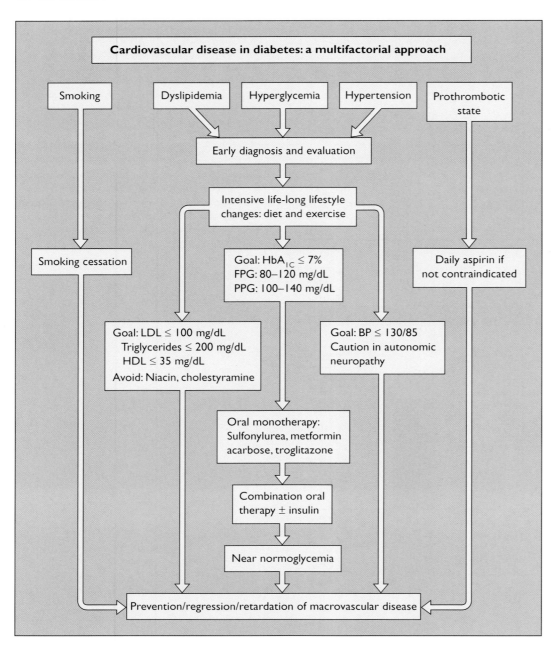

Cardiovascular disease in diabetes: a multifactorial approach

Smoking → Early diagnosis and evaluation

Dyslipidemia → Early diagnosis and evaluation

Hyperglycemia → Early diagnosis and evaluation

Hypertension → Early diagnosis and evaluation

Prothrombotic state

Early diagnosis and evaluation → Intensive life-long lifestyle changes: diet and exercise

Smoking cessation

Goal: HbA$_{1C}$ ≤ 7%
FPG: 80–120 mg/dL
PPG: 100–140 mg/dL

Daily aspirin if not contraindicated

Goal: LDL ≤ 100 mg/dL
Triglycerides ≤ 200 mg/dL
HDL ≤ 35 mg/dL
Avoid: Niacin, cholestyramine

Goal: BP ≤ 130/85
Caution in autonomic neuropathy

Oral monotherapy:
Sulfonylurea, metformin
acarbose, troglitazone

Combination oral therapy ± insulin

Near normoglycemia

Prevention/regression/retardation of macrovascular disease

FIGURE 7-17. A multifactorial approach to management of cardiovascular disease in diabetes. Multiple risk factors contribute to accelerated atherosclerosis and premature coronary artery disease (CAD) in diabetes. The cornerstone of prevention is aggressive intervention to identify and favorably modify established risk factors, including hyperglycemia, hyperlipidemia, and hypertension. Because of the extremely high risk of macrovascular disease in diabetes, the target low-density lipoprotein (LDL) cholesterol should be at least < 130 mg/dL and preferably < 100 mg/dL; the target high-density lipoprotein (HDL) cholesterol goal should be > 35 mg/dL; and the triglyceride goal should be < 200 mg/dL. Unless contraindicated, all diabetics should be on daily aspirin [21]. The importance of lifestyle changes and strict adherence to dietary and exercise recommendations should be emphasized at all times. BP—blood pressure; FPG—fasting plasma glucose; PPG—post-prandial plasma glucose

Economic Implications of Diabetic Complications

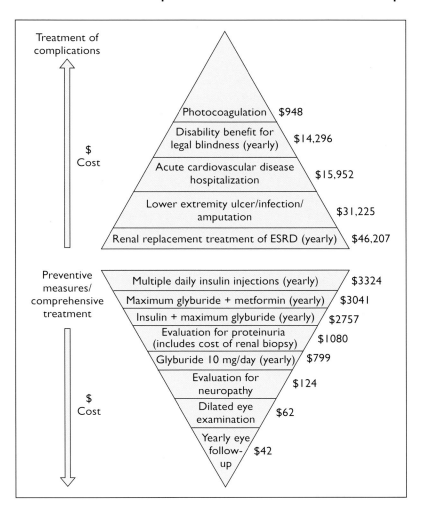

FIGURE 7-18. Dollar cost of diabetic complications: prevention versus treatment. The annual expense of treating diabetes and its complications in the United States (most of which is for treatment of type 2 diabetes) is estimated at about $100 billion [8]. Not only is type 2 diabetes costly, but it also causes excessive morbidity and mortality. Analysis of data has shown that prevention of this disease not only is preferable to treatment but also is more cost-effective. This figure compares the cost of comprehensive treatment of diabetes with medications and preventive measures with the monumental costs of treating disease complications such as retinopathy, nephropathy, neuropathy, foot disease, and cardiovascular disease. It has been estimated that comprehensive treatment of type 2 diabetes with HbA1C values maintained at 7.2% will reduce the cumulative incidence of blindness by 72%, end-stage renal disease by 87%, and lower extremity amputation by 67%. Cardiovascular disease risk is increased by 3%, and life expectancy is increased by 1.39 years. The estimated incremental cost per quality-adjusted life year (QALY) gained is $16,002. This efficiency of treating type 2 diabetes is similar to that for screening and treating hypertension and is in the range of interventions considered cost-effective. Treatment is more cost-effective for those with earlier onset of diabetes, minorities, and those with higher HbA1C under standard care. ESRD—end-stage renal disease. (*Data from* Eastman et al [22].)

Future Directions

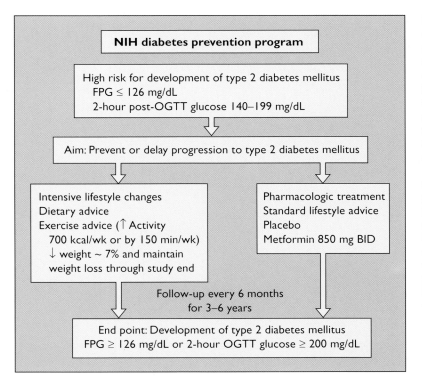

FIGURE 7-19. Prevention of type 2 diabetes. It is now clear that type 2 diabetes is not a milder form of diabetes. Its complications can be the same as or more severe than those in type 1 diabetes. Moreover, these complications occur early during the natural course of the disease, even before clinical onset. At the time of diagnosis of type 2 diabetes, 20% of patients have retinopathy, 8% have nephropathy, 9% have neuropathy [4], and up to 50% have underlying coronary artery disease (CAD) [18]. Treatment of hyperglycemia, hypertension, and hyperlipidemia may prevent or retard the progression of diabetic complications. However, even with early intervention and intensive treatment, there are significant morbidity and high costs. Preventing or delaying the onset of diabetes may be more cost-effective [4]. Impaired glucose tolerance (IGT with FPG: 110–125 mg/dL, or 2-hour post-OGTT glucose 140–199 mg/dL) has been shown to be a strong risk factor for development of type 2 diabetes and a possible risk factor for CAD. There are data to suggest that at this stage of IGT, patients are at high risk for diabetes and CAD, but have not yet developed end-organ disease. The Diabetes Prevention Program (DPP) supported by the National Institutes of Health (NIH) will determine if it is possible to prevent or delay the progression to type 2 diabetes in patients who have IGT. Possible treatment options include intensive lifestyle measures (diet and exercise) or pharmacologic means (metformin). The study, which commenced in 1996, will be completed in 2002. FPG—fasting plasma glucose; OGTT—oral glucose tolerance test.

References

1. Harris MI: Summary. In *Diabetes in America*. NIH Publication No. 95-1468. Edited by Harris MI, Cowie CC, Stern MP, *et al.* Washington, DC: US Government Printing Office; 1995:1–14.

2. De Fronzo RA: Lilly Lecture 1987: The triumvirate: β cell, muscle, liver. A collusion responsible for NIDDM. *Diabetes* 1988, 37:667–687.

3. Goldberg RB: Prevention of type 2 diabetes. *Med Clin North Am* 1998, 82:805–821.

4. Fagan TC, Deedwania PC: The cardiovascular dysmetabolic syndrome. *Am J Med* 1998, 105(1A):77S–82S.

5. King GL, Brownlee M: The cellular and molecular mechanisms of diabetic complications. *Endocrinol Metab Clin North Am* 1996, 25:255–270.

6. Aiello LP, Cavallerano J, Bursell S: Diabetic eye disease. *Endocrinol Metab Clin North Am* 1996, 25:271–291.

7. American Diabetes Association: Position statement: Diabetic retinopathy. *Diabetes Care* 1998, 21(suppl):S47–S49.

8. American Diabetes Association: *Direct and Indirect Costs of Diabetes in the United States in 1992.* Alexandria, VA: American Diabetes Association, 1993.

9. American Diabetes Association: Position statement: Diabetic nephropathy. *Diabetes Care* 1998, 21:S50–S53.

10. Marks JB, Raskin P: Nephropathy and hypertension in diabetes. *Med Clin North Am* 1998, 82:877–907.

11. Friedman E: Renal syndromes in diabetes. *Endocrinol Metab Clin North Am* 1996, 25:293–324.

12. Harati Y: Diabetes and the nervous system. *Endocrinol Metab Clin North Am* 1996, 25:325–359.

13. Boulton AJM, Malik RA: Diabetic neuropathy. *Med Clin North Am* 1998, 82:909–929.

14. Levin ME: Foot lesions in patients with diabetes mellitus. *Endocrinol Metab Clin North Am* 1996, 25:447–462.

15. American Diabetes Association: Position Statement: Foot care in diabetes. *Diabetes Care* 1998, 21(suppl):S54–S55.

16. Hakim LS, Goldstein I: Diabetic sexual function. *Endocrinol Metab Clin North Am* 1996, 25:379–400.

17. Zimmet PZ, Alberti KGMM: The changing face of macrovascular disease in NIDDM: An epidemic in progress. *Lancet* 1997, 350(SI):1–4.

18. Garber AJ: Vascular disease and lipids in diabetes. *Med Clin North Am* 1998, 82:931–948.

19. Krowelski AS, Warram JH, Valsania P, *et al.*: Evolving natural history of coronary artery disease in diabetes mellitus. *Am J Med* 1991, 90 (suppl 2A):56S–61S.

20. Kuusisito J, Mykannen L, Pyorala K, *et al.*: NIDDM and its metabolic control predict coronary artery disease in elderly subjects. *Diabetes* 1994, 43:960–967.

21. American Diabetes Association: Position statement: Management of dyslipidemia in adults with diabetes mellitus. *Diabetes Care* 1999, 22:556–559.

22. Eastman RC, Javitt JC, Herman WH, *et al.*: Model of complications in NIDDM: Analysis of the health benefits and cost-effectiveness of treating NIDDM with the goal of normoglycemia. *Diabetes Care* 1997, 20:735–744.

INSULIN RESISTANCE

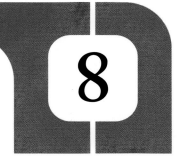

Ele Ferrannini

At the whole-body level, hormone response is the compounded result of secretory rate and cellular sensitivity. For many hormones, action is modulated through hormonal feedback (*eg,* corticotropin-releasing hormone [CRH] and adrenocorticotropic hormone [ACTH] for cortisol, gonadotrophin-releasing hormone and gonadotrophins for sex steroids). With this design, sensitivity is provided by the specific hormone receptors on target tissues as well as on the companion gland of the feedback loop. In the case of insulin, there is no major pituitary or hypothalamic relay; target tissues control secretion directly by determining the level of positive and negative stimuli. Thus, the circulating concentrations of substrates (mostly glucose, but also amino acids, free fatty acids [FFA], and ketone bodies), which result from insulin action on intermediary metabolism in different tissues, feed signals back to the β-cell. Sensitivity gating is provided by insulin receptors on target tissues (and on the β-cell itself). Possibly as a consequence of the peculiar system design, insulin resistance is a relatively common phenomenon in physiology as well as pathophysiology.

Insulin exerts multiple actions on many cell types, but the primary servoregulated signal for insulin release is the plasma glucose concentration. According to this construct, insulin resistance is a reduced sensitivity of glucose uptake to insulin stimulation sensed by the β-cell through elevated plasma glucose levels. Consequently, insulin resistance is defined as defective glucose disposal in the face of raised glucose and insulin concentrations.

Insulin sensitivity is set not only by the number and affinity of the insulin receptors but also by the functional state of the intracellular signaling pathways that transduce insulin binding to the various effectors (*eg,* glucose transport, phosphorylation and oxidation, glycogen synthesis, lipolysis, and ion exchange). Therefore, a massive reduction in the number of insulin receptors (or the presence of high titers of circulating anti-insulin or anti–insulin-receptor autoantibodies) is associated with a form of insulin resistance that is generalized and extreme (*ie,* all pathways are involved). These are, however, rare cases. More commonly, cellular resistance of the glucose pathway is caused by a malfunction of the signal transduction machinery. The various insulin effectors are, at least in part, independent of one another. As a consequence, cellular insulin resistance can be of any degree and usually is incomplete, or pathway-specific. In addition, resistance in the glucose pathway reinforces the insulin signal to other pathways (*eg,* protein turnover) via stimulation of β-cell activity. To the extent that they have preserved their sensitivity, other pathways are overly stimulated by the compensatory hyperinsulinemia. The pathophysiologic implication of this phenomenon is that, in insulin resistant states, any abnormality that is found to be associated with defective glucose metabolism (*eg,* dyslipidemia, higher blood pressure, platelet hypercoagulation, or prothrombotic changes) theoretically can be the result of either the insulin resistance itself or the chronic effects of the attendant hyperinsulinemia. This is the origin of the insulin resistance syndrome.

Definition and Measurement

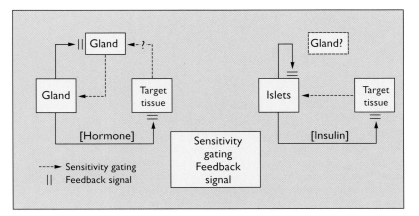

FIGURE 8-1. General organization of an endocrine system and peculiarity of the insulin system. For many protein and non-protein hormones, action is modulated by at least one, often two, hierarchical hormonal feedback paths (eg, corticotropin-releasing hormone and adrenocorticotropic hormone [ACTH] for cortisol, gonadotrophin-releasing hormone and gonadotrophins for sex steroids). Sensitivity is provided by the circulating hormone concentrations ([hormone]) acting upon specific hormone receptors located on target tissues as well as on the companion gland of the feedback loop. In the case of insulin, there is no major pituitary or hypothalamic relay; target tissues control secretion directly by determining the level of positive and negative stimuli. Thus, the circulating concentrations of substrates (mostly glucose, but also amino acids, free fatty acids [FFA], and ketone bodies), which result from insulin action on intermediary metabolism in different tissues, feed signals back to the β-cell. Sensitivity gating is provided by insulin receptors on target tissues; some degree of autoregulation is given by insulin receptors on the β-cell itself.

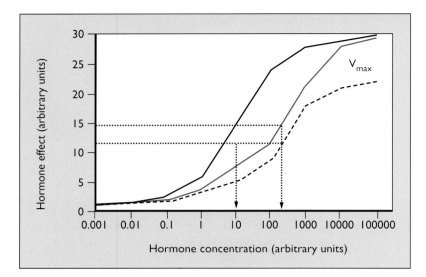

FIGURE 8-2. Shape and parameters of the dose-response curve for a hormone. In general, the relationship between concentration and action of a hormone is sigmoidal (*black line*): the response is sluggish in the low concentration range, then rises in an approximately linear manner, and then tapers off to saturation. Mathematically, this kind of dose-response relationship can be approximated by a Michaelis-Menten equation, in which the maximal effect is termed V_{max}, the hormone concentration at which the effect is half-maximal is termed K_m, and sensitivity is expressed by the ratio V_{max}/K_m. The figure exemplifies two types of abnormal response: reduced sensitivity, characterized by a 20-fold increase in K_m (*blue line*), and the same reduction in sensitivity coupled with an impaired maximal response (*dotted line*).

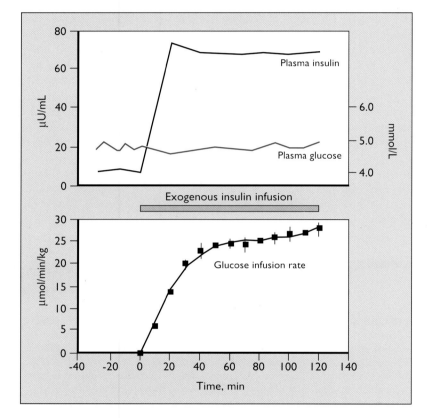

FIGURE 8-3. Euglycemic hyperinsulinemic insulin clamping. Euglycemic hyper-insulinemic insulin clamping is regarded as the gold standard for the measurement of insulin sensitivity in vivo [1,2]. Exogenous insulin is infused in a primed-constant format to raise plasma insulin concentrations to any desired level (in this figure, the postprandial range). As peripherally infused insulin is cleared rapidly from the plasma (at the rate of 0.6 to 1.4 L/min in nonobese healthy subjects [3]), a stable hyperinsulinemic plateau is reached within 20 minutes. Exogenous glucose is infused simultaneously to prevent insulin-induced hypoglycemia; the glucose infusion rate is adjusted every 5 to 10 minutes under the guidance of on-line plasma glucose measurements. During the second hour of a 2-hour clamp study, endogenous glucose release generally is suppressed, and the glucose infusion rate equals the total amount of glucose taken up by all tissues in the body. The *black squares* in the *lower panel* of the figure represent mean (± SEM) values of whole-body insulin-mediated glucose uptake (normalized for body weight) in 30 nondiabetic subjects of a range of ages and body weights.

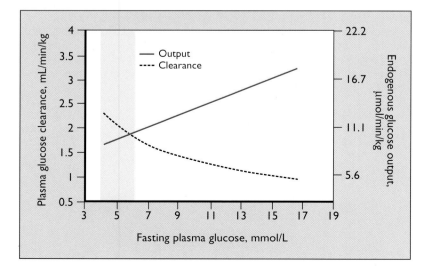

FIGURE 8-4. Glucose turnover in the fasting state. The use of a glucose isotope, either stable or radioactively labeled, allows one to measure the rate at which glucose is produced endogenously and cleared from the plasma in the fasting state. Following a prolonged primed-constant intravenous infusion, the tracer reaches isotopic equilibrium (*ie*, constant specific activity) throughout the body glucose space. Under these circumstances, the ratio of the tracer infusion rate to its steady-state plasma concentration measures whole-body glucose clearance (expressed in ml/min/kg of body weight). Endogenous glucose output (mostly from the liver) is then calculated as the product of glucose clearance by the fasting plasma glucose concentration and expressed in μmol/min per kg of body weight. The graph shows how glucose clearance and endogenous glucose output vary across a range of fasting plasma glucose concentrations, encompassing the normal (shaded area) and diabetic state. Whereas glucose clearance is reduced already for minor degrees of fasting hyperglycemia (<7 mmol/L), endogenous glucose output increases in approximate proportion to the severity of hyper-glycemia [4].

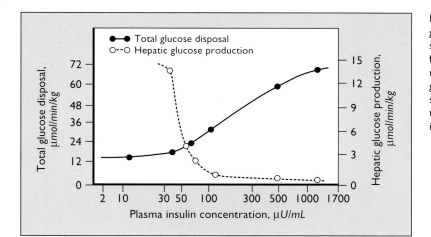

FIGURE 8-5. Insulin dose-response curves for stimulation of whole-body glucose uptake and inhibition of endogenous glucose production in healthy subjects. Curves were constructed by combining the insulin clamp technique at five insulin levels encompassing the physiologic and pharmacologic concentration range with tracer glucose infusion. The effect of insulin on endogenous (hepatic) glucose release is already maximal at plasma insulin concentrations that are submaximal for stimulation of glucose uptake [5]. Thus, under physiologic conditions, the earliest and most effective action of insulin to limit postprandial hyperglycemia is to suppress release of endogenous glucose into the systemic circulation.

Insulin Action

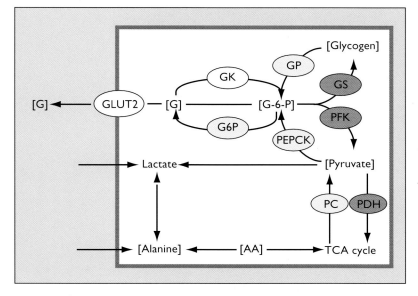

FIGURE 8-6. Hepatic glucose production. Simplified scheme of the main intracellular pathways of glucose production in the liver, glycogenolysis and gluconeogenesis (*thick lines*). Shaded boxes indicate key insulin-sensitive enzymes in the pathway. Substrate concentrations are in brackets; insulin-sensitive enzymes are inscribed in circles, shaded to indicate stimulatory action or hatched to indicate inhibitory action. Whereas glycogen breakdown directly increases the intracellular concentrations of glucose-6-phosphate, uptake of lactate, alanine, and other gluconeogenic amino acids provides 3-carbon precursors for de novo glucose-6-phosphate synthesis. G—free glucose; GP—glycogen phosphorylase; GS—glycogen synthase; G-6-P—glucose-6-phosphate; G6P—glucose-6-phosphatase; GK—glucokinase; PFK—phospofructokinase; PEPCK—phosphoenolpyruvate-carboxykinase; PC—pyruvate carboxylase; PDH—pyruvate dehydrogenase; AA—aminoacids; GLUT2—isoform 2 (non-insulin-sensitive) of the glucose transporter; TCA—tricarboxylic acids cycle.

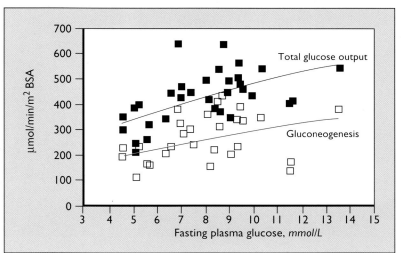

FIGURE 8-7. Contribution of gluconeogenesis to fasting plasma glucose concentration. Total endogenous glucose output (measured by the tracer dilution technique) and gluconeogenesis (determined by the deuterated water technique[6]) were simultaneously measured in fasting nondiabetic subjects and patients with type 2 diabetes mellitus. As expected (see Fig. 8-4), endogenous glucose output (*filled squares, solid line*) is related directly to the degree of hyperglycemia over a range of fasting plasma glucose concentrations. Gluconeogenesis (*empty squares, blue line*) makes up roughly one half of total glucose output in nondiabetic subjects, and is increased in diabetic patients, thereby contributing substantially to their fasting hyperglycemia (unpublished data). BSA—body surface area.

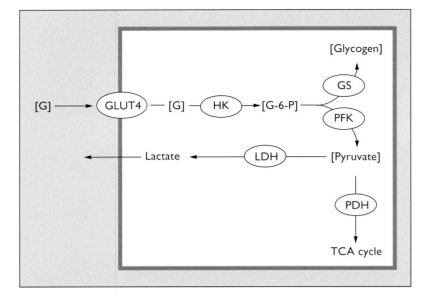

FIGURE 8-8. Peripheral glucose disposal. Simplified scheme of glycogen synthesis and glucose oxidation, the main pathways of intracellular glucose disposition in insulin target tissues. Shaded boxes indicate key insulin-sensitive enzymes in the pathway. G—free glucose; G-6-P— glucose-6-phosphate; GLUT4—isoform 4 (insulin-sensitive) of the glucose transporter; HK—hexokinase II; GS—glycogen synthase; PFK—phosphofructokinase; PDH—pyruvate dehydrogenase; LDH—lactic dehydrogenase; TCA—tricarboxylic acids cycle.

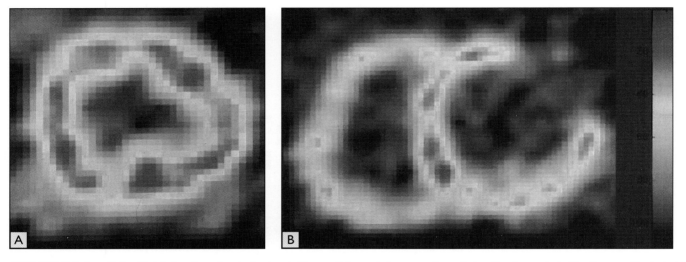

FIGURE 8-9. (see Color Plate) Insulin action in the heart. Myocardial muscle is insulin-sensitive. Whereas free fatty acids (FFA) represent the dominant fuel for cardiac muscle in the fasting state, an increase in circulating insulin concentrations inhibits lipolysis, thereby restraining FFA availability and promoting glucose uptake. By using ^{18}F-deoxyglucose (FDG), an analog of glucose (which is transported and phosphorylated in the same manner as D-glucose but not further metabolized) labeled with a short-lived radioactive isotope of fluorine (^{18}F), positron-emitting tomography (PET) detects a signal that is proportional to the rate of myocardial glucose uptake. The figure shows FDG images of human heart muscle during a euglycemic insulin clamp study like the one illustrated in Figure 8-3. The colors (with red being the most intense) indicate regions with different rates of glucose utilization. **A,** The left ventricle of a normal subject. **B,** The ventricular walls of a patient who suffered from an anterior myocardial infarction (MI) 6 months before the PET study. A "cold" area of missing glucose uptake is clearly visible at the upper right corner (the anterior wall of the left ventricle). Also evident is a diffuse decrease in insulin-mediated glucose uptake (insulin resistance) throughout the left ventricular wall, involving myocardial regions distant from the infarcted area and normally perfused (perfusion scan not shown) [7].

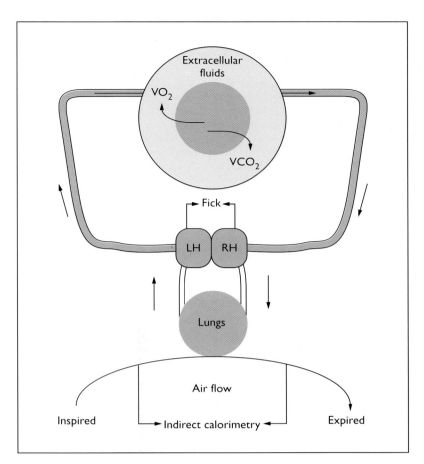

FIGURE 8-10. Measuring intracellular glucose disposition and energy expenditure in vivo via indirect calorimetry. The scheme illustrates the correspondence between indirect calorimetry (in which oxygen consumption = [O_2 in expired air - O_2 in inspired air] × air flow; carbon dioxide production = [CO_2 in expired air - CO_2 in inspired air] × air flow) and the Fick principle (by which oxygen consumption = (arterial blood O_2 - central venous blood O_2) × cardiac output; carbon dioxide production = (arterial blood CO_2 - venous blood CO_2) × cardiac output). With the use of calorimetric equations, net rates of oxidation of lipids and carbohydrates and of energy expenditure can be quantified at the whole-body as well as the organ level starting from gas-exchange data. LH—left heart; RH—right heart; VO_2—oxygen consumption; VCO_2—carbon dioxide production.

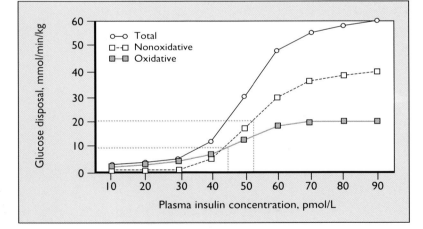

FIGURE 8-11. Dose-response curve for action of insulin on glucose oxidation and nonoxidative glucose disposal in the healthy subject. Indirect calorimetry can be combined with the insulin clamp technique to estimate glucose oxidation at various plasma insulin plateaus. Nonoxidative glucose disposal, consisting primarily of glycogen synthesis, is then obtained as the difference between total glucose uptake and net glucose oxidation. The figure presents data from healthy subjects studied over a range of plasma insulin levels; the dotted lines identify the K_m values for oxidative glucose disposal and glycogen synthesis. Glucose oxidation has a high sensitivity and low capacity; glycogen synthesis has lower sensitivity but higher capacity. Thus, under physiologic conditions, mild hyperinsulinemia stimulates glucose oxidation, whereas stronger insulinization promotes glucose storage into glycogen. Clamp studies combined with regional calorimetry have demonstrated that skeletal muscle is the insulin target tissue responsible for most (50% to 70%) of insulin-mediated glucose uptake and storage in vivo [8].

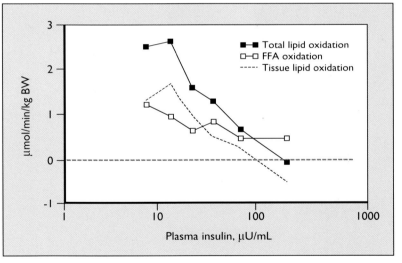

FIGURE 8-12. Dose-response curves for insulin action on lipid metabolism. Indirect calorimetry also yields estimates for total net lipid oxidation. The oxidation of circulating free fatty acid (FFA) can be measured by collecting labeled CO_2 in the expired air during the constant infusion of carbon-labeled palmitate. Tissue lipid oxidation is then defined as the difference between total lipid and FFA oxidation. In the clamp studies in normal subjects summarized in the figure, low insulin doses effectively inhibited both total lipid and FFA oxidation; high physiologic insulin doses (or chronic hyperinsulinemia) did not affect FFA oxidation any further, but caused net lipid synthesis (ie, negative values of lipid oxidation). (Data from Groop et al. [9].)

Insulin Resistance

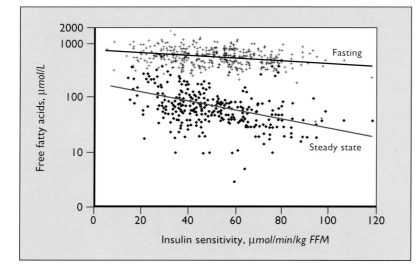

FIGURE 8-13. Relation between free fatty acid (FFA) concentrations and insulin sensitivity. In each of 450 nondiabetic subjects, plasma FFA concentrations measured in the fasting state and again at the end of a euglycemic insulin clamp (see Fig. 8-3) are plotted against the individual level of insulin sensitivity. The distance between the two regression lines measures the suppressive effect of insulin on lipolysis (*ie,* inhibition of tissue hormone-sensitive lipase). Lipolysis is resistant to insulin inhibition (in the fasting state as well as during insulinization) in subjects who are resistant to the effect of insulin on glucose uptake [10]. Thus, insulin sensitivity in lipolysis and glucose pathways is a coupled phenomenon.

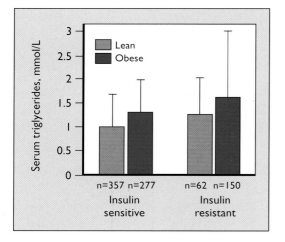

FIGURE 8-14. Insulin sensitivity and serum triglycerides. If the effect of insulin on lipolysis is deficient, both the peripheral tissues and the liver are exposed to an excess of circulating free fatty acids (FFA). In peripheral tissues, FFA impedes insulin-mediated glucose uptake (by substrate competition, according to Randle [11]); in the liver, FFA are incorporated into triglycerides at an increased rate. In accordance with the latter observation, serum triglyceride concentrations are higher in insulin-resistant individuals (*ie,* subjects in the lowest quartile of the distribution of insulin sensitivity) than in more insulin-sensitive subjects, whether they are obese or lean. The figure plots median and interquartile range for four groups: insulin-sensitive lean subjects; insulin-sensitive obese subjects; insulin-resistant lean subjects; and insulin-resistant obese subjects (unpublished data from the European Group for the Study of Insulin Resistance [EGIR] database [10]).

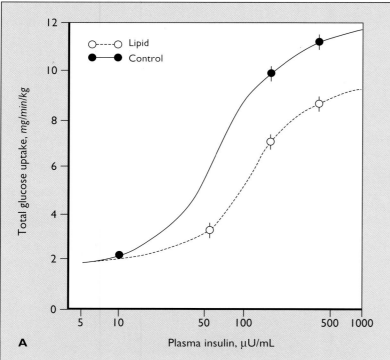

FIGURE 8-15. Experimental proof of substrate competition. Dose-response curves for total glucose uptake (**A**) and its main components,

(Continued on next page)

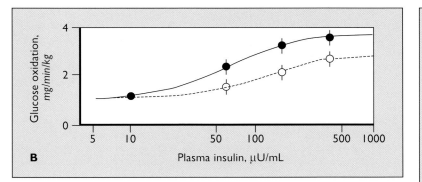

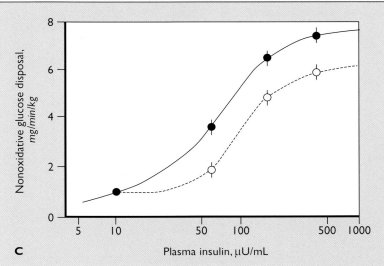

FIGURE 8-15. (*Continued*) glucose oxidation (**B**) and nonoxidative glucose disposal (**C**) (equivalent to glycogen synthesis), in healthy volunteers under control conditions (*solid lines*) and during the simultaneous infusion of Intralipid, a triglyceride emulsion (*dotted lines*). Provision of exogenous fatty substrates acutely impairs both total glucose uptake and its main components (glucose oxidation and glycogen synthesis), as predicated by substrate competition.

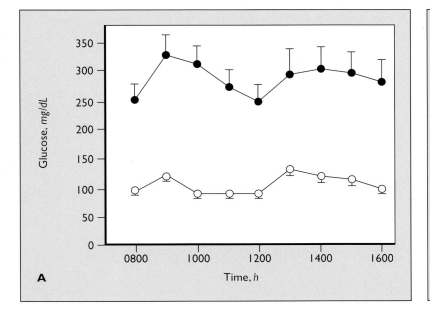

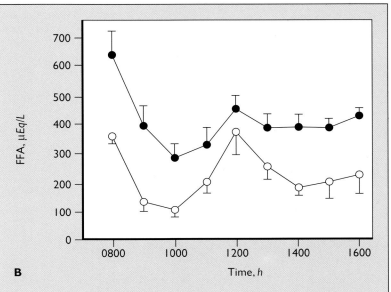

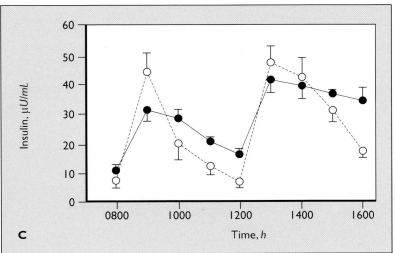

FIGURE 8-16. Day-long metabolic profile in type 2 diabetes. Plasma glucose (**A**), free fatty acids (FFA) (**B**), and insulin (**C**) concentrations in response to breakfast and lunch were measured in nondiabetic subjects (*empty circles*) and in type 2 diabetic patients (*filled circles*). Whereas average insulin levels were comparable in the two groups, both plasma glucose and FFA were markedly elevated in the diabetic patients [12]. Thus, patients with type 2 diabetes are resistant to insulin action on glucose disposal (*ie,* higher plasma glucose concentrations) as well as lipolysis (*ie,* higher plasma FFA levels) throughout the day. Consequently, insulin target tissues are exposed to chronically elevated FFA and may become laden with triglyceride deposits. (*From* Golay *et al.* [12]; with permission).

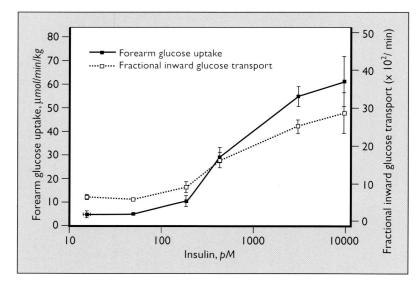

FIGURE 8-17. Glucose transport in vivo. In the human forearm, glucose transport can be measured under in vivo conditions by a triple-tracer method [13]. By this technique, the washout curves of three intra-arterially injected tracers (mannitol, to trace extracellular kinetics; 3-ortho-methylglucose, to trace glucose transport; and labeled glucose, to monitor intracellular glucose metabolism) are measured in a deep forearm vein that drains mostly muscle tissue. A compartmental model is then used on these data to calculate fractional inward glucose transport across the plasma membrane of skeletal muscle. The dose-response curve for glucose transport in the human forearm tissues was measured in healthy subjects by the triple tracer technique during graded hyperinsulinemia created by the insulin clamp technique. The graph also shows the parallelism between inward glucose transport and total glucose uptake in forearm tissues.

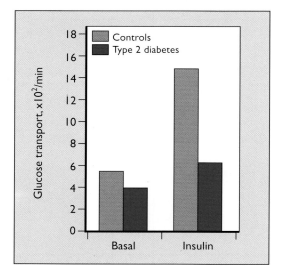

FIGURE 8-18. Defective glucose transport in type 2 diabetes. Inward glucose transport was measured by the triple-tracer technique in the basal state (overnight fast) and during euglycemic hyperinsulinemia in matched groups of patients with type 2 diabetes and nondiabetic controls. Diabetes is associated with a marked defect in the ability of insulin to stimulate glucose transport in skeletal muscle tissues [14].

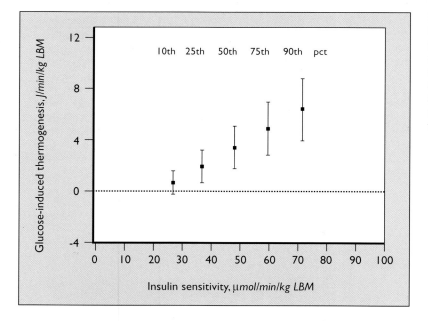

FIGURE 8-19. Insulin resistance and thermogenesis. One of the actions of insulin in vivo is to stimulate energy expenditure (*ie*, thermogenesis). Glucose-induced thermogenesis (GIT) is the change in energy expenditure observed during euglycemic hyperinsulinemia, as measured by indirect calorimetry during an insulin clamp in this case. The figure shows point estimates (± SEM) of GIT at different percentiles (pct) of insulin sensitivity in 322 nondiabetic subjects after statistical adjustment by gender, age, and body mass index. Insulin-resistant subjects show a defect in glucose-induced thermogenesis that is proportional to the degree of insulin resistance (unpublished data). LBM—lean body mass.

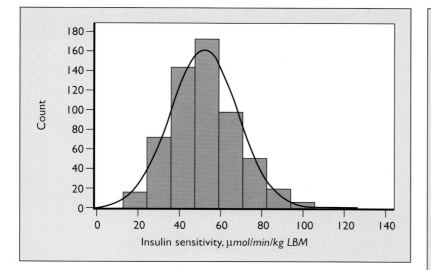

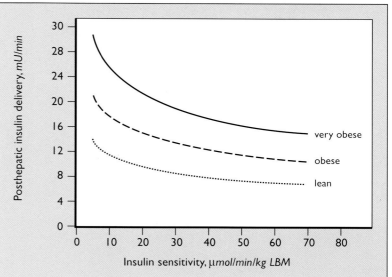

FIGURE 8-20. Insulin sensitivity in the general population. The graph shows the frequency distribution plot of insulin sensitivity (as measured by the euglycemic insulin clamp) in a cohort of 580 nondiabetic, nonobese (BMI ≤25 kg/m²) white subjects of both sexes. The distribution is significantly different from the normal distribution. The graft is skewed to the left as a result of an excess of insulin-resistant individuals (data from the EGIR study [15]). There is, however, no evidence to suggest a bimodal or multimodal distribution of this trait. In general terms, this distribution is compatible with a model in which genetic drive is influenced by powerful environmental factors. LBM—lean body mass.

FIGURE 8-21. Relation between insulin sensitivity and insulin secretion. In a cohort of 1200 nondiabetic white subjects of both sexes, the relationship between insulin sensitivity (by the insulin clamp technique) and insulin secretion (estimated from the clamping data as the posthepatic insulin delivery rate) is highly curvilinear (hyperbolic), such that in insulin-resistant individuals small changes in insulin sensitivity are associated with large (compensatory) changes in insulin secretion. The plot also shows the impact of obesity as an independent factor that greatly amplifies insulin secretion at any given level of insulin resistance. Thus, any degree of insulin hypersecretion (and, therefore, of hyperinsulinemia) can be described as the sum of a component that is secondary (compensatory) to insulin resistance and a part that is primary. The primary component is particularly common in obese individuals. (*Data from* Ferrannini *et al.*[16].)

FIGURE 8-22. Impact of age on insulin sensitivity. In nondiabetic, otherwise healthy subjects, aging has a marginal effect on insulin resistance [15]. Thus, the aging population tends to be insulin-resistant because it is enriched with individuals with impaired glucose tolerance, essential hypertension, or obesity rather than as a result of senescence itself.

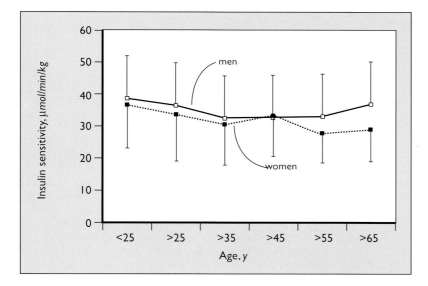

Insulin Resistance Syndrome

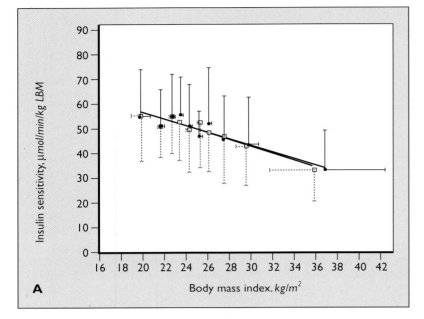

A

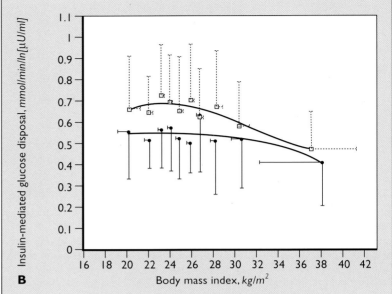

B

FIGURE 8-23. Insulin resistance and obesity. The dependence of insulin sensitivity on obesity (expressed as the body mass index) is expressed in two ways in this figure. When total insulin-mediated glucose uptake is normalized by lean body mass (**A**), insulin sensitivity declines linearly with body mass, equally in men (*dotted lines*) and women (*solid bars*). However, when insulin-mediated glucose disposal is expressed in absolute terms (**B**) (in mmol/min, corrected for the steady-state plasma insulin concentration achieved during the clamp), the negative impact of obesity is seen only in very obese individuals (BMI >32 kg/m²). Thus, in the obese person, each unit mass of lean tissue (mostly skeletal muscle) is resistant to the action of insulin in direct proportion to the excess body fatness. However, the expanded body mass of the moderately obese person compensates for the reduced insulin sensitivity and contributes to the maintenance of glucose tolerance [16].

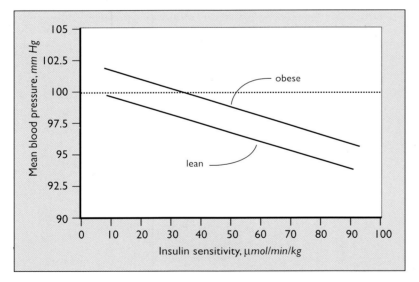

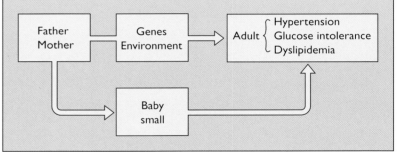

FIGURE 8-25. Insulin resistance and intrauterine development. Low birthweight has been found to be associated with the emergence in adulthood of hypertension, impaired glucose tolerance, and dyslipidemia, all states of impaired insulin action. Therefore, in addition to genes and environmental factors, insulin sensitivity may be modulated by changes that occur during intrauterine development. Thus, intrauterine growth retardation, possibly caused by maternal insulin resistance, may exert negative effects on the development of β-cells, insulin sensing in target tissues, and the vasculature.

FIGURE 8-24. Insulin resistance and blood pressure. Patients with essential hypertension are, as a group, insulin-resistant. This is not a special feature of essential hypertension, however, but the extension of a physiologic link into the disease domain. In fact, insulin resistance is associated with higher blood pressure levels in the normotensive population. The graph shows the significant inverse relationship between mean blood pressure and insulin sensitivity (as measured by the clamping technique) in 450 nondiabetic subjects in the EGIR cohort. The regression lines are adjusted by gender and age, and are drawn across the observed range of insulin sensitivity. The lower line (*lean*) is the predicted dependence in a subjects with a body mass index of 25 kg/m², whereas the upper line (*obese*) is the function for an individual with a body mass index of 35 kg/m². The dotted line is an arbitrary threshold for clinical hypertension. Obesity and insulin resistance work together to raise arterial blood pressure [17].

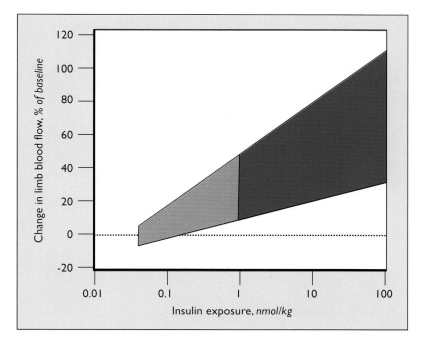

FIGURE 8-26. Hemodynamic actions of insulin: I. Insulin induces dilatation of peripheral (forearm, leg, or calf) vasculature as a function of exposure (dose of insulin × length of exposure, expressed as total nmol/kg of body weight). The darker area represents the physiologic insulin exposure, over which the average vasodilatory response is in the range 15% to 30%. The scheme is a compilation of a number of published studies. (*Adapted from* Yki-Järvinen and Utriainen [18]; with permission).

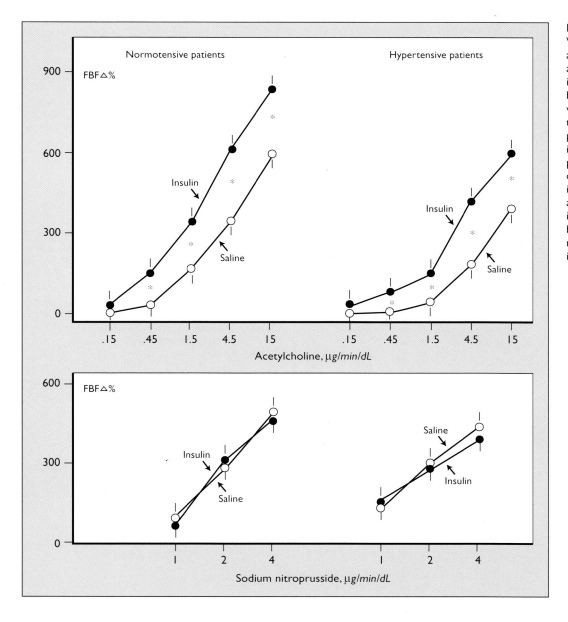

FIGURE 8-27. Hemodynamic actions of insulin: II. When infused locally (ie, through the brachial artery) at physiologic doses, insulin potentiates acetylcholine-induced (*top*), but not nitroprusside-induced (*bottom*), vasodilatation in humans [19], both in normotensive subjects (*left*) and in patients with essential hypertension (*right*). These data suggest that insulin vasodilatation is an endothelium-dependent phenomenon. In addition, the potentiating effect of insulin was similar in healthy subjects and hypertensive patients (who were resistant to the effect of insulin on glucose uptake), suggesting that the actions of insulin on the vasculature and glucose metabolism are largely independent of each other. *Asterisks* indicate mean values that are significantly different between insulin and saline infusion. *Asterisks* indicate mean values that are significantly different between insulin and saline infusion. FBF—forearm blood flow.

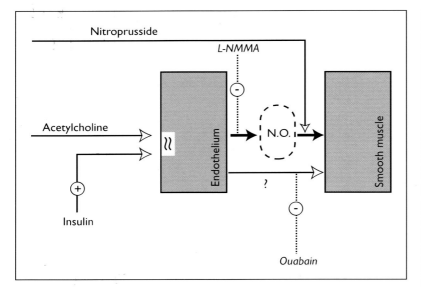

FIGURE 8-28. Hemodynamic actions of insulin: III. Insulin receptors are present on endothelial as well as on smooth muscle cells; thus, both types of cells are potential targets for insulin action. Insulin-induced vasodilatation [20] and insulin potentiation of acetylcholine-induced vasodilatation can both be blocked by L-monomethyl-arginine (L-NMMA), a competitive inhibitor of nitric oxide (NO) synthase [19], indicating that a likely mechanism for this effect of insulin is NO release from the endothelium. Direct provision of NO with nitroprusside bypasses the endothelial step. Furthermore, both insulin-induced vasodilatation [21] and insulin potentiation of acetylcholine-induced vasodilatation [19] can be blocked by ouabain, an inhibitor of sodium-potassium ATPase, suggesting that cell membrane hyperpolarization is an alternative mechanism for this action of insulin. Insulin-induced hyperpolarization can be exerted directly on the smooth muscle cell or involve the release of an unidentified hyperpolarizing factor from the endothelium.

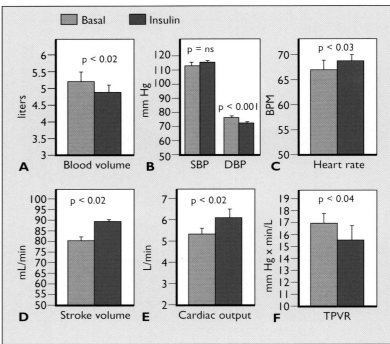

FIGURE 8-29. Hemodynamic actions of insulin: IV. Vasodilatation is not the only vascular action of insulin. Following physiologic hyperinsulinemia established by insulin clamping, blood volume is reduced (**A**); diastolic blood pressure (DBP) falls slightly, whereas systolic blood pressure (SBP) increases somewhat (**B**); heart rate goes up (**C**); stroke volume and cardiac output increase (**D** and **E**); and total peripheral vascular resistances (TPVR) decrease (**F**). This hemodynamic picture is compatible with a direct effect of insulin to reduce vascular resistance (vasodilatation) and a simultaneous effect of insulin to stimulate adrenergic activity (enhanced cardiac contractility). bpm—beats per minute.

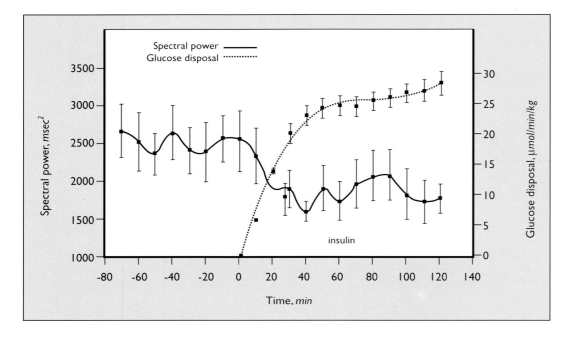

FIGURE 8-30. Hemodynamic actions of insulin: V. Spectral analysis of heart rate variability provides information on the autonomic nervous control of cardiac function. Total spectral power reflects parasympathetic and adrenergic inputs related to baroreflex control of heart rate; these inputs are mediated through the central nervous system. During a standard euglycemic insulin clamp, insulin causes a prompt and marked decline in total spectral power, which is temporally and quantitatively unrelated to insulin stimulation of glucose disposal [22]. This effect is partially independent of changes in heart rate, and therefore reflects direct desensitization of the autonomic neural reflex arch. In addition, the effect is more marked on the parasympathetic component of the autonomic arch (parasympathetic withdrawal), thereby giving rise to relative sympathetic dominance.

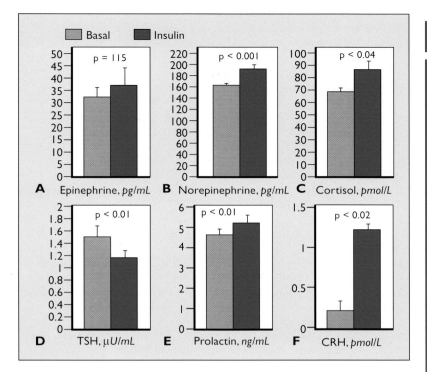

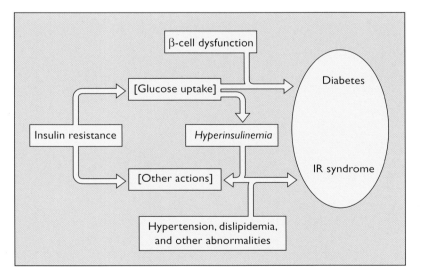

FIGURE 8-31. Insulin action and the central nervous system. Physiologic euglycemic hyperinsulinemia is associated with a rise in the circulating levels of epinephrine and norepinephrine (**A** and **B**), cortisol (**C**), prolactin (**E**), and corticotropin releasing hormone (CRH) (**F**) and a decrease in thyroid stimulating hormone (TSH) (**D**) [22]. This pattern of hormonal responses is compatible with a moderate stress reaction orchestrated by CRH. Thus, the hemodynamic, autonomic nervous, and hormonal responses to peripheral hyperinsulinemia coherently indicate that insulin acts in the central nervous system, most probably following transport from the plasma across the blood-brain barrier [23].

NATIVE AND EXPERIMENTAL INSULIN RESISTANCE

Physiologic	Nonendocrine
Puberty	Essential hypertension
Pregnancy	Chronic uremia
Bed rest	Liver cirrhosis
Contraceptives	Rheumatoid arthritis
High-fat diet	Acanthosis nigricans
Metabolic	Chronic heart failure
Type 2 diabetes	Myotonic dystrophia
Uncontrolled type 1 diabetes	Trauma, burns, sepsis
Diabetic ketoacidosis	Surgery
Obesity	Neoplastic cachexia
Severe malnutrition	Experimental
Hyperuricemia	Short-term hyperglycemia
Insulin-induced hypoglycemia	Short-term hypoglycemia
Excessive alcohol consumption	Short-term hyperinsulinemia
Endocrine	Short-term hypoinsulinemia
Thryotoxicosis	Fat infusion
Hypothyroidism	Amino acid infusion
Cushing syndrome	Infusion of counterregulatory
Pheochromocytoma	hormones
Acromegaly	Acidosis

FIGURE 8-32. Native and experimental insulin resistance. This table lists conditions that have been found to be associated with insulin resistance or under which insulin resistance can be produced experimentally.

FIGURE 8-33. Insulin action and the insulin resistance syndrome: a working hypothesis. Insulin resistance (IR) in the glucose pathway combines with β-cell dysfunction to produce the hyperglycemia of diabetes. Insulin resistance also induces compensatory hyperinsulinemia. Insulin pathways other than glucose metabolism (lipids, blood pressure, endothelial function, autonomic nervous system) may themselves be resistant or, if normally sensitive, be overly stimulated by the hyperinsulinemia. The signs and symptoms of the insulin resistance syndrome develop from these pathways.

References

1. DeFronzo RA, Tobin J, Andres R: Glucose clamp technique: a method for quantifying insulin secretion and resistance. *Am J Physiol* 1979, 237:E214–E223.

2. Ferrannini E, Mari A: How to measure insulin sensitivity. *J Hypertens* 1998, 16:895–906.

3. Iozzo P, Beck-Nielsen H, Laakso M, *et al.*: Independent influence of age on basal insulin secretion in nondiabetic humans. *J Clin Endocrinol Metab* 1999, 84:863–868.

4. DeFronzo RA, Simonson D, Ferrannini E: Hepatic and peripheral insulin resistance: a common feature of insulin-independent and insulin-dependent diabetes. *Diabetologia* 1982, 23:313–320.

5. DeFronzo RA, Ferrannini E, Hendler R, *et al.*: Regulation of splanchnic and peripheral glucose uptake by insulin and hyperglycemia in man. *Diabetes* 1983, 32:35–45.

6. Landau BR, Wahren J, Chandramouli V, *et al.*: Use of 2H2O for estimating rates of gluconeogenesis. Application to the fasted state. *J Clin Invest* 1995, 95:172–178.

7. Paternostro G, Camici PG, Lammerstma AA, *et al.*: Cardiac and skeletal muscle insulin resistance in patients with coronary artery disease: a study with positron-emitting tomography. *J Clin Invest* 1996, 98:2094–2099.

8. Kelley DE, Mokan M, Simoneau JA, Mandarino LJ: Interaction between glucose and free fatty acid metabolism in human skeletal muscle. *J Clin Invest* 1993, 92:91–98.

9. Groop LC, Saloranta C, Schenk M, *et al.*: The role of free fatty acid metabolism in the pathogenesis of insulin resistance in obesity and non-insulin dependent diabetes mellitus. *J Clin Endocrinol Metab* 1991, 72:96–102.

10. Ferrannini E, Camastra S, Coppack SW, *et al.*: Insulin action and non-esterified fatty acids. *Proc Nutr Soc* 1997, 56:753–761.

11. Randle PJ, Garland PB, Hales CN, Newsholme EA: The glucose fatty acid cycle: its role in insulin sensitivity and the metabolic disturbances of diabetes mellitus. *Lancet* 1963, i:785–789.

12. Golay A, Swilocky AL, Chen YD, Reaven GM: Relationship between plasma free fatty acid concentration, endogenous glucose production, and fasting hyperglycemia in normal and non-insulin-dependent diabetic individuals. *Metabolism* 1987, 36:692–696.

13. Bonadonna RC, Saccomani MP, Seely L, *et al.*: Glucose transport in human skeletal muscle: the in vivo response to insulin. *Diabetes* 1993, 42:191–198.

14. Bonadonna RC, Del Prato S, Cobelli C, *et al.*: Transmembrane glucose transport in skeletal muscle of patients with non-insulin dependent diabetes. *J Clin Invest* 1993, 92:486–492.

15. Ferrannini E, Vichi S, Beck-Nielsen H, *et al.*: Insulin action and age. *Diabetes* 1996, 45:947–953.

16. Ferrannini E, Natali A, Bell P, *et al.*: Insulin resistance and hypersecretion in obesity. *J Clin Invest* 1997, 100:1166–1173.

17. Ferrannini E, Natali A, Capaldo B, *et al.*: Insulin resistance, hyperinsulinemia, and blood pressure. Role of age and obesity. *Hypertension* 1997, 30:1144–1149.

18. Yki-Järvinen H, Utriainen T: Insulin-induced vasodilatation: physiology or pharmacology? *Diabetologia* 1998, 41:369–379.

19. Taddei S, Virdis A, Mattei P, *et al.*: Effect of insulin on acetylcholine-induced vasodilation in normotensive subjects and patients with essential hypertension. *Circulation* 1995, 92:2911–2920.

20. Steinberg HO, Brechtel G, Johson A, *et al.*: Insulin-mediated skeletal muscle vasodilatation is nitric oxide dependent. A novel action of insulin to increase nitric oxide release. *J Clin Invest* 1994, 94:1172–1179.

21. Tack CJJ, Lutterman JA, Vervoot G, *et al.* Activation of the sodium-potassium pump contributes to insulin-induced vasodilatation in humans. *Hypertension* 1996, 28:426–432.

22. Muscelli E, Emdin M, Natali A, *et al.* Autonomic and hemodynamic responses to insulin in lean and obese humans. *J Clin Endocrinol Metab* 1998, 83:2084–2090.

23. Schwartz MW, Figlewicz DP, Baskin DB, Woods SC, Porta D, Jr: Insulin in the brain: a hormonal regulator of energy balance. *Endocr Rev* 1992, 13:81–113.

HYPOGLYCEMIA

F. John Service

Hypoglycemia is a clinical syndrome, arising from diverse causes, in which low levels of plasma glucose eventually lead to neuroglycopenia. Symptoms of hypoglycemia begin at plasma glucose levels of approximately 60 mg/dL, and impairment of brain function begins at levels of approximately 50 mg/dL. The rate of decrease in plasma glucose levels does not influence the occurrence of symptoms. The symptoms of hypoglycemia have been classified into two major groups: autonomic and neuroglycopenic. The latter have been identified from experimental studies as the following: dizziness, confusion, difficulty in speaking, headache, inability to concentrate, warmth, weakness, confusion or difficulty in thinking, and fatigue or drowsiness. In a retrospective analysis of 60 patients with insulinoma, 85% of patients had various combinations of diplopia, blurred vision, sweating, palpitations, and weakness; 80% had confusion or abnormal behavior; 53% had amnesia or coma; and 12% had generalized seizures. Symptoms of hypoglycemia differ among patients but are consistent from episode to episode for each patient. Symptoms do not evolve in a consistent chronologic order; autonomic symptoms (sweating, trembling, anxiety, palpitation, hunger, tingling) do not always precede the neuroglycopenic symptoms. Many patients experience only neuroglycopenic symptoms. Persons with recurrent hypoglycemia may develop varying degrees of hypoglycemia unawareness analogous to that observed in persons with insulin-dependent diabetes. None of these symptoms is specific for hypoglycemia; the presence of one of several may be from other causes.

The long-established classification of hypoglycemia as either food-deprived (composed of organic diseases and manifested by neuroglycopenic symptoms) or food-stimulated (arising from functional disturbances and manifested by autonomic symptoms) is no longer useful.

Persons with insulinomas, the archetypical food-deprived hypoglycemic disorder, may have symptoms after eating (and in rare instances only at this time) as well as during fasting. Persons with factitious hypoglycemia have erratically occurring symptoms that are independent of food ingestion. Food-stimulated hypoglycemias, such as galactosemia, hereditary fructose intolerance, and ackee-fruit poisoning, result in neuroglycopenic symptoms. The disorders that supposedly arise from a functional disturbance of glucose homeostasis and produce only autonomic symptoms—functional hypoglycemia, early diabetes hypoglycemia, and alimentary hypoglycemia—were predicated on the now-discredited 5-hour oral glucose-tolerance test and have no scientific support.

A more useful approach is a classification based on clinical characteristics. Persons who appear healthy are likely to have hypoglycemic disorders different from those experienced by ill persons. Hospitalized patients are at additional risk for hypoglycemia, often from iatrogenic factors. Hypoglycemia may occur from accidental drug ingestion in healthy persons, the mistaken dispensing of a sulfonylureaa, or the idiosyncratic actions of some of the drugs used to treat seriously ill patients. The occurrence of hypoglycemia in a patient with an illness known to be associated with this condition requires little, if any, investigation of its cause, only a recognition of the association of the disease with the risk for hypoglycemia. Healthy-appearing persons of all ages and both sexes are at risk for insulinomas. Factitious hypoglycemia due to self-administered insulin is often seen in female health care workers. These clinical patterns facilitate the differential diagnosis and help direct the diagnostic evaluation. Asymptomatic patients may have artifactual hypoglycemia because of leukemia or severe hemolysis or may have adapted to lifelong hypoglycemia caused by glycogen storage disease [1].

Symptoms, Classification, and Glucose Behavior in Hypoglycemic Disorders

CLINICAL CLASSIFICATION OF HYPOGLYCEMIC DISORDERS

Patient appears healthy*

No coexistent disease
  Drugs
    Ethanol
    Salicylates
    Quinine
    Haloperidol
  Insulinoma
  Insulin or sulfonylurea factitial hypoglycemia
  Severe exercise
  Ketotic hypoglycemia

Compensated coexistent disease
  Drugs
    Dispensing error
    Disopyramide
    Beta-adrenergic blocking agents
    Sulfhydryl- or thiol-containing drugs with autoimmune insulin syndrome
    Unripe ackee fruit and undernutrition

Patient appears ill

Drugs
  Pentamidine and *Pneumocystis carinii* pneumonia
  Trimethoprim–sulfamethoxazole and renal failure
  Propoxyphene and renal failure
  Quinine and cerebral malaria
  Quinine and malaria
  Topical salicylates and renal failure

Predisposing illness
  Children
    Small-for-gestational-age infant
    Beckwith-Wiedemann syndrome
    Erythroblastosis fetalis
    Infant of diabetic mother
    Glycogen storage disease
    Defects in amino acid and fatty acid metabolism
    Reye's syndrome
    Cyanotic congenital heart disease
    Hypopituitarism
    Isolated growth hormone deficiency
    Isolated adrenocorticotropic hormone deficiency
    Addison's disease
    Galactosemia
    Hereditary fructose intolerance
    Carnitine deficiency
    Defective type I glucose transporter in the brain
  Adults
    Acquired severe liver disease
    Large non–beta-cell tumor
    Sepsis
    Renal failure
    Congestive heart failure
    Lactic acidosis
    Starvation
    Anorexia nervosa
    Following removal of pheochromocytoma
    Insulin receptor antibody hypoglycemia
    Mutations in the beta-cell sulfonylurea receptor gene
    Glutamate dehydrogenase gene
    Glucokinase gene

Hospitalized patient
  Diseases predisposing to hypoglycemia
  Total parenteral nutrition and insulin therapy
  Questran interference with glucocorticoid absorption
  Shock

*Mutations in the β-cell sulfonylurea receptor gene, glutamate dehydrogenase gene, and glucokinase gene are rare causes of hyperinsulinemic hypoglycemia usually manifested in infancy or childhood.

FIGURE 9-1. Clinical classification of hypoglycemic disorders.

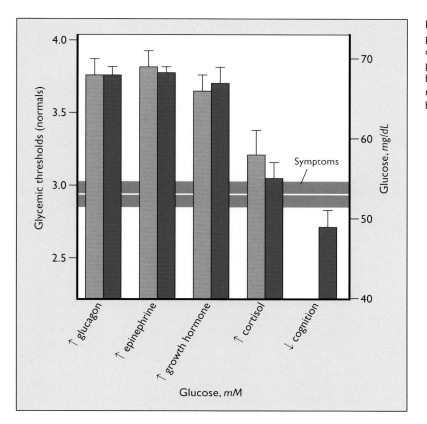

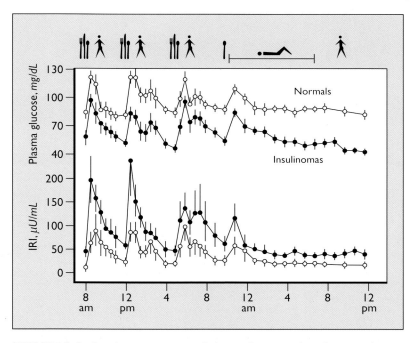

FIGURE 9-2. Mean arterialized venous glycemic thresholds of increments in plasma levels of glucagon, epinephrine, growth hormone, and cortisol for symptoms of hypoglycemia and for impairment of cognitive function during decrements in plasma glucose levels in normal humans from two independent studies. Light blue bars represent data from a report by Series in 1995 [2]; dark blue bars represent data from a chapter by Series in 1989 [3]). Error bars are the upper bound of the standard error. (*Adapted from* Cryer [4].)

FIGURE 9-3. Plasma glucose responses to a mixed meal. *Triangles* represent responses in healthy persons; *white* (fasting hypoglycemia profile) and *black* (postprandial hypoglycemia profile) *circles* represent responses in persons with insulinoma. Postprandial hypoglycemia with spontaneous resumption of normoglycemia can infrequently be seen in patients with this disorder. Therefore, categorization of patients by timing of hypoglycemic symptoms may not be useful for diagnosing the cause of the hypoglycemic disorder. (*From* Service [2]; with permission.)

FIGURE 9-4. Serial measurements of plasma glucose and insulin were done in normal persons and patients with insulinoma. Although plasma glucose levels increased after meal ingestion (represented by the knife, fork, and spoon symbol), it declined to hypoglycemic levels in the postabsorptive state and during fasting. Insulinomas were persistently hyperinsulinemic in the absorptive, postabsorptive, and fasting states (the striding symbol represents exercise, and the reclining symbol represents sleep). (*From* Service *et al.* [5]; with permission.)

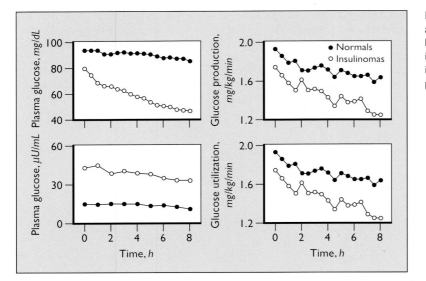

FIGURE 9-5. Glucose turnover was isotopically measured in normal persons and patients with insulinoma during food deprivation. Insulinomas became hypoglycemic primarily as a result of decreased glucose production rather than increased glucose utilization. Thus, the primary effect of persistent hyperinsulinemia in insulinomas is to turn off hepatic glucose production. (*From* Rizza [6]; with permission.)

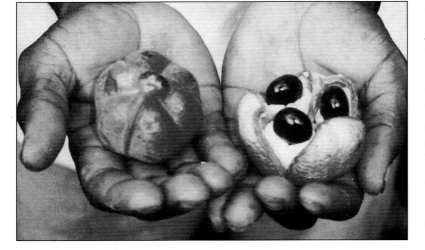

FIGURE 9-6. (*see* Color Plate) The ackee fruit in its unripe form (*left*) and ripe form (*right*). The ackee tree, indigenous to west Africa, was introduced to Jamaica in 1778 by Thomas Clarke. In Jamaica it is considered a dietary staple. It is well known in west Africa and Jamaica that the fruit may be poisonous during certain stages in its development.

Outbreaks of a disorder commonly called Jamaica vomiting sickness tend to occur during the colder months of the year, when other food is scarce and the fruit is still unripe. The major clinical features of this disorder, caused by ingestion of an unripe ackee fruit, include the sudden onset of vomiting and violent retching, which is preceded by generalized epigastric discomfort lasting 2 hours to 3 days. After a period of prostration averaging 10 hours, the second bout of vomiting may occur, followed by convulsions and sometimes death. The most striking finding is marked hypoglycemia. Well-nourished people may never develop manifestations of the disease, whereas those with chronic malnutrition, especially children between 2 and 5 years of age, are much more likely to become symptomatic. Hypoglycins A and B mediate the illness: They inhibit transport of long-chain fatty acids into the mitochondria, thereby suppressing their oxidation and resulting in depression of gluconeogenesis [3].

FIGURE 9-7. Protocol for prolonged 72-hour fast.

PROTOCOL FOR PROLONGED SUPERVISED FAST

1. Date the onset of the fast as of the last ingestion of calories. Discontinue use of all nonessential medications.

2. Allow the patient to drink calorie-free and caffeine-free beverages.

3. Ensure that the patient is active during waking hours.

4. Measure plasma levels of glucose, insulin, C-peptide, and, if an assay is available, proinsulin in the same specimen: repeat measurements every 6 hours until the plasma glucose level is < 60 mg/dL. At this point, the interval should be reduced to every 1 to 2 hours.

5. End the fast when the plasma glucose level is < 45 mg/dL and the patient has symptoms or signs of hypoglycemia.

6. At the end of the fast, measure plasma levels of glucose, insulin, C-peptide, proinsulin, β-hydroxy-butyrate, and sulfonylurea in the same specimen. Then inject 1 mg of glucagon intravenously and measure plasma glucose level after 10, 20, and 30 minutes. At this point the patient can be fed.

7. When a deficiency is suspected, measure plasma levels of cortisol, growth hormone, or glucagon at the beginning and end of the fast [7].

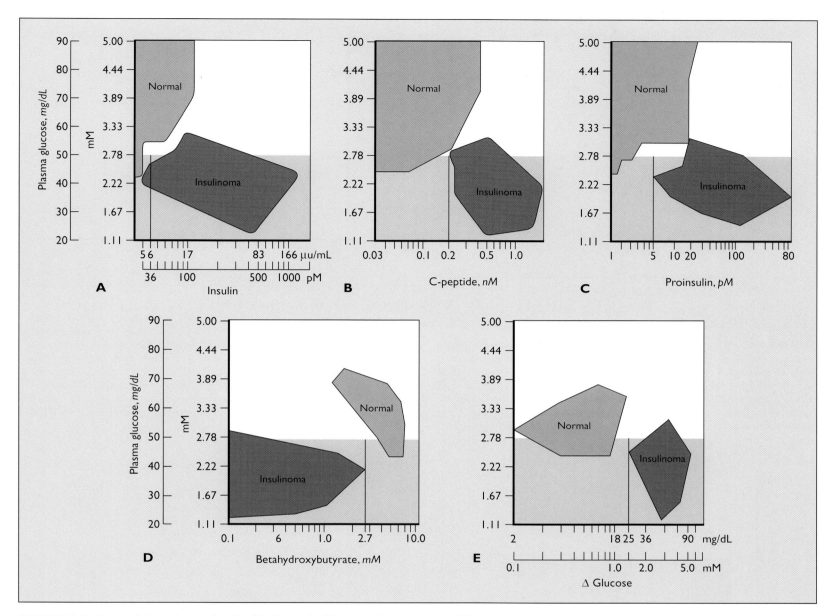

FIGURE 9-8. Limits of plasma levels of insulin (**A**), C-peptide (**B**), proinsulin (**C**), and β-hydroxybutyrate (**D**) and changes in plasma glucose levels (**E**) in response to intravenous glucagon, according to 1) plasma glucose levels at the end of a 72-hour fast in 25 normal persons and 2) the point at which the features of Whipple's triad were noted in 40 patients with histologically confirmed insuli-nomas. The shaded areas represent plasma glucose levels (50 mg/dL (2.8 mmol/L). The vertical lines represent the diagnostic criteria for insulinoma: insulin level of at least 6 micro units per mL (36 pmol/L), C-peptide level of at least 0.2 nmol/L, proinsulin level of at least 5 pmol/L, beta-hydroxybutyrate level 2.7 mmol/L or less, and change in glucose level of at least 25 mg/dL (1.4 mmol/L).

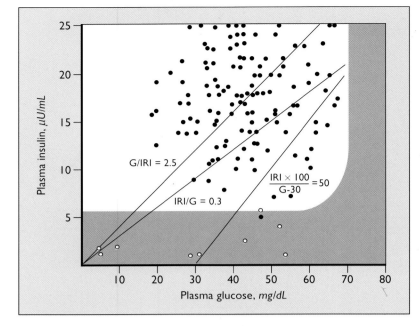

FIGURE 9-9. Plasma insulin (IRI) concentrations in patients with insulinoma (*black circles*) and patients with non–insulin-mediated hypoglycemic disorders (*white circles*) plotted against concurrent plasma glucose (G) levels. Various ratios relating these two variables are shown. None of the ratios is as useful as the absolute insulin value of 6 micro units/mL (36 pmol/L) for separating insulin-mediated from non–insulin-mediated hypoglycemia when the insulin level is within the normal overnight fasting range. (*From* Service [3]; with permission.)

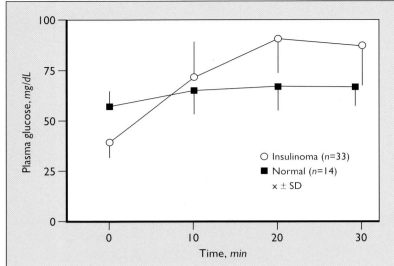

FIGURE 9-10. Plasma glucose responses to glucagon, 1 mg, administered intravenously at the end of the prolonged fast (0 minutes) are greater in patients with insulinoma than in normal persons. The rationale for this procedure is that insulin is glycogenic and antiglycogenolytic and therefore results in persistence of hepatic glycogen despite fasting. Patients with insulin-mediated hypoglycemia have a maximum increment of at least 25 mg/dL above the terminal fasting plasma glucose levels, whereas others (normal persons or those with non–insulin-mediated hypoglycemia whose hepatic glycogen has been depleted by fasting) have lower increments [7]. Error bars represent the standard deviation. (*From* Service et al. [5]; with permission.)

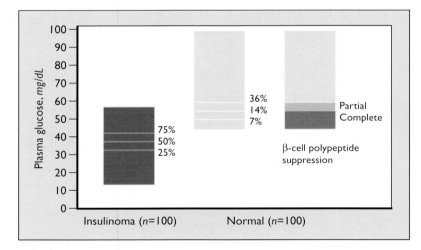

FIGURE 9-11. Plasma glucose levels at the end of a 72-hour fast. The yellow panel depicts the range (57 to 44 mg/dL) at the termination of the prolonged 72-hour fast (Whipple's triad) in 100 patients with insulinoma (the fast was terminated well before the 72-hour point because of the occurrence of symptomatic hypoglycemia confirmed biochemically). The 75th percentile (42 mg/dL), 50th percentile (38 mg/dL), and 25th percentile (33 mg/dL) are also shown. The red panel shows the plasma glucose levels at the 72-hour point in 100 normal persons who underwent the 72-hour fast. Thirty-six percent of patients had a plasma glucose level of 60 mg/dL or less, 14% had a level of 55 mg/dL or less, and 7% had a level of 50 mg/dL or less. Two patients had terminal plasma glucose levels of 44 mg/dL. The blue panel depicts suppression of beta-cell polypeptides in normal persons at the end of the 72-hour fast. One or two of the three beta-cell polypeptides (insulin, C-peptide, and proinsulin) were suppressed below our diagnostic criteria for hyperinsulinemia in the range 60 to 55 mg/dL, and all three were suppressed when the plasma glucose level was 55 mg/dL or lower.

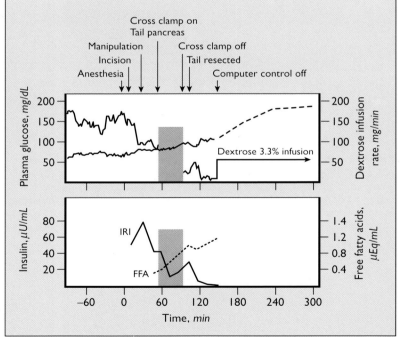

FIGURE 9-12. The Biostator (Life Science Instruments, Elkharst, IN) has been used by some practitioners to maintain euglycemia in the preoperative and intraoperative period. A reduction in the glucose infusion rate after removal of the insulinoma indicates that all hyperfunctioning tissue has been removed. An alternate approach is to conduct frequent serial measurements of plasma glucose levels in the operating room. Patients are taken to the operating room without glucose running, and the plasma glucose level is permitted to decrease to a modestly hypoglycemic range. After tumor removal, an increase in the plasma glucose level can be expected within 30 minutes in most patients. In some patients, the plasma glucose level is increasing as a result of stress before tumor removal. Also after removal of the tumor, the slope of the elevation in the glucose level increases distinctly. (*From* Kudlow *et al.* [8]; with permission.)

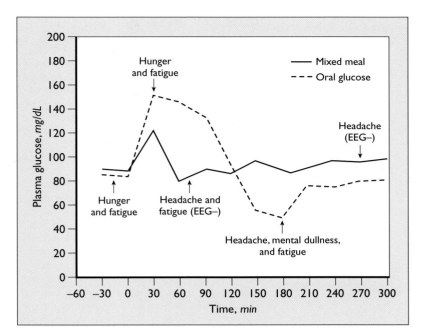

FIGURE 9-13. The oral glucose tolerance test has been used to evaluate patients with suspected reactive hypoglycemia. Unfortunately, this test is of no use because a high percentage of normal persons have a post–oral glucose testing nadir of 50 mg/dL or less. The preferred assessment is a mixed-meal test. As shown in this figure, individual symptoms occurred throughout the oral glucose tolerance test, both at the nadir and at the apogee. In addition, symptoms were present during the mixed-meal test when no evidence of hypoglycemia was noted. These observations provide strong evidence that symptoms could not be ascribed to hypoglycemia. (*From* Service [3]; with permission.)

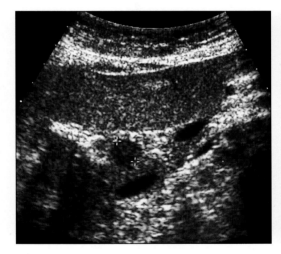

FIGURE 9-14. The ultrasonographic characteristic of insulinoma is hypoechogenicity. The insulinoma is marked with white crosses and is distinctly hypoechogenic in contrast to surrounding tissue.

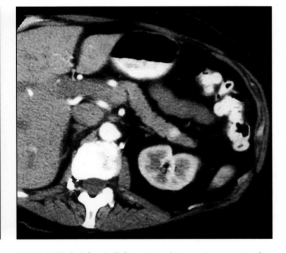

FIGURE 9-15. (*see* Color Plate) Color Doppler analysis shows the hypervascularity of the insulinoma noted in Figure 9-14.

FIGURE 9-16. A 0.8-cm insulinoma is seen in the arterial phase of the spiral computed tomographic scan, which was obtained by using triple-phase agent.

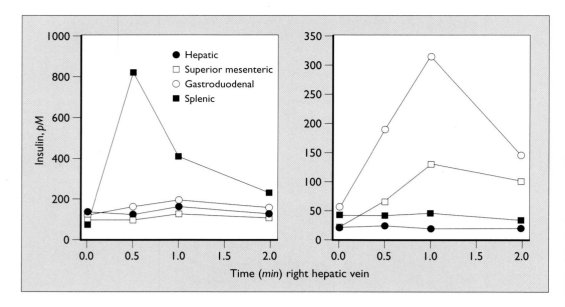

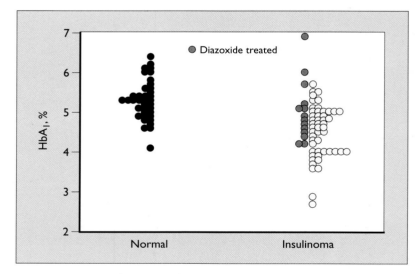

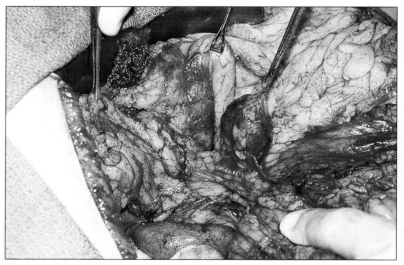

FIGURE 9-17. The selective arterial calcium stimulation test is both a localization (actually a regionalization) procedure and a dynamic test. The principle of this procedure is that hyperfunctioning beta cells release insulin in response to the injection of a small dose of calcium intra-arterially, whereas normal beta cells do not. During this procedure, the insulin level is measured before and at fixed time sequences after the injection of 0.025 mEq of calcium per kg of body weight sequentially into the splenic, gastroduodenal, and superior mesenteric arteries. A two- to three-fold increment in the level of insulin in the right hepatic vein indicates hyperfunctioning beta cells—either insulinoma or hypertrophic islets—in the arterial distribution of the injected artery. In the left panel, the positive response after injection into the splenic artery indicates that hyperfunctioning beta cells (presumably an insulinoma) are present in the tail of the pancreas. In the right panel, the positive responses to injections into the superior mesenteric and gastroduodenal arteries suggests that the insulinoma is likely to be in the head of the pancreas. (*From* Doppman *et al.* [9]; with permission.)

FIGURE 9-18. Glycated hemoglobin values (measured by affinity chromatography) are shown for normal persons evaluated for potential hypoglycemic disorder and insulinomas, some of whom had been treated with diazoxide. Although glycated hemoglobin values are lower in patients with insulinoma than in normal persons, the values overlap too much to allow a diagnostic level to be established. Twenty-five percent of the patients with insulinoma had glycated hemoglobin values of 4.1% or less; this was at the lower limit of values observed in normal persons. (*From* Hassoun *et al.* [10]; with permission.)

FIGURE 9-19. (*see* Color Plate) Insulinomas vary in size, from a few millimeters to several centimeters. The median is 1.5 cm. This figure shows a 4-cm tumor. In a large series of patients (*n* = 224) observed at the Mayo Clinic from 1927 to 1986 [11], 86.6% of patients had a single benign tumor, 5.9% had malignant tumors, 8.9% had multiple tumors, and 7.6% had multiple endocrine neoplasia type syndrome. The estimated incidence in the northern European population is 4 cases per 1 million patient-years. The median age in the Mayo Clinic series was 47 years (range, 8 to 82 years), and 59% of patients were women. During the study period, one patient had islet hyperplasia.

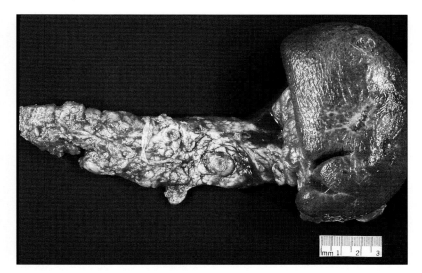

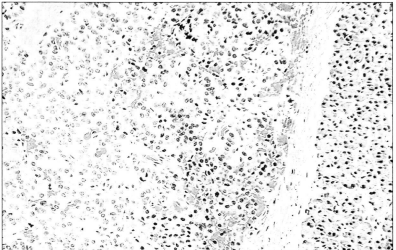

FIGURE 9-20. (*see* Color Plate) This specimen shows removal of the distal pancreas and spleen in a patient with multiple islet cell tumors as part of the multiple endocrine neoplasia (MEN) I syndrome. Insulinoma constitutes the second most common pancreatic tumor in the MEN I syndrome. In a study from the Mayo Clinic [11], more than 50% of patients with insulinoma as part of MEN I syndrome had multiple tumors. The associated endocrinopathies have primarily been hyperparathyroidism, prolactinoma, gastrinoma, and Cushing disease. The standard operative approach is to enucleate tumors in the head of the pancreas and, if tumors are present in the rest of the pancreas, to conduct a partial pancreatectomy.

FIGURE 9-21. (*see* Color Plate) This low-power view of pancreatic tissue shows normal exocrine pancreas on the right side of the figure. The left side of the figure shows an islet-cell tumor composed of uniform cells with round nuclei and eosinophilic cytoplasm. The tumor is highly vascular, and small clusters of red blood cells are present throughout the neoplasm. Mitotic figures are not identified, and there is no invasive growth of the neoplasm. These findings suggest that this tumor is probably benign. (Hematoxylin and eosin; original magnification, × 6).

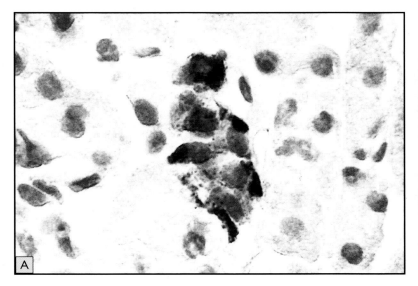

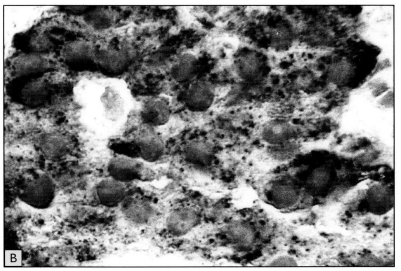

FIGURE 9-22. (*see* Color Plate) Higher magnification of an insulin-producing islet-cell tumor after immunostaining. **A,** Normal exocrine and endocrine pancreatic tissues. An islet cell staining positively for insulin is present in the middle of the pancreatic exocrine tissue. **B,** An insulinoma with strong diffuse positive immunoreactivity after staining with an insulin antibody. The tumor cells reveal diffuse granular cytoplasmic staining. The blue staining of the nuclei is from the hematoxylin counterstain. (×40)

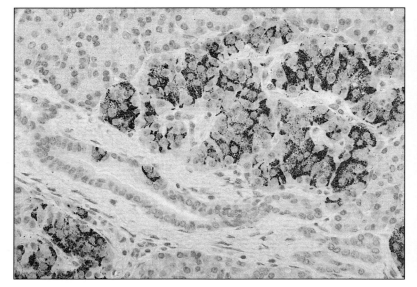

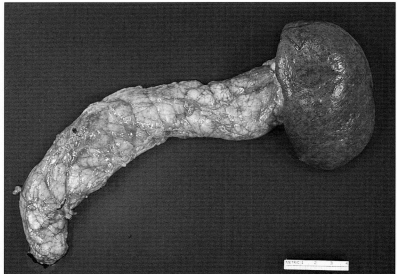

FIGURE 9-23. (*see* Color Plate) Islet hyperplasia/nesidioblastosis is a rare cause of hyperinsulinemic hypoglycemia in adults. This slide shows large islets immunostained with insulin, as well as two beta cells budding from the acinar duct. The latter is the characteristic of nesidioblastosis [12]. (×150)

FIGURE 9-24. (*see* Color Plate) When hyperinsulinemic hypoglycemia in an adult is suspected to be due to islet hyperplasia/nesidioblastosis and an insulinoma cannot be identified by intraoperative ultrasonography or complete mobilization and palpation of the pancreas, gradient-guided partial pancreatectomy is indicated. In this patient, a selective arterial calcium stimulation test indicated hyperfunctioning beta cells in the region of the splenic and gastroduodenal arteries. As a result, resection was performed to the right of the superior mesenteric vein [12].

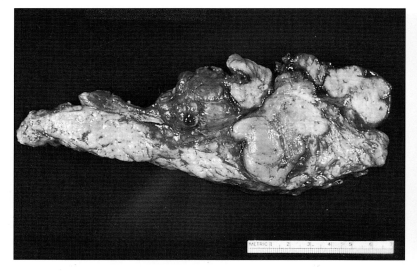

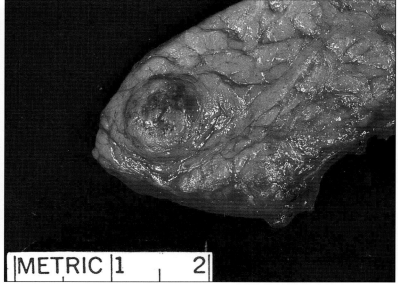

FIGURE 9-25. (*see* Color Plate) Islet-cell carcinoma in the body of the pancreas. The tail of the pancreas is to the right. The tumor has a paler appearance than the surrounding pancreas. In addition, the tumor involves adjacent nodes shown on the inferior portion of the resected tissue. In general, islet-cell carcinomas are larger than benign tumors and metastasize regionally to nodes. The life expectancy of patients with islet-cell carcinoma is considerably longer than that of patients with acinar-cell pancreatic carcinoma [11].

FIGURE 9-26. (*see* Color Plate) Solitary insulinoma slightly less than 2 cm in diameter embedded in the tail of the pancreas. The pancreatic duct is adjacent to the tumor, and the proximity of the tumor to the duct mandated distal pancreatectomy. Insulinomas áre reddish-brown or gray, which distinguishes them from normal pancreatic tissue. In this case, the tumor is reddish-brown. These tumors also have a firmer consistency than normal pancreatic tissue.

Survival Rates and Recurrence

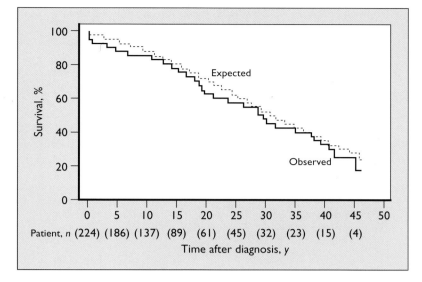

FIGURE 9-27. Survival after diagnosis of insulinoma (Mayo clinic patients: 1927–1986). Among 224 patients whose initial surgery resulted in removal of an insulinoma at the Mayo Clinic, the overall survival rate (including the small number of patients with malignant insulinoma) was no different from the rate expected for the general population. (*From* Service *et al.* [11]; with permission).

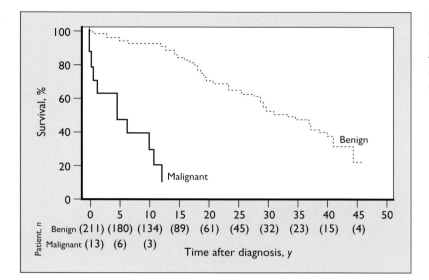

FIGURE 9-28. Survival rates for malignant insulinoma diagnosed on the basis of the presence of metastases at the time of pancreatic exploration (Mayo Clinic patients: 1927–1986). The 10-year rate was approximately 40%. Although this is far less than the survival rate seen in patients with benign insulinoma, it does exceed the rate associated with acinar-cell pancreatic carcinoma. (*From* Service *et al.* [11]; with permission.)

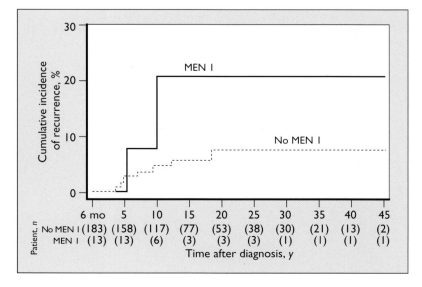

FIGURE 9-29. Recurrence rates in 224 patients whose initial surgery resulted in the removal of an insulinoma at the Mayo Clinic observed over a 60-year period (1927 to 1986) and followed for 45 years. Insulinomas did not recur within the first 4 years of follow-up, indicating that subsequent hyperinsulinemic hypoglycemia was not caused by persistent insulinoma. The recurrence rates were 7% for patients without multiple endocrine neoplasia (MEN) I syndrome and 21% for those with MEN I syndrome. No patient had a documented recurrence 20 years after the initial surgery. (*From* Service *et al.* [11]; with permission.)

References

1. Service FJ: Hypoglycemic disorders. *N Engl J Med* 1995, 332:1144–1152.

2. Service FJ: Hypoglycemias. In: *Cecil's Textbook of Medicine, Update 4*. Edited by Smith LH Jr. Philadelphia: WB Saunders; 1989.

3. Service FJ: Clinical presentations and laboratory evaluation of hypo-glycemic disorders in adults. In: *Hypoglycemic Disorder: Pathogenesis, Diagnosis and Treatment*. Edited by Service FJ. Boston: GK Hall; 1983:73–95.

4. Cryer PE: Glucose counter-regulation: the physiological mechanisms that prevent or correct hypoglycemia. In: *Hypoglycaemia and Diabetes: Clinical and Physiological Aspects*. Edited by Frier BM, Fisher BM. London: Edward Arnold; 1993:34–55.

5. Service FJ, Nelson RL: Insulinoma. *Compr Ther* 1980, 6:70–74.

6. Rizza RA, Haymond MW, Verdonk CA, *et al.*: Pathogenesis of hypoglycemia in insulinoma patients: suppression of hepatic glucose production by insulin. *Diabetes* 1981, 30:377–381.

7. O'Brien T, O'Brien PC, Service FJ: Insulin surrogates in insulinoma. *J Clin Endocrinol Metab* 1993, 77:448–451.

8. Kudlow JE, Albisser AM, Angel A, *et al.*: Insulinoma resection facilitated by the artificial endocrine pancreas. *Diabetes* 1978, 27:774–777.

9. Doppman JL, Chang R, Fraker DL, *et al.*: Localization of insulinomas to regions of the pancreas by intra-arterial stimulation with calcium. *Ann Intern Med* 1995, 123:269–273.

10. Hassoun AAK, Service FJ, O'Brien PC: Glycated hemoglobin in insulinoma. *Endocr Pract* 1998, 4:181–183.

11. Service FJ, O'Brien PC, Kao PC, *et al.*: C-peptide suppression test: effects of gender, age and body mass index. Implications for the diagnosis of insulinoma. *J Clin Endocrinol Metab* 1992, 74:204–210.

12. Service FJ, Natt N, Thompson GB, *et al.*: Non-insulinoma pancreatogenous hypoglycemia: a novel syndrome of hyperinsulinemic hypoglycemia in adults independent of mutations in Kir6.2 and SUR1 genes. J Clin Endocrin Metab 1999, 84 (5): 1582-1589.

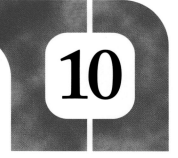

MECHANISMS OF HYPERGLYCEMIC DAMAGE IN DIABETES

Michael Brownlee

In the 1990s, the central therapeutic problem in diabetes mellitus is not management of its acute metabolic derangements but prevention and treatment of its chronic complications. In the United States, diabetes is the leading cause of new blindness in people 20 through 74 years old, and the leading cause of end-stage renal disease. Diabetics are the fastest growing group of renal dialysis and transplant recipients. The life expectancy for patients with diabetic end-stage renal failure is only three or four years. Over 60% of diabetics are affected by neuropathy, which includes distal symmetrical polyneuropathy, mononeuropathies, and a variety of autonomic neuropathies causing erectile dysfunction, urinary incontinence, gastroparesis, and nocturnal diarrhea. Approximately 60% of type 2 diabetics have hypertension. Accelerated lower extremity arterial disease in conjunction with neuropathy makes diabetes account for 50% of all nontraumatic amputations in the United States. Diabetics have a death rate from coronary heart disease that is two to four times that of nondiabetics. A similar increased risk occurs with stroke. Heart disease in diabetics appears earlier in life and is more often fatal. Life expectancy is about seven to ten years shorter than for people without diabetes [1].

Epidemiological studies show a strong relationship between glycemia and diabetic complications in both type 1 and type 2 diabetes. There is a continuous relationship between level of glycemia and the risk of development and progression of complications. In this chapter, we review the mechanisms of hyperglycemic damage in diabetes. The discussion includes the specificity of target organ damage, the major mechanisms of hyperglycemic tissue damage, the relationship of various mechanisms to each other, the potential role of insulin resistance, the genetics of complication susceptibility, and the development of complications during post-hyperglycemic euglycemia.

Target-Organ Specificity of Hyperglycemic Damage

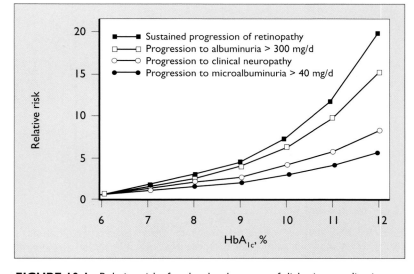

FIGURE 10-1. Relative risks for the development of diabetic complications at different levels of mean hemoglobin A$_{1c}$ (HbA$_{1c}$, glycated hemoglobin), obtained from the Diabetes Control and Complications Trial. Patients with insulin-dependent diabetes whose intensive insulin therapy resulted in HbA$_{1c}$ values 2% lower than those receiving conventional insulin therapy had a 76% lower incidence of retinopathy, a 54% lower incidence of nephropathy, and a 60% reduction in neuropathy. A relationship between level of chronic hyperglycemia and diabetic macrovascular disease has also been found in several recent studies. Thus, hyperglycemia is the primary initiating factor in the pathogenesis of diabetic complications. (*Adapted from* Skyler [1].)

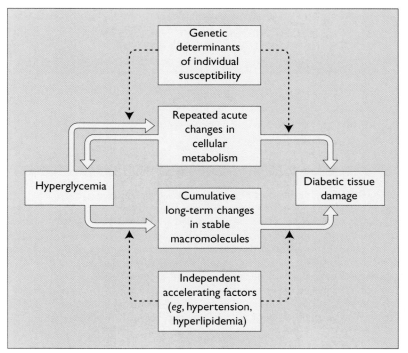

FIGURE 10-2. The mechanisms by which hyperglycemia and independent risk factors interact to cause chronic diabetic complications. One group of mechanisms involves repeated acute changes in cellular metabolism that are reversible when euglycemia is restored. Another group of mechanisms involves cumulative changes in long-lived macromolecules that persist despite restoration of euglycemia. These mechanisms are influenced by genetic determinants of susceptibility or resistance to hyperglycemic damage and by independent risk factors such as hypertension. (*Adapted from* Giardino and Brownlee [2]; with permission.)

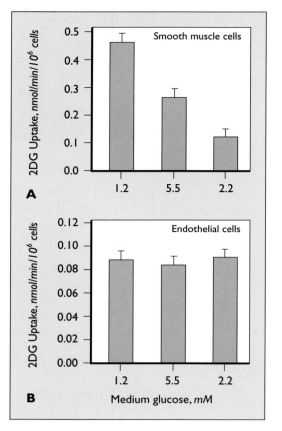

A

B

FIGURE 10-3. Lack of downregulation of glucose transport in cells affected by diabetic complications. Vascular smooth muscle cells, which are not damaged by hyperglycemia, show an inverse relationship between glucose concentration and glucose transport measured as 2-deoxyglucose uptake (**A**). In contrast, vascular endothelial cells, a major target of hyperglycemic damage, show no significant change in glucose transport when the glucose level is elevated (**B**). Thus, intracellular hyperglycemia appears to be the major determinant of diabetic tissue damage. (*Adapted from* Kaiser *et al.* [3]; with permission.)

Major Mechanisms of Hyperglycemic Damage

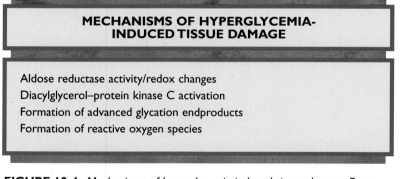

MECHANISMS OF HYPERGLYCEMIA-INDUCED TISSUE DAMAGE

Aldose reductase activity/redox changes

Diacylglycerol–protein kinase C activation

Formation of advanced glycation endproducts

Formation of reactive oxygen species

FIGURE 10-4. Mechanisms of hyperglycemia-induced tissue damage. Four major hypotheses about how hyperglycemia causes diabetic complications have generated extensive data, as well as several clinical trials based on specific inhibitors of these mechanisms. No unifying hypothesis links these four mechanisms, but either polyol pathway-induced redox changes (decreased ratios of the reduced form of nicotinamide adenine dinucleotide phosphate to the oxidized form of nicotinamide adenine dinucleotide phosphate and increased ratios of the reduced form of nicotinamide adenine dinucleotide to the oxidized form of nicotinamide adenine dinucleotide) or hyperglycemia-induced formation of reactive oxygen species may account for all of the other biochemical abnormalities.

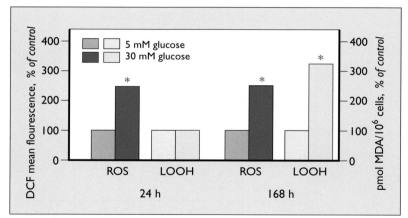
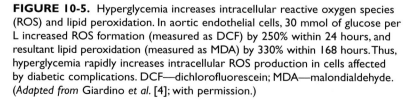

FIGURE 10-5. Hyperglycemia increases intracellular reactive oxygen species (ROS) and lipid peroxidation. In aortic endothelial cells, 30 mmol of glucose per L increased ROS formation (measured as DCF) by 250% within 24 hours, and resultant lipid peroxidation (measured as MDA) by 330% within 168 hours. Thus, hyperglycemia rapidly increases intracellular ROS production in cells affected by diabetic complications. DCF—dichlorofluorescein; MDA—malondialdehyde. (*Adapted from* Giardino *et al.* [4]; with permission.)

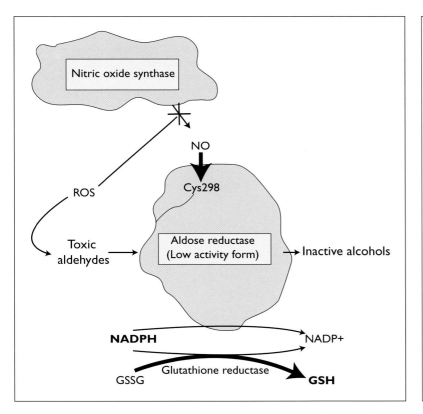

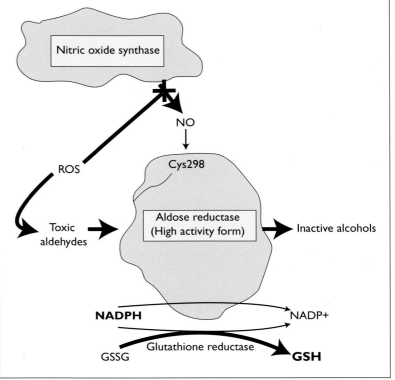

FIGURE 10-6. Potential function of aldose reductase in nondiabetic cells. The enzyme aldose reductase converts a variety of toxic aldehydes (such as 2-oxo-aldehydes and those derived from lipid peroxidation) to inactive alcohols. The reduced form of nicotinamide adenine dinucleotide phosphate is the cofactor in both this reaction and in the regeneration of glutathione by glutathione reductase. Reactive oxygen species (ROS) appear to reduce nitric oxide levels. The activity of aldose reductase is reversibly downregulated by nitric oxide modification of a cysteine residue in the enzyme's active site. (*Adapted from* Chandra *et al.* [5], Pieper *et al.* [6], and King and Brownlee [7].)

FIGURE 10-7. Potential function of aldose reductase in nondiabetic cells under oxidative stress. In a euglycemic environment, reactive oxygen species (ROS) increase the concentration of toxic aldehydes. At the same time, nitric oxide levels are reduced, thereby converting aldose reductase to a high activity form. Glutathione levels are unaffected. (*Adapted from* Chandra *et al.* [5], Pieper *et al.* [6], and King and Brownlee [7].)

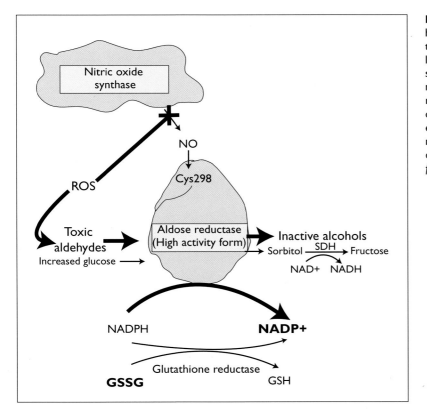

FIGURE 10-8. Potential function of aldose reductase in diabetic cells. In a hyperglycemic environment, reactive oxygen species (ROS) are increased, with the same consequences described in Figure 10-7. In addition, increased intracellular glucose levels result in increased enzymatic conversion to the polyalcohol sorbitol and in concomitant decreases in levels of the reduced form of nicotinamide adenine dinucleotide phosphate and glutathione. In cells where aldose reductase activity is sufficient to deplete glutathione, hyperglycemia-induced oxidative stress would be augmented. Sorbitol is oxidized to fructose by the enzyme sorbitol dehydrogenase (SDH). In cells where SDH activity is high, this may result in an increased ratio of the reduced form of nicotinamide adenine dinucleotide to the oxidized form of nicotinamide adenine dinucleotide. (*Adapted from* Chandra *et al.* [5], Pieper *et al.* [6], and King and Brownlee [7].)

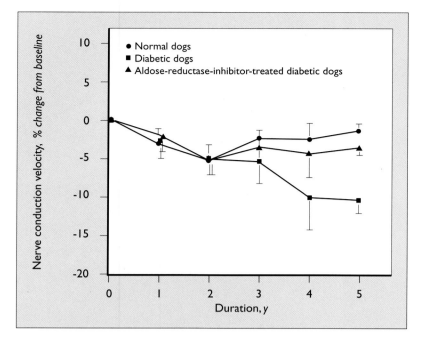

FIGURE 10-9. Effect of aldose reductase inhibition on diabetes-induced decreases in nerve conduction velocity. In diabetic dogs, conduction became significantly less than normal within 42 months. Conduction velocity in dogs treated with aldose reductase inhibitors remained statistically equal to normal throughout the 5-year study. In contrast, aldose reductase inhibition had no effect on the development of diabetic retinopathy. (*Adapted from* Engerman *et al.* [8]; with permission.)

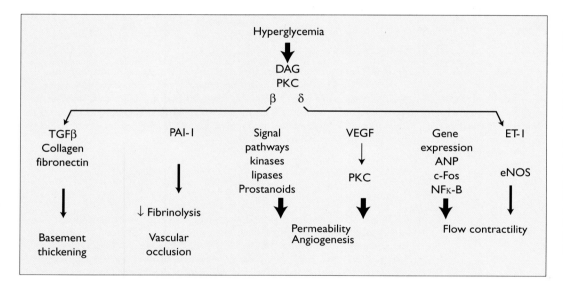

FIGURE 10-10. Potential consequences of hyperglycemia-induced diacylglycerol-protein kinase C activation. Hyperglycemia increases diacylglycerol (DAG) content, in part by de novo synthesis, and possibly also by phosphatidylcholine hydrolysis. Increased DAG activates protein kinase C (PKC), primarily the beta and delta isoforms. Activated PKC increases the production of cytokines and extracellular matrix, the fibrinolytic inhibitor PAI-1, and the vasoconstrictor endothelin-1. Protein kinase C is also a mediator of vascular endothelial growth factor (VEGF) activity. These changes would contribute to basement membrane thickening, vascular occlusion, increased permeability, and activation of angiogenesis. ANP— atrial natriuretic peptide; eNOS—endothelial nitric oxide synthetase; ET-1—endothelin-1; TGF—transforming growth factor. (*Adapted from* Koya and King [9]; with permission.)

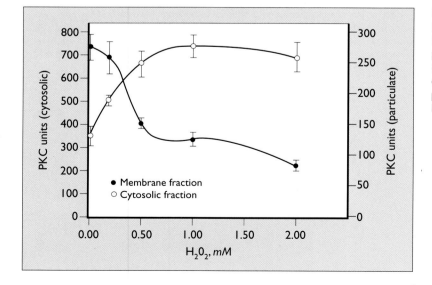

FIGURE 10-11. Reactive oxygen species (ROS) activate protein kinase C (PKC) in vascular endothelial cells. As ROS-producing H_2O_2 increases, it activates PKC. The mechanism appears to involve direct or indirect activation of phospholipase D, which hydrolyzes phosphatidylcholine to produce diacylglycerol (DAG). Reactive oxygen species could also increase DAG through increased de novo synthesis resulting from ROS inhibition of the enzyme glyceraldehyde phosphate dehydrogenase. (*Adapted from* Taher *et al.* [10] and Schuppe-Koistinen *et al.* [11].)

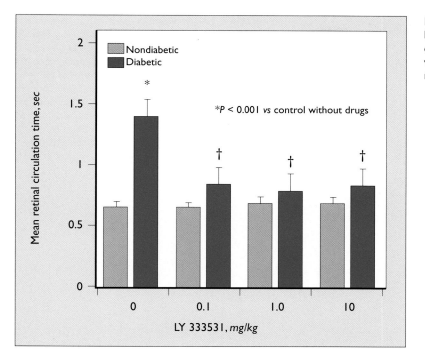

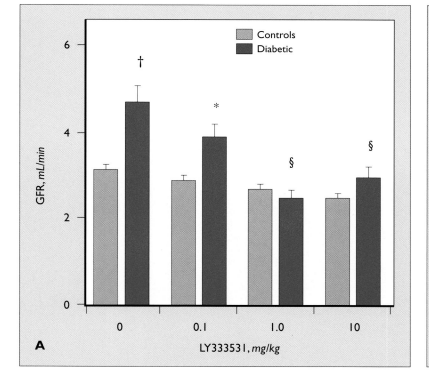

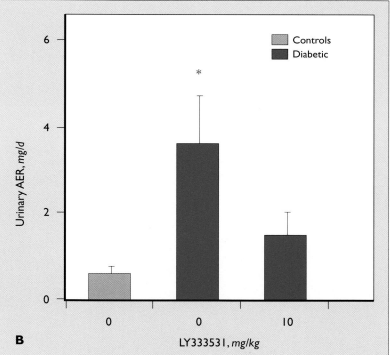

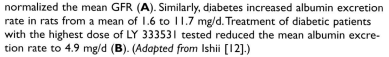

FIGURE 10-12. Amelioration of diabetes-induced retinal vascular dysfunction by an inhibitor of protein kinase C beta. In rats, diabetes increased mean retinal circulation time from 0.67 seconds to 1.40 seconds. In diabetic patients, treatment with the highest dose of the protein kinase C beta inhibitor LY 333531 tested reduced the time to 0.87 seconds. (*Adapted from* Ishii *et al.* [12]; with permission.)

FIGURE 10-13. Amelioration of diabetes-induced renal dysfunction by an inhibitor of protein kinase C (PKC) beta. In rats, diabetes increased glomerular filtration rate (GFR) from a mean of 3.0 to 4.6 mL/min. In diabetic patients, treatment with the highest dose of the PKC beta inhibitor LY 333531 tested normalized the mean GFR (**A**). Similarly, diabetes increased albumin excretion rate in rats from a mean of 1.6 to 11.7 mg/d. Treatment of diabetic patients with the highest dose of LY 333531 tested reduced the mean albumin excretion rate to 4.9 mg/d (**B**). (*Adapted from* Ishii [12].)

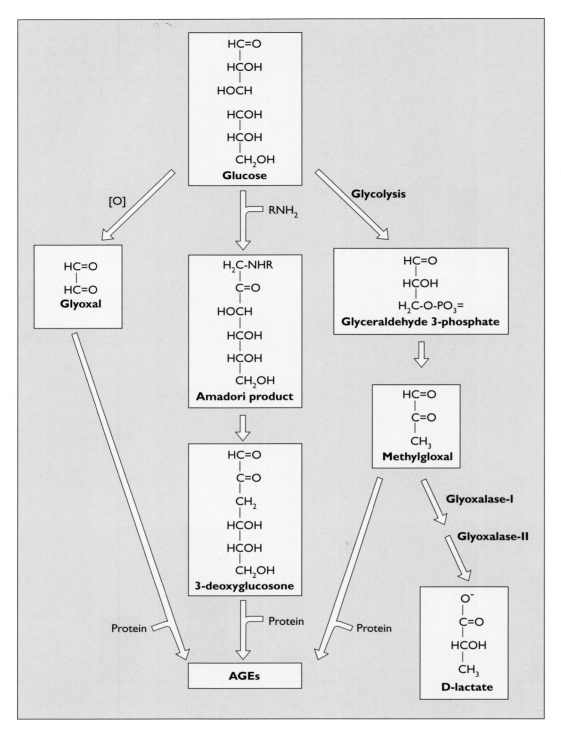

FIGURE 10-14. Potential pathways leading to the formation of advanced glycation endproducts (AGEs). The latter can arise from autoxidation of glucose to glyoxal, decomposition of the Amadori product to 3-deoxyglucosone, and fragmentation of glyceraldehyde-3-phosphate to methylglyoxal. These reactive dicarbonyls react with amino groups of proteins to form AGEs. Methylglyoxal and glyoxal are detoxified by the glyoxalase system. All three AGE precursors are also substrates for other reductases. (*Adapted from* Shinohara *et al.* [13] and Vander Jagt *et al.* [14]; with permission.)

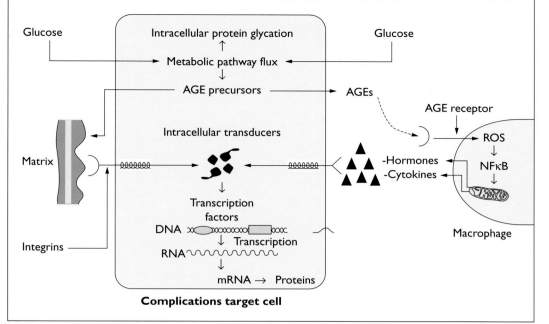

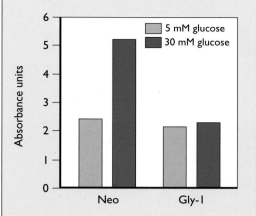

FIGURE 10-15. Intracellular production of advanced glycation endproduct (AGE) precursors damages target cells by three general mechanisms. First, intracellular protein glycation alters protein function. Second, extracellular matrix modified by AGE precursors has abnormal functional properties. Third, plasma proteins modified by AGE precursors bind to AGE receptors on adjacent cells, such as macrophages, thereby inducing receptor-mediated production of reactive oxygen species (ROS). The latter, in turn, activates NFκB and expression of pathogenic gene products, including cytokines and hormones. mRNA—messenger RNA. (*Adapted from* Brownlee [15]; with permission.)

FIGURE 10-16. Intracellular protein glycation by the advanced glycation endproduct precursor methylglyoxal increases macromolecular endocytosis in endothelial cells. After exposure to 30 mmol of glucose per L, macromolecular endocytosis by GM7373 endothelial cells that were stably transfected with neomycin resistance gene (neo) were increased 2.2-fold. In contrast, when increased methylglyoxal accumulation was prevented by overexpressing the enzyme glyoxalase I (gly-1) in these cells, 30 mmol of glucose per L did not increase macromolecular endocytosis. (*Adapted from* Shinohara et al.[13].)

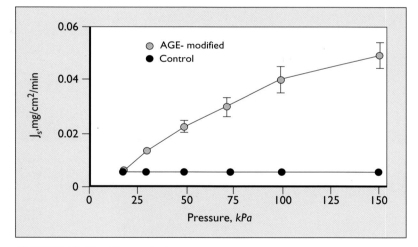

FIGURE 10-17. Glomerular basement membrane modified by advanced glycation endproducts (AGEs) has increased permeability to albumin. Ultrafiltration of albumin (Js) by AGE-modified glomerular basement membrane is significantly increased compared with ultrafiltration of albumin by unmodified glomerular basement membrane over a range of different filtration pressures. (*Adapted from* Cochrane and Robinson [16].)

PROTEINS THAT BIND ADVANCED GLYCATION ENDPRODUCTS

RAGE

p60 (oligosaccharyltransferase-48)

p90 (80K-H, protein kinase C substrate)

Galectin-3

Scavenger receptor (type II)

FIGURE 10-18. Advanced glycation endproduct (AGE)–binding proteins and putative receptors. Five AGE-binding proteins have been identified. 1) RAGE is a novel member of the immunoglobulin superfamily; its ligation generates reactive oxygen species and activates the pleiotropic transcription factor NFκB; 2) p60 exhibits 95% identity to OST-48, a component of the oligosachharyltransferase complex in microsomal membranes; 3) p90 has significant sequence homology with human 80K-H, a substrate of protein kinase C; 4) galectin-3, a carbohydrate-binding protein, also binds AGEs; 5) the type II macrophage scavenger receptor binds AGEs and mediates their uptake by endocytosis. RAGE—receptor for AGE. (*Adapted from* Yan et al. [17], Li et al. [18], Vlassara et al. [19], and Araki et al. [20].)

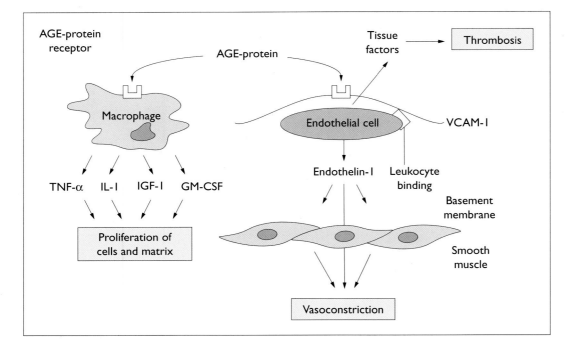

FIGURE 10-19. The mechanisms by which advanced glycation endproduct (AGE)–modified protein binding to specific receptors on macrophages and endothelial cells may cause pathologic changes in diabetic blood vessels. On macrophages and mesangial cells, binding stimulates production of tumor necrosis factor (TNF)-alpha, interleukin-1 (IL-1), insulin-like growth factor-1 (IGF-1), and granulocyte-macrophage colony-stimulating factor (GM-CSF) at levels that increase proliferation of smooth muscle cells and increase matrix production. On endothelial cells, binding induces procoagulatory changes in gene expression and increased expression of leukocyte-binding vascular adhesion molecule-1 (VAMC-1). (*Adapted from* Brownlee [21]; with permission.)

EFFECT OF AMINOGUANIDINE TREATMENT ON DIABETIC TARGET TISSUE

Variable	Nondiabetic Persons	DiabeticPersons	Diabetic Persons Receiving AminoguanidineTreatment
Retinal acellular capillaries, *mm²*	9 ±2	167±27	33±11
Retinal microaneurysms, *% positive*	0	37.5	0
Urinary albumin excretion, *mg/24 h*	2.4±1.3	38.9±1.4	5.1±1.5
Mesangial volume fraction, %	12.5±2.5	18.8±2.5	13.7±0.6
Motor nerve conduction velocity, *m/sec*	65.5. ±2	52.4±3	64±2
Nerve action potential amplitude, %	100	63	97
Arterial elasticity, *nL/mm Hg/mm*	–	7.5±1.5	10.8±3
Arterial fluid filtration, *nL/mm*	–	0.9	0.45

FIGURE 10-20. Amelioration of abnormalities in diabetic target tissues by an advanced glycation endproduct inhibitor. The effects of this inhibitor (aminoguanidine) on diabetic abnormalities have been investigated in the retina, kidney, nerve, and artery. In experimental animals, the development of all pathognomonic abnormalities examined was inhibited by 85% to 90%. (*Adapted from* Brownlee [15]; with permission.)

Interrelationship of Mechanisms of Hyperglycemic Damage

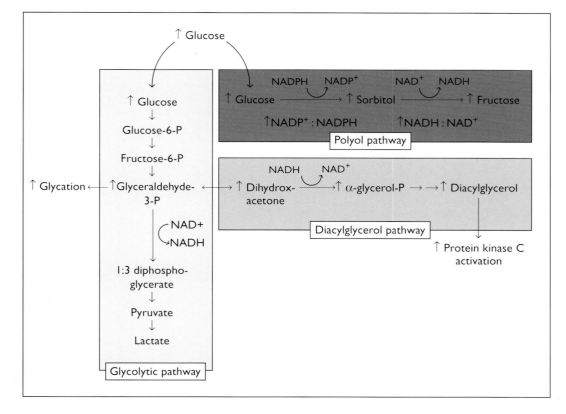

FIGURE 10-21. Potential relationship between polyol pathway–induced redox changes and the three other biochemical mechanisms underlying complications. Increased glucose flux through this pathway could increase the ratio of the oxidized form of nicotinamide adenine dinucleotide phosphate ($NADP^+$) to the reduced form of nicotinamide adenine dinucleotide phosphate to (NADPH), thereby reducing glutathione reductase activity and increasing oxidative stress. Increased sorbitol flux through this pathway could also increase the ratio of the reduced form of nicotinamide adenine dinucleotide (NADH) to the oxidized form of nicotinamide adenine dinucleotide (NAD^+), thereby blocking glycolysis at the level of triose phosphates and increasing formation of alpha-glycerol phosphate, a precursor of diacylglycerol. In addition, increased triose phosphate concentrations would produce more of the most potent advanced glycation endproduct precursor, methylglyoxal. In experiments, however, aldose reductase inhibitors have no effect on hyperglycemia-induced increases in endothelial cell diacylglycerol. (*Adapted from* Ruderman *et al.* [22] and Xia *et al.* [23]; with permission.)

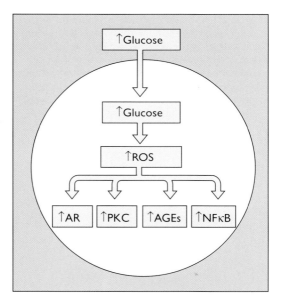

FIGURE 10-22. Potential relationship between hyperglycemia-induced reactive oxygen species and the three other biochemical mechanisms underlying complications. Reactive oxygen species may activate aldose reductase, induce diacylglycerol, activate protein kinase C, induce advanced glycation endproduct formation, and activate the pleiotropic transcription factor NFκB. (*Adapted from* Chandra *et al.* [5], Pieper *et al.* [6], Taher *et al.* [10], Giardino *et al.* [4], Elgawish *et al.*al [24], and Piette *et al.* [25].)

Potential Role of Insulin Resistance

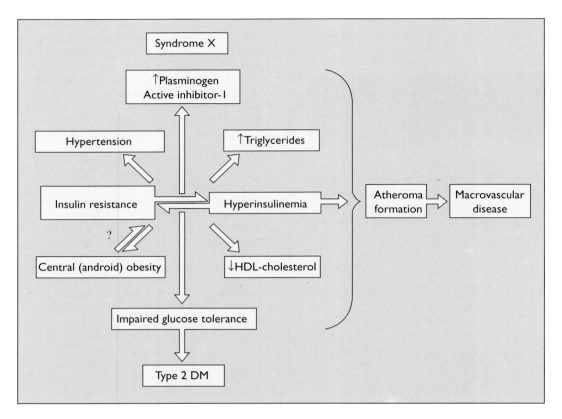

FIGURE 10-23. Insulin resistance may exacerbate known risk factors for vascular damage. Insulin resistance or hyperinsulinemia is associated with atherogenic changes in plasma lipoproteins, increased plasminogen activator inhibitor-1 levels, and hypertension. This association has been termed "syndrome X." HDL—high-density lipoprotein. (*Adapted from* Gray and Yudkin [26]; with permission.)

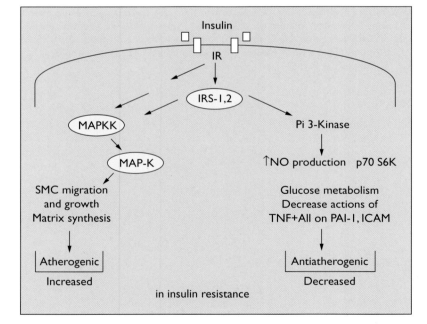

FIGURE 10-24. Insulin resistance (IR) in vascular cells may promote damage by inhibiting antiatherogenic gene expression. Selective resistance to insulin action in the phosphatidyl inositol 3-kinase signaling pathway may reduce antiproliferative nitric oxide (NO) production and interfere with insulin's inhibitory effect on tumor necrosis factor (TNF) and the stimulation of PAI-1 and intracellular adhesion molecule (ICAM) expression by angiotensin II. IRS—insulin receptor substrate; MAP-K—mitogen-activated protein kinase; MAPKK—mitogen-activated protein kinase kinase; PI—phosphatidyl inositol; SMC—smooth muscle cell. (*Adapted from* King and Brownlee [7]; with permission.)

Genetics of Susceptibility to Complications

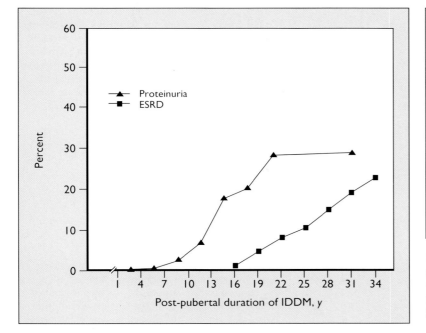

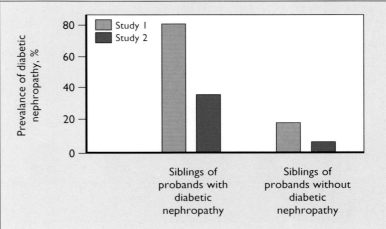

FIGURE 10-26. Familial clustering of diabetic nephropathy suggests a major genetic effect. In one study, the risk for nephropathy was 83% in diabetic siblings of an affected patient compared with 16% in diabetic siblings of an unaffected patient. In another study, the risks were 33% and 10%, respectively. (*Adapted from* Trevisan *et al.*[28].)

FIGURE 10-25. Prevalence of clinically significant diabetic nephropathy in patients with insulin-dependent diabetes according to diabetes duration. The cumulative incidence of overt proteinuria levels off at 27%. After 34 years of diabetes, the cumulative incidence of end-stage renal disease is 21.4%. These data suggest that only a subset of patients are susceptible to the development of clinical nephropathy. (*Adapted from* Krolewski *et al.*[27].)

Development of Complications During Posthyperglycemic Euglycemia

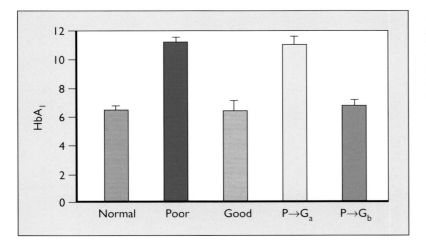

FIGURE 10-27. Development of retinopathy during posthyperglycemic normoglycemia ("hyperglycemic memory"). Shown are mean hemoglobin $_{AI}$ values for dogs in one study [29]. Normal dogs were compared to diabetic dogs that had had poor control for 5 years, good control for 5 years, or poor control for 2.5 years ($P \rightarrow G_a$) followed by good control for the next 2.5 years ($P \rightarrow G_b$). Values for both the good control group and the $P \rightarrow G_b$ group were identical to those in the normal group. (*Adapted from* Engerman and Kern [29].)

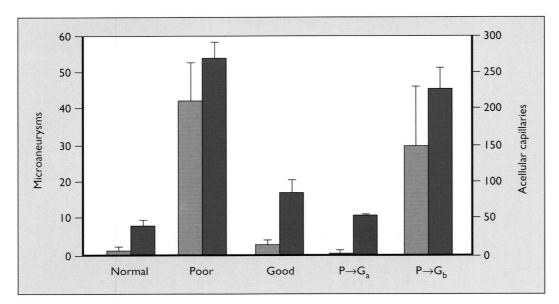

FIGURE 10-28. Development of retinopathy during posthyperglycemic normoglycemia ("hyperglycemic memory"). Shown is quantitation of retinal microaneurysms and acellular capillaries in one study [29]. Lesions of diabetic retinopathy developed during 5 years of poor control. Good control almost always prevented this abnormality. After 2.5 years of poor control, retinopathy was absent. However, despite the institution of good control in this group after 2.5 years, retinopathy developed over the next 2.5 years to an extent almost equal to that seen in the 5-year poor control group. (Adapted from *Engerman and Kern [29].*)

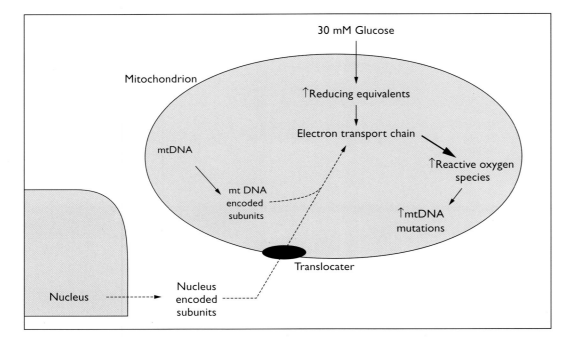

FIGURE 10-29. Potential mechanism for hyperglycemic memory. Hyperglycemia-induced increases in reactive oxygen species may be a consequence of increased reducing equivalents generated from increased glucose metabolism flowing through the mitochondrial electron transport chain. The increased production of reactive oxygen species would not only increase aldose reductase activity, protein kinase C activity, and formation of advanced glycation endproducts but would also induce mutations in mitochondrial DNA (mtDNA). (*Adapted from* Wei [30] and Nishikawa *et al.* [31].)

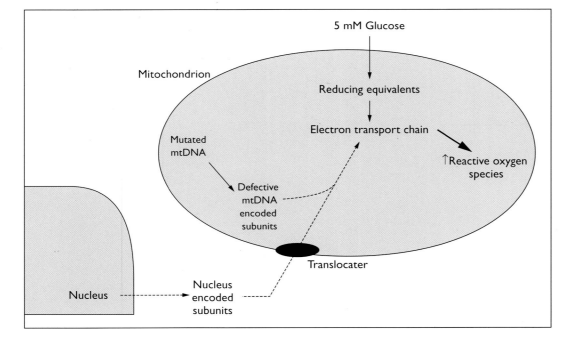

FIGURE 10-30. Potential mechanism for hyperglycemic memory. Mitochondrial DNA (mtDNA) mutated by hyperglycemia-induced reactive oxygen species would encode defective electron transport chain subunits. These defective subunits would cause increased production of reactive oxygen species by the electron transport chain at physiologic concentrations of glucose and glucose-derived reducing equivalents. (*Adapted from* Wei [30] and Nishikawa *et al.* [31].)

References

1. Skyler J: Diabetic complications: the importance of glucose control. In: *Endocrinology and Metabolism Clinics of North America.* Edited by Brownlee MB, King GL. Philadelphia: WB Saunders; 1996.

2. Giardino J, Brownlee M: Mechanisms of chronic diabetic complications. In: *Textbook of Diabetics,* vol 1. Edited by Pickup JC, Williams G. London: Blackwell Scientific; 1997.

3. Kaiser N, Sasson S, Feener EP: Differential regulation of glucose transport and transporters by glucose in vascular endothelial and smooth muscle cells. *Diabetes* 1993, 42:80–89.

4. Giardino I, Edelstein D, Brownlee M: BCL-2 expression or antioxidants prevent hyperglycemia-induced formation of intracellular advanced glycation endproducts in bovine endothelial cells. *J Clin Invest* 1996, 97:1422–1428.

5. Chandra A, Srivastava S, Petrash JM: Active site modification of aldose reductase by nitric oxide donors. *Biochim Biophys Acta* 1997, 131:217–222.

6. Pieper GM, Langenstroer P, Siebeneich W: Diabetic-induced endothelial dysfunction in rat aorta: role of hydroxyl radicals. *Cardiovasc Res* 1997, 34:145–156.

7. King GL, Brownlee MB: The cellular and molecular mechanisms of diabetic complications. In: *Endocrinology and Metabolism Clinics of North America.* Edited by Brownlee MB, King GL. Philadelphia: WB Saunders; 1996.

8. Engerman RL, Kern TS, Larson ME: Nerve conduction and aldose reductase inhibition during 5 years of diabetes or galactosaemia in dogs. *Diabetologia* 1994, 37:141–144.

9. Koya D, King GL: Protein kinase C activation and the development of diabetic complications. *Diabetes* 1998, 47:859–867.

10. Taher MM, Garcia JG, Natarajian V: Hydroperoxide-induced diacylglycerol formation and protein kinase C activation in vascular endothelial cells. *Arch Biochem Biophys* 1993, 303:260–266.

11. Schuppe-Koistinen I, Modéus P, et al.: S-thiolation of human endothelial cell glyceraldehyde-3-phosphate dehydrogenase after hydrogen peroxide treatment. *Eur J Biochem* 1994, 221:1033–1037.

12. Ishii H, Jirousek MR, et al.: Amelioration of vascular dysfunctions in diabetic rats by an oral PKC beta inhibitor. *Science* 1996, 272:728–731.

13. Shinohara M, Thornalley PJ, et al.: Overexpression of glyoxalase-1 in bovine endothelial cells inhibits intracellular advanced glycation endproduct formation and prevents hyperglycemia-induced increases in macro-molecular endocytosis. *J Clin Invest* 1998, 1142–1147. volume number

14. Vander Jagt DL, Torres JE, Hunsaker LA, et al.: Physiological substrates of human aldose and aldehyde reductases. *Adv Exp Med Biol* 1997, 414:491–497.

15. Brownlee M: Glycation and diabetic complications. *Diabetes* 1994, 43:836–841.

16. Cochrane SM, Robinson GB: In vitro glycation of glomerular basement membrane alters its permeability: a possible mechanism in diabetic complications. *FEBS Lett* 1995, 375:41–44.

17. Yan SD, Schmidt AM, et al.: Enhanced cellular oxidant stress by the inter-action of advanced glycation end products with their receptors/binding proteins. *J Biol Chem* 1994, 269:9889–9897.

18. Li YM, Mitsuhashi T, et al.: Molecular identity and cellular distribution of advanced glycation endproduct receptors: relationship of p60 to OST-48 and p90 to 80K-H membrane proteins. *Proc Natl Acad Sci U S A* 1996, 93:11047–11052.

19. Vlassara H, Li YM, et al.: Identification of galectin-3 as a high-affinity binding protein for advanced glycation end products (AGE): a new member of the AGE-receptor complex. *Mol Med* 1995, 1:634–646.

20. Araki N, Higashi T, et al.: Macrophage scavenger receptor mediates the endocytic uptake and degradation of advanced glycation end products of the Maillard reaction. *Eur J Biochem* 1995, 230:408–415.

21. Brownlee M: Advanced glycation end products in diabetic complications. *Curr Opin Endocrinol Diabetes* 1998, 3:291–297.

22. Ruderman NB, Williamson JR, et al.: Glucose and diabetic vascular disease. *FASEB J* 1992, 6:2905–2914.

23. Xia P, Inoguchi T, et al.: Characterization of the mechanism for the chronic activation of diacylglycerol-protein kinase C pathway in diabetes and hypergalactosemia. *Diabetes* 1994, 43:1122–1129.

24. Elgawish A, Glomb M, Friedlander M, et al.: Involvement of hydrogen peroxide in collagen cross-linking by high glucose in vitro and in vivo. *J Biol Chem* 1996, 271:12964–12972.

25. Piette J, Piret B, Bonizzi G, et al.: Multiple redox regulations in NF-κB transcription factor activation. *Biol Chem* 1997, 378:1237–1245.

26. Gray RP, Yudkin JS: Cardiovascular disease in diabetic mellitus. In: *Textbook of Diabetes*, vol. 1. Edited by Pickup JC, Williams G. London: Blackwell Scientific; 1997.

27. Krolewski SA, Warram JH, et al.: Epidemiology of late diabetic complications: a basis for the development and evaluation of prevention programs. In: *Endocrinology and Metabolism Clinics of North America.* Edited by Brownlee MB, King GL. Philadelphia: WB Saunders; 1996.

28. Trevisan R, Barnes DJ, et al.: Pathogenesis of diabetic nephropathy. In: *Textbook of Diabetes*, vol. 2. Edited by Pickup JC, Williams G. London: Blackwell Scientific; 1997.

29. Engerman RL, Kern TS: Progression of incipient diabetic retinopathy during good glycemic control. *Diabetes* 1987, 36:808–812.

30. Wei Y: Oxidative stress and mitochondrial DNA mutations in human aging. *Soc Exp Biol Med* 1998, 217:53–63.

31. Nishikawa T, Edelstein D, et al.: Reversal of hyperglycemia-induced PKC activation, intracellular AGE formation, and sorbitol accumulation by inhibition of electron transport complex II. *Diabetes* 1999, 48(Suppl).

Eye Complications of Diabetes

Lloyd Paul Aiello

Diabetic retinopathy is a well-characterized, sight-threatening, chronic, ocular disorder that eventually develops to some degree in nearly all patients with diabetes mellitus. With experienced ophthalmic evaluation, diabetic retinopathy can be detected in its early stages. Existing therapies are remarkably effective when administered at the appropriate time in the disease process. In addition, improvement of systemic glycemic control is associated with a delay in onset and slowing of progression of diabetic retinopathy. Nevertheless, diabetic retinopathy is the leading cause of new cases of legal blindness among Americans between the ages of 20 and 74 years. The pathologic changes associated with diabetic retinopathy are similar in types 1 and 2 diabetes mellitus, although there is a higher risk of more frequent and severe ocular complications in type 1 diabetes [1]. However, because more patients have type 2 than type 1 disease, patients with type 2 disease account for a higher proportion of those with visual loss.

Most visual loss associated with diabetes results from either new vessel growth on the retina (proliferative diabetic retinopathy [PDR]) or increased retinal vascular permeability (macular edema). The retinopathic stages associated with the greatest risk of visual loss are called high-risk PDR and clinically significant macular edema (CSME). In the United States, an estimated 700,000 persons have proliferative diabetic retinopathy (PDR), 130,000 have high-risk PDR, 500,000 have macular edema, and 325,000 have CSME [2–5]. An estimated 63,000 cases of PDR, 29,000 of high-risk PDR, 80,000 of macular edema, 56,000 of CSME, and 5000 new cases of legal blindness occur yearly as a result of diabetic retinopathy [1,6]. Blindness has been estimated to be 25 times more common in persons with diabetes than in those without the disease [7,8].

Estimates of the medical and economic impact of retinopathy-associated morbidity have been performed using computer simulations. The models predict that if patients with type 1 disease receive treatment as recommended in the clinical trials in the absence of good glycemic control, a savings of $624 million and 173,540 person-years of sight would be realized [3,4]. The Diabetes Control and Complication Trial (DCCT) showed that the rate of development of any retinopathy and, once present, the rate of retinopathic progression were significantly reduced after 3 years of intensive insulin therapy [9,10]. Applying DCCT intensive insulin therapy to all persons with insulin-dependent diabetes mellitus in the United States would result in a gain of 920,000 person-years of sight, although the costs of intensive therapy are three times that of conventional therapy [11,12].

An understanding of the pathogenesis, natural history, and available treatment options for patients with diabetic retinopathy is critical for all health care providers, because current therapeutic options can be remarkably effective at preventing severe visual loss when administered in an appropriate and timely manner. Indeed, with appropriate medical and ophthalmologic care, over 90% of visual loss resulting from diabetic retinopathy can be prevented [13,14].

Anatomy, Symptoms, and Pathology

FIGURE 11-1. Normal ocular anatomy. This schematic cross section shows the normal anatomy of the human eye. Diabetes can affect almost all ocular structures (*see* Fig. 11-2). However, the characteristic and most common changes occur in the retina and are termed *diabetic retinopathy*. Most of the severe sight-threatening complications involve either pathologic growth of vessels (neovascularization) in the retina or increased retinal vessel permeability [14]. These conditions are termed *proliferative diabetic retinopathy* and *diabetic macular edema*, respectively. Neovascularization also can arise at the iris, potentially leading to neovascular glaucoma.

OCULAR STRUCTURES AFFECTED BY DIABETES

Ocular Structure	Diabetes-Associated Pathology
Lids, nerves, and muscles	Palsy of cranial nerves III, IV, or VI
Cornea	Reduced sensitivity
	Increased susceptibility to corneal erosions
	Increased susceptibility to infection (corneal ulcers)
Anterior chamber	Hyphema (blood)
	Shallowing with longer disease duration
Iris	Neovascularization
	Depigmentation
Lens	Increased susceptibility to cataract
Vitreous	Vitreous hemorrhage
	Early posterior vitreous detachment
	Asteroid hyalosis
Retina	Retinal hemorrhages
	Microaneurysms
	Venous beading
	Intraretinal microvascular abnormalities
	Capillary vessel loss
	Neovascularization
	Edema
	Lipid deposits
Optic disc	Neovascularization
	Diabetic papillopathy (swelling)
Sclera and other tissues	Delayed wound healing

FIGURE 11-2. Diabetes can affect most structures of the human eye [15]. Diabetes-induced ischemia of cranial nerves III, IV, and VI can result in drooping of the lids, ocular motility abnormalities, or both as a result of impaired enervation of the ocular muscles. Corneal erosions, corneal ulcers, cataracts, and delayed wound healing also reflect the general diabetic state. However, most visual loss associated with diabetes arises from complications involving neovascularization of the retina (or iris) or increased vasopermeability of the retinal vasculature.

CLINICAL PRESENTATIONS OF DIABETIC EYE COMPLICATIONS

Diabetes-Associated Pathology	Clinical Symptoms
Palsy of cranial nerves III, IV, VI	Diplopia: binocular
	Ptosis
	Anisocoria
	"Blurred vision": binocular
Reduced corneal sensitivity or corneal erosions or corneal infections	Ocular pain
	Ocular discharage
	Corneal opacification
	Decreased vision
Hyphema	Decreased vision
	Blood layering in anterior chamber
Angle closure glaucoma	Ocular pain
	"Halos" around lights
	Decreased vision
Iris neovascularization	Ocular pain
	Decreased vision
	Blood layering in anterior chamber
Cataract	Decreased vision
	Glare with bright lights
Vitreous hemorrhage	"Spots," "cobwebs," "lines" in vision (floaters)
	Decreased vision
Macular edema	Moderately decreased vision
	Image distortion
Proliferative diabetic retinopathy	Symptoms associated with vitreous hemorrhage and macular edema
Retina detachment	Photopsia
	Floaters
	Scotoma
	Decreased vision
	Image distortion
Diabetic papillopathy	Visual field change

FIGURE 11-3. Clinical presentations associated with diabetic eye complications. Each of the numerous diabetes-associated ocular pathologies can present with a diverse array of symptoms. Only a partial list is presented here. It is important to realize that serious diabetic eye disease may exist *without any discernible symptoms*. This fact underscores the essential need for regular, routine, lifelong follow-up regardless of the presence or absence of visual symptoms.

OCULAR PATHOLOGY ASSOCIATED WITH RETINOPATHY PROGRESSION

Disease Stage	Common Pathologic Changes
Preclinical stages	Alterations in retinal blood flow
	Loss of retinal pericytes
	Thickening of basement membranes
Early stages: Mild NDPR	Retinal vascular microaneurysms and blot hemorrhages
	Increased retinal vascular permeability
	Cotton wool spots
Middle stages: Moderate NPDR	Venous caliber changes or beading
	IRMAs
Severe NPDR	Retinal capillary loss
Very severe NPDR	Retinal ischemia
	Extensive intraretinal hemorrhages and microaneurysms
Advanced stages: PDR	Neovascularization of the disc
	Neovascularization elsewhere
	Neovascularization of the iris
	Neovascular glaucoma
	Pre-retinal and vitreous hemorrhage
	Fibrovascular proliferation
	Retinal traction, retinal tears, retinal detachment

FIGURE 11-4. Ocular pathology associated with progression of diabetic retinopathy. Diabetic retinopathy generally progresses through well-characterized stages. Each stage is associated with typical pathologic changes. Some degree of clinically apparent retinopathy occurs in nearly all patients with diabetes of 20 or more years' duration, although preclinical alterations in blood flow, pericyte number, and basement membrane thickness can occur much earlier [16]. The clinical stages before the development of neovascularization are termed *nonproliferative diabetic retinopathy* (NPDR). NPDR is subdivided into mild, moderate, severe, or very severe categories, depending on the type and extent of clinical pathology present. Increased vascular permeability can occur at this or any later stage. As the disease progresses, gradual loss of the retinal microvasculature results in retinal ischemia. Venous caliber abnormalities, intraretinal microvascular abnormalities (IRMAs), and more severe vascular leakage are common reflections of this increasing retinal nonperfusion (see Fig. 11-7). Once ischemia-induced neovascularization occurs, the disease is referred to as proliferative diabetic retinopathy (PDR) (see Fig. 11-9). Neovascularization can arise at the optic disc (neovascularization of the disc) or elsewhere in the retina (neovascularization elsewhere). The new vessels are fragile and prone to bleeding, resulting in vitreous hemorrhage. With time, the neovascularization tends to undergo fibrosis and contraction, resulting in retinal traction, retinal tears, vitreous hemorrhage, and retinal detachment (see Fig. 11-13). New vessels also can arise on the iris, resulting in neovascular glaucoma (see Fig. 11 -14). (*Adapted from* Aiello, *et al.* [14]; with permission.)

Nonproliferative Diabetic Retinopathy

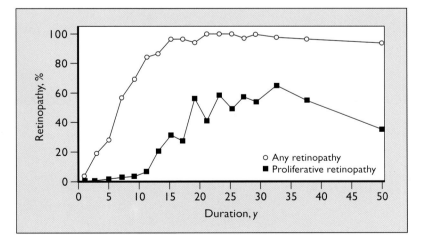

FIGURE 11-5. Incidence of diabetic retinopathy by duration of diabetes. The percentage of patients developing either any diabetic retinopathy or proliferative diabetic retinopathy is presented as a function of duration of type 1 diabetes in years. Note that almost all patients have some evidence of diabetic retinopathy once the duration of diabetes exceeds 15 years. In addition, the incidence of proliferative diabetic retinopathy (PDR) is negligible within 5 years of the onset of diabetes, although nearly 60% of patients eventually will develop PDR. These observations serve as the foundation for clinical care recommendations concerning the appropriate timing of initial ophthalmologic evaluation, as detailed in Figure 11-6. (*Adapted from* Krolewski *et al.* [17]; with permission.)

INITIAL OPHTHALMOLOGIC EXAMINATION SCHEDULE

Age at Onset of Diabetes Mellitus	Recommended First Examination	Minimum Routine Follow-up*
29 years or younger	Within 3–5 years after diagnosis of diabetes Once patient is age 10 years or older	Yearly
30 years or older	At time of diagnosis of diabetes	Yearly
Patient becomes pregnant	Before conception and during first trimester	Physician discretion pending results of first trimester examination

*Abnormal findings necessitate more frequent follow-up.

FIGURE 11-6. Only about 25% of patients with type 1 diabetes will have any retinopathy after 5 years, although most eventually will develop the disease (*see* Fig. 11-5) [18]. The prevalence of PDR is less than 2% at 5 years. For patients with type 2 disease, however, the onset date of diabetes frequently is not known precisely, and thus, more severe disease can be observed soon after diagnosis. Up to 3% of patients first diagnosed after aged 30 may have clinically significant macular edema or high-risk PDR at the time of initial diagnosis of diabetes [19]. Thus, in patients over aged 10, the initial ophthalmic examination is recommended beginning 5 years after the diagnosis of type 1 diabetes mellitus and on diagnosis of type 2 diabetes mellitus [14]. The onset of vision-threatening retinopathy is rare in children before puberty, regardless of the duration of diabetes; however, if diabetes is diagnosed between the ages of 10 and 30 years, significant retinopathy may arise within 6 years [2]. Puberty can accelerate the progression of retinopathy. Thus, the initial ophthalmic evaluation is recommended within 3 to 5 years of diagnosis, once the patient is aged 10 years or older [14,20]. Diabetic retinopathy also can become particularly aggressive during pregnancy in women with diabetes [21]. Ideally, patients with diabetes who are planning pregnancy should have an eye examination within 1 year of conception. Pregnant women should have a comprehensive eye examination in the first trimester of pregnancy. Close follow-up throughout pregnancy is indicated, with subsequent examinations determined by the findings present at the first trimester examination. This guideline does not apply to women who develop gestational diabetes because they are not at increased risk of developing diabetic retinopathy. (*Adapted from* Aiello *et al.* [14]; with permission.)

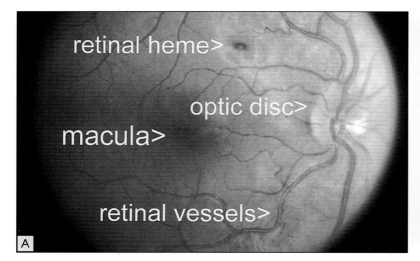 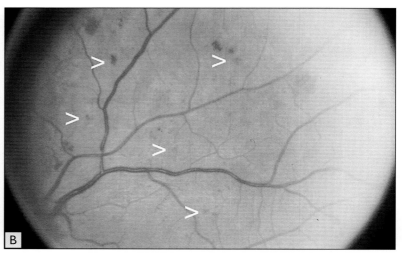

FIGURE 11-7. (*see* Color Plate) Characteristic findings in nonproliferative diabetic retinopathy (NPDR). The classic findings associated with NPDR are demonstrated. **A,** The central region of the human retina is called the macula and is responsible for detailed vision. This patient's right eye has minimal diabetic retinopathy, and the retina is normal except for a single retinal hemorrhage (retinal heme). The optic disc is located nasal to the macula, and the retinal vessels emanate from the optic nerve and surround the macula. **B,** Retinal blot hemorrhages (*arrows*) and microaneurysms, which are saccular dilations of the vessel wall. These lesions often are two of the earliest clinically observed abnormalities. The patient has severe NPDR when hemorrhages and microaneurysms of this extent or greater in all four quadrants of the retina are observed.

(Continued on next page)

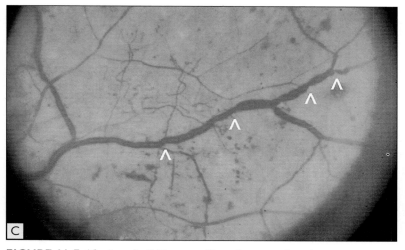

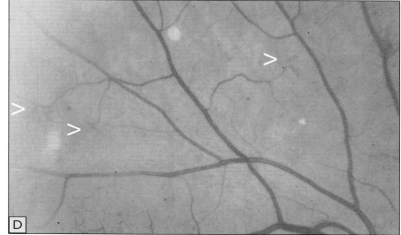

FIGURE 11-7. *(Continued)* **C,** Venous caliber changes referred to as *venous beading.* This finding often represents more advanced retinopathy, as is evident in this photograph *(arrows).* Two or more retinal quadrants of any venous beading (not necessarily as pronounced as here) signify severe NPDR. **D,** *Arrows* show intraretinal microvascular abnormalities (IRMAs). IRMAs are abnormalities within the retina and may be a harbinger of early retinal neovascularization. IRMAs often are associated with more advanced NPDR, and only one or more retinal quadrants of IRMAs of this or greater extent represent severe NPDR. Note that the clinical findings associated with severe NPDR therefore may be quite subtle. Any two or more of the findings associated with severe NPDR place the patient in the very severe category of NPDR. (Panels *B, C,* and *D from* The Early Treatment Diabetic Retinopathy Study Research Group [22]; with permission.)

Proliferative Diabetic Retinopathy and Macular Edema

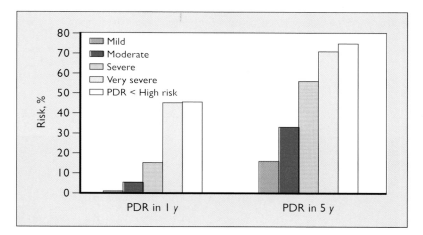

FIGURE 11-8. Progression to high-risk proliferative diabetic retinopathy (PDR) becomes more likely as the severity of nonproliferative diabetic retinopathy increases (NPDR). Demonstrated is the likelihood of developing high-risk PDR (*see* Fig. 11-9) within 1 or 5 years for patients with mild, moderate, severe, and very severe levels of NPDR or PDR with less than high-risk characteristics. High-risk PDR is associated with the greatest incidence of severe and irreversible visual loss. Each increase in NPDR severity level is associated with an increase in progression to the sight-threatening proliferative stage of the disease. The known progression rates permit determination of appropriate intervals between follow-up ocular evaluations for patients with differing levels of diabetic retinopathy. Typically, follow-up ocular evaluations are performed as follows: annually for no retinopathy, every 6 to 12 months for mild to moderate NPDR, every 3 to 4 months for severe to very severe NPDR, and every 2 to 4 months for PDR that is less than high risk [14]. (*Adapted from* The Early Treatment Diabetic Retinopathy Study Research Group [23]; with permission.)

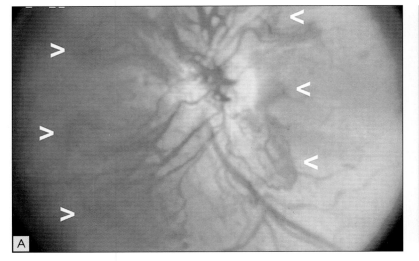

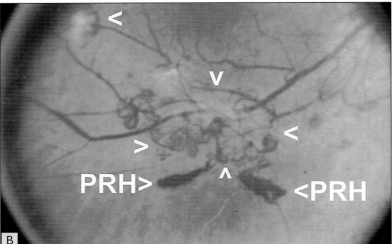

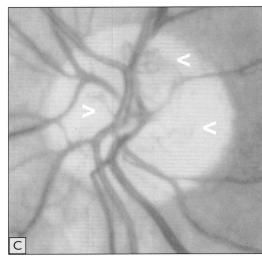

FIGURE 11-9. (*see* Color Plate) Characteristic clinical manifestations of proliferative diabetic retinopathy (PDR). When any neovascularization is present, diabetic retinopathy is termed *proliferative diabetic retinopathy*. The extent and location of neovascularization determine whether the PDR is considered to be high risk or less than high risk. Neovascularization at the optic disc (NVD), larger areas of vessels, and the presence of concurrent vitreous hemorrhages are the critical findings. Without laser photocoagulation, patients with high-risk PDR have a 28% risk of severe visual loss (< 5/200, which is worse than legally blind) within 2 years. This risk compares with a 7% risk of severe visual loss after 2 years for patients with PDR without the high-risk characteristics [24,25]. **A**, Extensive NVD. **B**, Extensive neovascularization at an area remote (>1500 m) from the optic disc, referred to as neovascularization elsewhere (NVE). Pre-retinal hemorrhage (PRH) also is present. **C**, NVD approximately equal to one third to one fourth of the disc area. The following are the risk factors: presence of any neovascularization within the eye, NVD, pre-retinal (or vitreous) hemorrhage, and large areas of neovascularization. NVD equal to or greater than that shown in *Panel C* is considered large. NVE greater than or equal to half of the disc area is considered large. When three or more of the risk factors listed previously are present, the patient has PDR with high-risk characteristics (PDR-HRC). Thus, the patient in *Panel A* has PDR-HRC because neovascularization is present, located at the disc, and large in extent. The patient in *Panel B* also has PDR-HRC because neovascularization is present, the extent of NVE is large, and pre-retinal hemorrhage is present. *Panel C* represents the minimal amount of NVD required for PDR-HRC. (Parts *B* and *C from* The Early Treatment Diabetic Retinopathy Study Research Group [22]; with permission.)

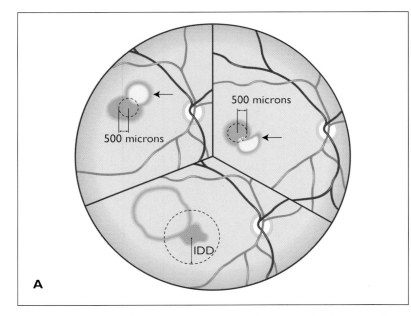

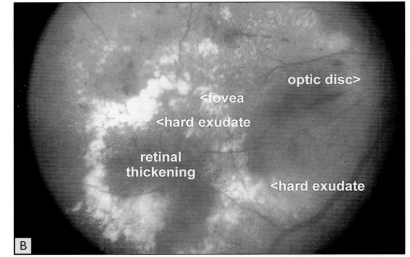

FIGURE 11-10. (*see* Color Plate) Clinical manifestations of diabetic macular edema. Increased permeability of the retinal microvasculature can result in transudation of serum and other blood components into the substance of the retina, often with deposition of lipid in the form of hard exudates. Retinal edema and thickening result. Macular edema may be present at any level of diabetic retinopathy and is defined as retinal thickening within 3000 μm of the center of the macula (fovea). Macular edema that threatens the center of vision is termed *clinically significant macular edema* (CSME) [23,26]. **A**, Situations in which macular edema (*white*) is of sufficient extent and correct location to be termed *CSME*. Specifically, edema qualifies as CSME when it is at or within 500 μm of the fovea; associated with hard exudates (*arrows*) at or within 500 μm of the fovea; or one disc area in size, with any part of the edema at or within 1500 μm of the fovea. **B**, CSME owing to extensive hard exudate and thickening involving the fovea and surrounding retina. 1DD—one disk diameter. (*Panel A* adapted from Cavallerano [27]; with permission.)

Complications and Causes of Visual Loss

CAUSES OF VISUAL LOSS IN DIABETIC RETINOPATHY

Complication Threatening Vision	Common Therapeutic Approach
Clinically significant macular edema	Focal or grid laser photocoagulation surgery
Macular capillary nonperfusion	No currently effective therapy
High-risk proliferative diabetic retinopathy	Scatter (panretinal) laser photocoagulation surgery (PRP)
Vitreous hemorrhage	Careful observation or vitrectomy
Traction, rhegmatogenous retinal detachment, or both	Vitrectomy
Traction distorting the macula	Careful observation or vitrectomy
Fibrovascular tissues obscuring the retina	Careful observation or vitrectomy
Neovascular glaucoma	PRP, cryotherapy plus intraocular pressure management, or both

FIGURE 11-11. Diabetic retinopathy can result in permanent and irreversible visual loss by several mechanisms. Long-standing CSME induces moderate visual loss from edema in the foveal region (see Fig. 11-10). If extensive capillary closure occurs in the macular region, vision can be permanently and irreversibly affected from the loss of blood supply to the fovea (see Fig. 11-12). Untreated high-risk proliferative diabetic retinopathy (PDR) primarily causes severe visual loss either by vitreous hemorrhage or retinal traction. Vitreous hemorrhage can reduce vision markedly owing to obscuration of the visual axis by blood (see Fig. 11-12). However, because the blood itself is relatively benign, vision will be recovered (in the absence of other ocular damage) once the hemorrhage clears either spontaneously or, when not resolving, after vitrectomy surgery (see Fig. 11-19). In contrast, neovascularization eventually tends to undergo a scarring process with fibrosis and contraction, resulting in retinal traction (see Fig. 11-13). Such traction can cause visual loss by distorting the macula; tearing the retina; or precipitating retinal detachment, further vitreous hemorrhage, or both. Rarely, fibrovascular tissue itself may obscure the visual axis (see Fig. 11-12). If neovascularization of the iris occurs, neovascular glaucoma may result and lead to permanent visual loss (see Fig. 11-14). (*Adapted from* Aiello *et al.* [14]; with permission.)

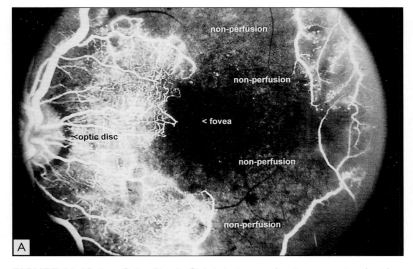

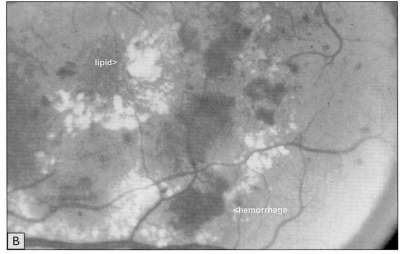

FIGURE 11-12. (*see Color Plate*) Ophthalmic complications associated with visual loss in diabetic retinopathy. Visual loss associated with diabetic retinopathy can arise from multiple complications of the disease. If the characteristic progressive capillary loss eventually involves a large portion of the central macula, then visual acuity is compromised. **A,** Fluorescein angiogram showing extensive macular capillary nonperfusion. Fluorescent dye (fluorescein) was injected into the patient's antecubital vein, and photographs were taken of the retina as the dye was passing through the retinal vessels. This technique, called *fluorescein angiography*, allows excellent visualization of the retinal vasculature. In this instance, the dye in the retinal vessels appears white, and the photograph shows nearly complete loss of the retinal vasculature perfusion in the macular region. These anatomic changes and their visual sequelae are irreversible. **B,** Extensive retinal vascular leakage into the macular region with retinal thickening, lipid deposits, and retinal hemorrhage. This patient has severe macular edema, with associated visual loss.

(*Continued on next page*)

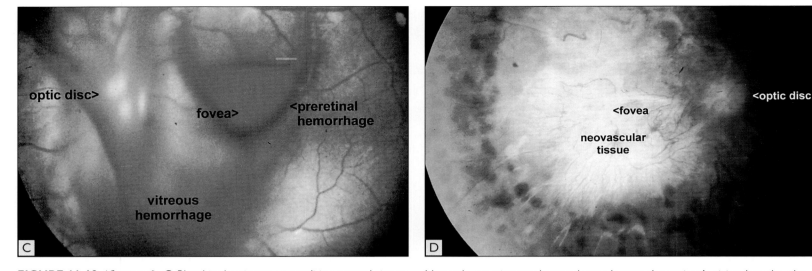

FIGURE 11-12. (*Continued*) **C**, Blood in the vitreous, a condition termed *vitreous hemorrhage* or *preretinal hemorrhage*. Preretinal hemorrhage refers specifically to blood immediately in front of the retina, whereas vitreous hemorrhage may be anywhere in the vitreous cavity. Vitreous hemorrhages are common in diabetic retinopathy owing to the fragility of new vessels and traction often exerted on these vessels by progressive retinal fibrosis. Although the hemorrhages usually clear spontaneously, surgical intervention may be required if they persist (*see* Fig. 11-19).

Not only can vitreous hemorrhage obscure the patient's vision but also the ophthalmologist's view of the retina, which may necessitate evaluation of the retinal anatomy using ultrasonography if the hemorrhage is severe (*see* Fig. 11-13). **D**, A rare form of visual loss in diabetes in which a sheet of neovascular tissue obscures the visual axis. Removal of the tissue by vitrectomy surgery often can restore useful vision (*see* Fig. 11-19). (*Courtesy of* The Wilmer Ophthalmological Institute.)

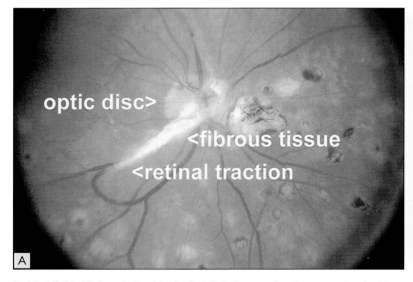

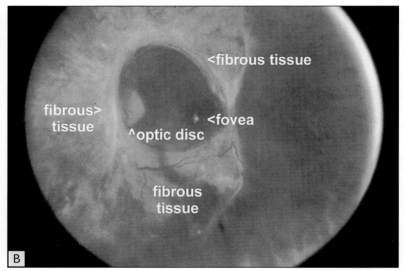

FIGURE 11-13. (*see* Color Plate) Ophthalmic complications associated with retinal traction in diabetic retinopathy. Some of the most severe visual losses associated with diabetic retinopathy result from the complications of traction exerted on the retina by fibrosing neovascular tissue. Initially, the traction can result in localized retinal detachment that when distant from the critical areas of the retina has little visual significance. **A**, A localized traction retinal detachment from the optic disc to an inferior retinal vessel. Note the elevation and distortion

of the retinal vessel at the area of traction. As seen here, the detachment does not threaten the macula but should be examined carefully at regular intervals for progression toward the fovea. **B**, More extensive fibrovascular tissue and traction along the vascular arcades of the retina surrounding the macula. This configuration is typical of retinal traction in diabetic retinopathy because of the predilection for fibrovascular tissues to form along the vascular arcades. This configuration has been termed *wolf-jaw* owing to its apparent imminent "bite" on the macula.

(*Continued on next page*)

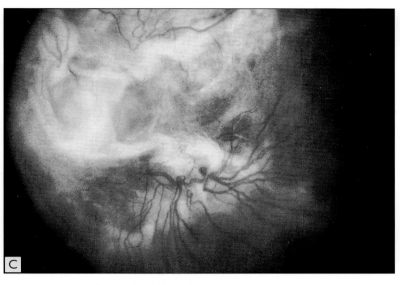

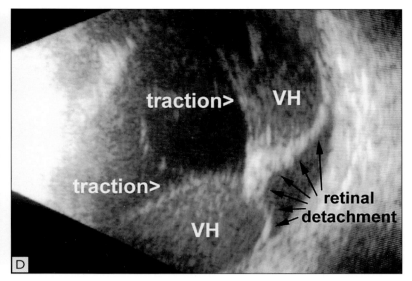

FIGURE 11-13. *(Continued)* **C,** A nearly total retinal detachment with extensive fibrovascular proliferation. Large retinal detachments also may occur when the tractional forces are sufficient to tear a hole in the retina, allowing vitreous fluid to pass into the subretinal space (rhegmatogenous detachment). If vitreous hemorrhage obscures the view of the retina, ultrasonography is indicated to monitor ocular status. **D,** Ultrasonography of vitreous hemorrhage (VH), retinal traction, and traction retinal detachment. When traction retinal detachment threatens the macula, vitrectomy surgery usually is indicated *(see* Fig. 11-19). (Panel D *courtesy of* R. Calderon, OD.)

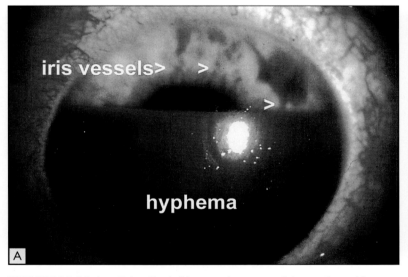

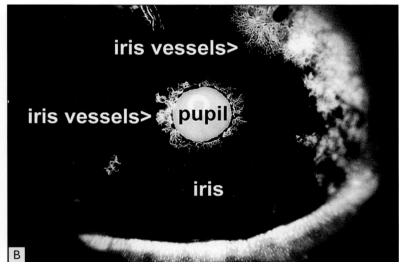

FIGURE 11-14. *(see Color Plate)* Neovascularization of the iris. In proliferative diabetic retinopathy, neovascularization can occur not only on the retina but also on the iris. Neovascularization of the iris sometimes is referred to as *rubeosis iridis.* If the neovascularization progresses to the base of the iris, the normal outflow channels for the aqueous fluid from the anterior chamber can become occluded and the intraocular pressure can increase dramatically. This condition, called *neovascular glaucoma,* can result in severe and permanent visual loss. Treatment involves prompt scatter laser photocoagulation as done for proliferative diabetic retinopathy *(see* Fig. 11-15). **A,** Neovascularization of the iris with hemorrhage into the aqueous chamber, called *hyphema,* that sometimes occurs from these vessels. When present, hyphema usually is not this severe. **B,** Iris neovascularization using fluorescein angiography *(see* Fig. 11-12A). Fluorescein dye in the iris vessels *(white)* demonstrates the extent of the neovascularization on the iris.

Treatment

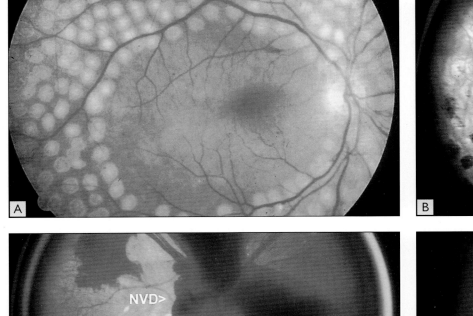

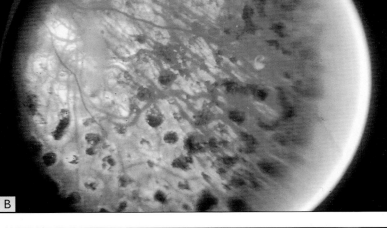

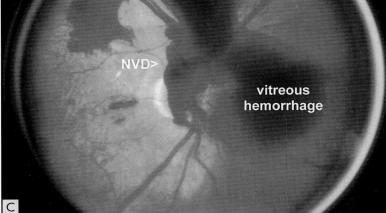

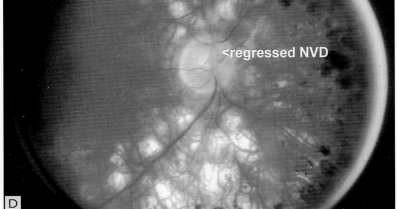

FIGURE 11-15. (*see* Color Plate) Panretinal laser photocoagulation for proliferative diabetic retinopathy (PDR). The primary therapy for PDR is scatter (panretinal) laser photocoagulation. However, cryotherapy or vitrectomy with endophotocoagulation may be effective when photocoagulation is not feasible. Treatment entails using a laser to place multiple burns throughout the midperiphery of the retina in an attempt to reduce the risk of visual loss. In general, prompt treatment is advised for patients with high-risk PDR. Some patients with PDR that is less than high-risk or with severe or very severe NPDR also may benefit from panretinal photocoagulation, depending on factors such as type of diabetes, medical status, access to care, compliance with follow-up, status and progression of the fellow eye, and family history [23,28]. **A**, Clinical appearance of the retina shortly after panretinal photocoagulation in PDR. The 500-micron-diameter retinal burns appear moderately white in intensity and one-half burn width apart. Laser burns are not placed over the retinal vessels, optic disc, or within the macular region. A total of 1200 to 1800 retinal burns generally are applied over two to three sessions occurring a few days to weeks apart. The procedure is done on an outpatient basis and generally requires only topical anesthesia. **B**, Panretinal photocoagulation scars as they appear months to years after their application. Note the areas of increased retinal pigmentation, atrophy, and spreading of the area of each retinal scar. **C**, PDR, neovascularization of the disk, and vitreous hemorrhage before laser panretinal photocoagulation. **D**, The same patient 2 years after panretinal photocoagulation. Note the resolution of the vitreous hemorrhage and regression of the neovascularization with only a small, fibrotic, nonperfused remnant of the original neovascular frond at the optic disc. Such remnants often do not regress completely and usually do not threaten vision. NVD—neovascularization at the disk. (Parts B, C, and D *from* The American Academy of *Ophthalmology* Diabetes 2000 Diabetic Retinopathy Course; with permission.)

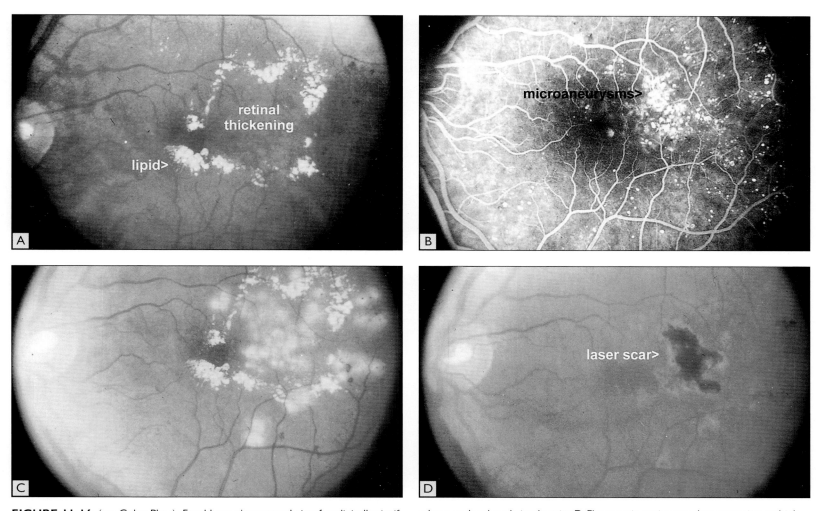

FIGURE 11-16. (*see* Color Plate) Focal laser photocoagulation for clinically significant diabetic macular edema. The primary therapy for clinically significant diabetic macular edema is focal laser photocoagulation. Treatment entails placing light 50- to 100-μm-diameter burns focally over leaking microaneurysms or in a grid pattern if retinal leakage is diffuse. Once the need for treatment is determined clinically, fluorescein angiography often is used to identify the type of leakage and specific microaneurysms for treatment. If treatment is successful, resolution of the macular edema may be expected 3 or more months after therapy. Treatment may be reapplied if the edema persists or recurs. **A**, Circinate lipid deposits, clinically significant macular edema, and reduced visual acuity. **B**, Fluorescein angiogram demonstrating multiple microaneurysms in the area of thickening within the circinate ring. **C**, Clinical appearance of the retina immediately after focal laser photocoagulation to the leaking microaneurysms. The retinal burns applied in this case are more intense than is optimal. **D**, Clinical appearance of the eye several months after laser therapy. The lipid and edema have resolved, and no thickening of the retina is present. Likewise, visual acuity has improved. The residual scarring of the retina is heavier than desired owing to the intensity of the initial laser burns. (*Adapted from* the American Academy of Ophthalmology Diabetes 2000 Program; with permission.)

THERAPEUTIC EFFICACY IN THE TREATMENT OF DIABETIC RETINOPATHY

Indication	Treatment	Efficacy
Clinically significant macular edema	Focal laser photocoagulation	50% reduction in moderate visual loss* after 3 y
High-risk proliferative diabetic retinopathy (PDR)	Scatter photocoagulation	60% reduction in severe visual loss** after 3 y
Development of high-risk PDR	Scatter photocoagulation	87% reduction in severe visual loss** after 3 y
		97% reduction in bilateral severe visual loss** after 3 y
		90% reduction in legal blindness after 5 y
Severe PDR and severe vitreous hemorrhage***	Vitrectomy	60% increased chance of 20/40 or better after 2 y
Severe PDR and vision 10/200 or better***	Vitrectomy	34% increased chance of 20/40 or better after 2 y
No diabetic retinopathy	Intensive glycemic control	76% reduction in onset of retinopathy
Nonproliferative diabetic retinopathy	Intensive glycemic control	63% reduction in retinopathy progression
		47% reduction in severe nonproliferative diabetic retinopathy and PDR
		26% reduction in development of macular edema
		51% reduction in need for laser treatment

FIGURE 11-17. The only patient-initiated efforts proved to reduce the risk of visual loss include maintenance of optimal glycemic control and insistence on routine ophthalmologic evaluation [9,29]. Once visually significant complications of diabetes have arisen, the mainstay of therapy is laser photocoagulation. Scatter (panretinal) photocoagulation for the treatment of proliferative diabetic retinopathy is remarkably effective in preventing severe visual loss when patients at risk receive therapy in an appropriate and timely manner. Indeed, with appropriate medical and ophthalmologic care, over 95% of visual loss resulting from diabetic retinopathy can be prevented [13]. Focal photocoagulation for the treatment of clinically significant macular edema is somewhat less effective, although half of moderate visual loss can be prevented in this manner. If the application of laser photocoagulation is not possible or is ineffective, pars plana vitrectomy surgery also is useful in preventing visual impairment (see Fig. 11-19). *Moderate visual loss is defined as at least doubling of the visual angle (eg, 20/40 to 20/80). **Severe visual loss is defined as best corrected acuity of 5/200 or worse on two consecutive visits 4 months apart. ***For patients with type 1 diabetes only; no benefit was observed in the group having adult-onset diabetes. (Adapted from Aiello et al. [14]; with permission.)

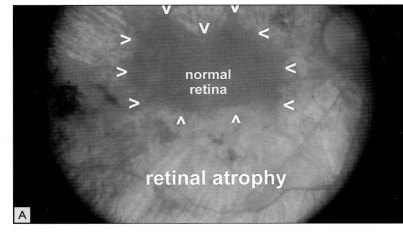

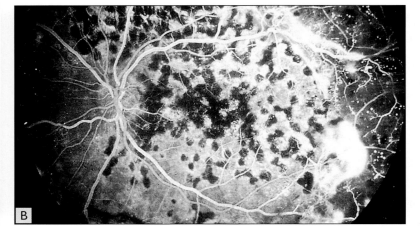

FIGURE 11-18. (see Color Plate) Side effects and complications of laser photocoagulation. Although laser photocoagulation is remarkably effective at preventing the visual loss associated with diabetic retinopathy, the therapy itself is inherently destructive. Each retinal laser burn destroys a portion of previously viable retina in an attempt to maintain better visual function than would be achieved without treatment. Thus, the therapy itself is associated with unavoidable side effects, most notably constriction of peripheral visual field and reduced night vision. These symptoms result from the selective destruction of the retinal midperiphery that subserves these functions. Unexpected complications also can arise from laser photocoagulation. **A,** Appearance of the retina several years after excessive laser panretinal photocoagulation. Note that the atrophy resulting from individual laser scars has spread to the point at which confluent loss of the peripheral retina occurs. Only the central aspect of the macula (arrows) remains intact. As expected, this patient has severe constriction of the visual field and significant difficulty with night vision. **B,** Fluorescein angiogram of panretinal photocoagulation mistakenly applied directly through the macula. The dark laser scars in this macular area, which is critical for detailed vision, cause permanent blind spots in the center of vision and reduced visual acuity.

(Continued on next page)

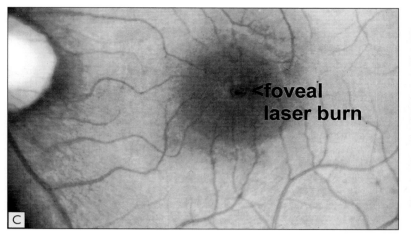

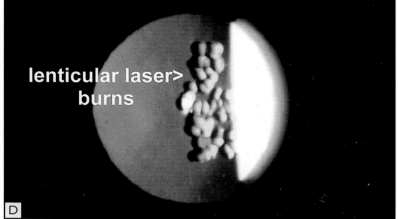

FIGURE 11-18. (*Continued*) **C,** A single laser burn mistakenly applied to the fovea. This area of retina subserves central vision, accounting for the large central blind spot and poor detailed vision experienced by this patient, who now is legally blind. **D,** Laser photocoagulation focused too far anteriorly may result in vaporization of the crystalline lens, as observed in this retroilluminated photograph of the human lens. Visual loss associated with this rare complication can be corrected by cataract surgery. (*Panels B–D courtesy of* the Wilmer Ophthalmological Institute.)

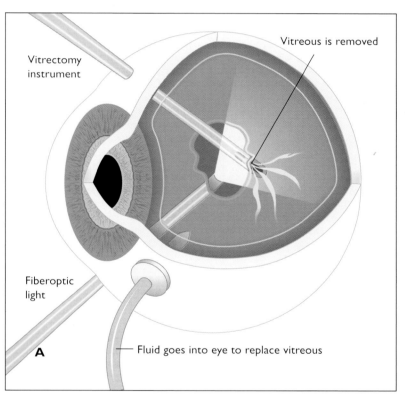

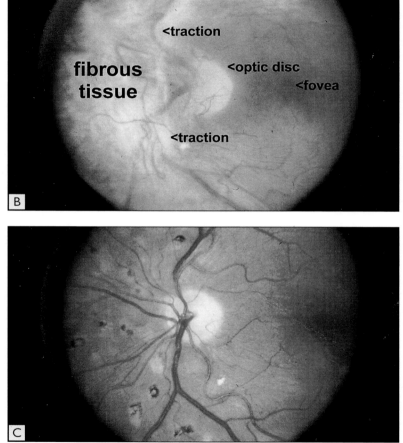

FIGURE 11-19. (*see Color Plate*) Pars plana vitrectomy surgery. Instances occur when high-risk proliferative diabetic retinopathy (PDR) is not amenable to laser photocoagulation and may arise as a result of the following: advanced disease, poor retinal visualization (*ie*, severe vitreous hemorrhage or cataract), active neovascularization despite complete laser treatment, traction-macular detachment, or combined traction-rhegmatogenous retinal detachment. In such cases, pars plana vitrectomy surgery may offer a therapeutic option. Vitrectomy surgery has the potential for serious complications, including profound visual loss and permanent pain and blindness. Thus, surgery should be undertaken only after careful consideration of the potential risks and benefits [30]. Vitrectomy performed by an experienced vitreoretinal surgeon, however, often can maintain vision in patients who otherwise almost certainly would have severe visual loss. **A,** Schematic representation of the pars plana vitrectomy procedure. Three openings are made from the outside of the eye into the vitreous cavity. An infusion line is placed in one opening to maintain pressure within the eye during surgery. The other two openings are used for the variety of instruments that can manipulate the vitreous and retina. Fiber optic instruments allow for illumination, and the surgery is monitored by visualization through the pupil using an operating microscope. **B,** PDR and extensive fibrovascular neovascularization before vitrectomy surgery. Note the fibrous tissue surrounding the optic disc that is exerting traction on the major superior and inferior retinal vessels, dragging them nasally. **C,** The same retina after vitrectomy surgery. Note the removal of the fibrous tissue that had surrounded the optic disc with return of the major retinal vessels to a more normal anatomic position after removal of the traction. (*Panel A from* "For my patient: retinal detachment and vitreous surgery," The Retina Research Fund; *panels B and C from* the American Academy of *Ophthalmology* Diabetic Retinopathy Vitrectomy Study course; with permission.)

Growth Factors and Potential Novel Therapies

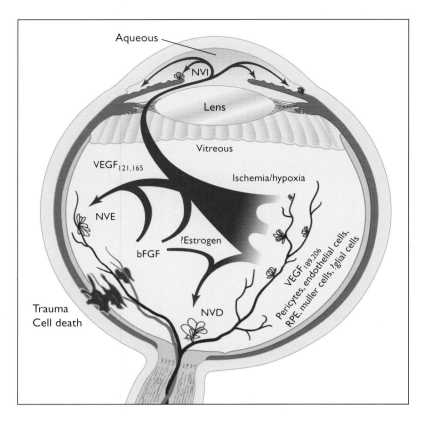

FIGURE 11-20. Model of growth factor action in diabetic retinopathy. For the past half century, investigators have recognized that numerous ischemic retinopathies result in retinal neovascularization and vascular leakage similar to that observed in diabetic retinopathy. These findings have suggested that common inciting events and mediating factors may be responsible for these complications. The potential role of growth factors in mediating retinal neovascularization was first suggested by Michaelson in 1948 and later refined by numerous investigators [31]. A schematic representation of the growth factor model of intraocular neovascularization is shown. Damage to the retinal tissues, probably caused by capillary loss and subsequent hypoxia in the case of diabetes, results in the release of growth factors from the retina. These growth factors are secreted by a variety of retinal cell types and may act locally to produce neovascularization and vascular permeability or may diffuse through the vitreous cavity to induce these complications at distant sites. The presence of two or more growth factors may actually augment the induction of neovascular activity, as is the case with basic fibroblast growth factor (bFGF) and vascular endothelial growth factor (VEGF). In addition, the growth factors may diffuse down a concentration gradient from the vitreous cavity into the aqueous cavity where they are eventually cleared through the trabecular meshwork at the base of the iris. This diffusion path would account for neovascularization observed at the iris. Numerous growth factors have been implicated in this process. Molecules that probably contribute to the neovascularization in diabetic retinopathy include basic fibroblast growth factor, growth hormone, insulin-like growth factor 1, and vascular endothelial growth factor. Of these, VEGF is the only molecule that possesses all the expected characteristics for a major mediator of intraocular neovascularization and vasopermeability. The relative growth factor concentrations and angiogenic potency are represented by arrow width. NVD—neovascularization at the disc; NVE—neovascularization elsewhere; NVI—neovascularization at the iris; RPE–retinal pigment epithelium. (*Adapted from* Aiello *et al.* [32]; with permission.)

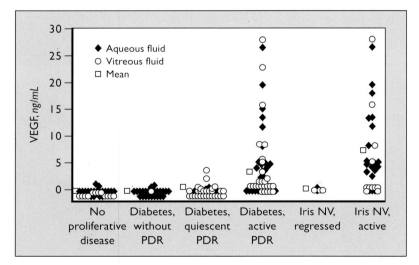

FIGURE 11-21. For a growth factor to mediate intraocular neovascularization in diabetic retinopathy, it should be present at elevated concentrations during or shortly before the onset of active neovascularization. Demonstrated are the results of a study in which intraocular fluids were obtained from 136 patients with diabetes who were undergoing intraocular surgery. The concentration of vascular endothelial growth factor (VEGF) in the intraocular fluids was evaluated and the results plotted by extent of retinopathy. Concentrations of VEGF were low in patients who did not have diabetes or who had diabetes but no proliferative diabetic retinopathy (PDR). However, when patients had active neovascularization either of the retina or iris, concentrations of VEGF were greatly elevated. Once neovascularization had become quiescent, concentrations of vascular endothelial factor returned to baseline. The study also demonstrated the predicted concentration gradient between the vitreous and aqueous cavities and a 75% decrease in VEGF levels after successful laser panretinal photocoagulation. NV–neovascularization. (*Adapted from* Aiello *et al.* [33]; with permission.)

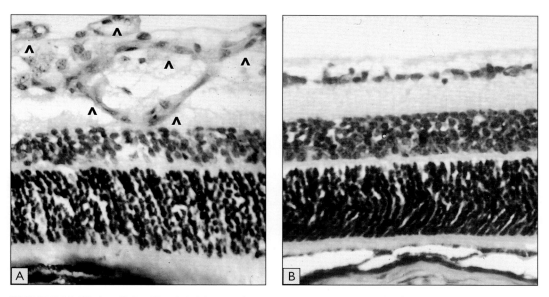

FIGURE 11-22. (see Color PLate) Inhibition of vascular endothelial growth factor (VEGF) suppresses retinal neovascularization in animals. If vascular endothelial growth factor is responsible for a significant portion of the neovascular response in ischemic retinopathies, then inhibition of this molecule should result in suppression of retinal neovascularization. Several investigators have now evaluated this causal relationship. Inhibition of VEGF using three different techniques has resulted in suppression of retinal and iris neovascularization in murine and primate models [34–36]. Demonstrated are the results from one of these studies using the chimeric receptor antagonists in a murine model of ischemia-induced retinopathy [34,37]. When these inhibitors of VEGF are injected into the neonatal eye at the time when the retinas become hypoxic, suppression of subsequent retinal neovascularization occurs in 95% to 100% of animals. The magnitude of inhibition is approximately 50%. **A,** Histologic cross section of a neonatal mouse retina that received an intraocular injection of an inactive control compound. The *arrows* show the extensive inner retinal neovascularization. **B,** Corresponding area of retina in the contralateral eye of the same animal that received an active inhibitor of VEGF. Note the suppression of inner retinal neovascularization and normal appearance of the retina by light microscopic examination without evidence of retinal toxicity. These data suggest that growth factor inhibitors eventually may prove useful as novel therapies for diabetic retinopathy and macular edema. Such therapeutic approaches theoretically would eliminate the side effects inherent in the retinal-destructive treatments in use today (see Figs. 11-15 and 11-18). VEGF inhibitory agents currently are being tested in clinical trials. (*Adapted from* Aiello [38]; with permission.)

Acknowledgments

The excellent technical and editorial assistance of Jerry D. Cavallerano, OD, PhD, is gratefully acknowledged.

Portions of this chapter are adapted from Aiello, et al. [14] and the American Academy of Opthalmology Diabetes 2000 Diabetic Retinopathy Course.

References

1. Klein R, BE Klein, Moss SE: Visual impairment in diabetes. *Ophthalmology* 1984, 91:1–9.
2. Klein R, Klein BE, Moss SE, Cruickshanks KJ: The Wisconsin Epidemiologic Study of Diabetic Retinopathy. XV. The long-term incidence of macular edema. *Ophthalmology* 1995, 102:7–16.
3. Javitt JC, Aiello LP, Bassi LJ, et al.: Detecting and treating retinopathy in patients with type I diabetes mellitus. Savings associated with improved implementation of current guidelines. American Academy of Ophthalmology. *Ophthalmology* 1991, 98:1565–1573.
4. Javitt JC, Aiello LP, Chiang Y, et al.: Preventive eye care in people with diabetes is cost-saving to the federal government. Implications for health-care reform. *Diabetes Care* 1994, 17:909–917.
5. Javitt JC, Aiello LP: Cost-effectiveness of detecting and treating diabetic retinopathy [see comments]. *Ann Intern Med* 1996, 124:164–169.
6. Javitt, JC, Canner JK, Sommer A: Cost effectiveness of current approaches to the control of retinopathy in type I diabetics. *Ophthalmology* 1989, 96:255–264.
7. Kahn HA, Hiller R: Blindness caused by diabetic retinopathy. *Am J Ophthalmol* 1974, 78:58–67.
8. Palmberg PF: Diabetic retinopathy. *Diabetes* 1977, 26:703–709.
9. The Diabetes Control and Complications Trial Research Group: The effect of intensive treatment of diabetes on the development and progression of long-term complications in insulin-dependent diabetes mellitus [see comments]. *N Engl J Med* 1993, 329:977–986.
10. Anonymous: The relationship of glycemic exposure (HbA1c) to the risk of development and progression of retinopathy in the Diabetes Control and Complications Trial. *Diabetes* 1995, 44:968–983.
11. Anonymous: Lifetime benefits and costs of intensive therapy as practiced in the Diabetes control and complications trial. The Diabetes Control and Complications Trial Research Group [see comments] *JAMA* 1996 276:1409–1415; published erratum, *JAMA* 1997, 278:25.
12. Anonymous: Resource utilization and costs of care in the Diabetes Control and Complications Trial. *Diabetes Care* 1995, 18:1468–1478.
13. Ferris FL: How effective are treatments for diabetic retinopathy? *JAMA* 1993, 269:1290–1291.
14. Aiello LP, Gardner TW, King GL, et al.: Diabetic retinopathy: technical review. *Diabetes Care* 1998, 21:143–156.
15. National Diabetes Data Group: Diabetes in America. US Government Printing Office, Washington, DC, 1995.
16. Bursell SE, Clermont AC, Kinsley BT, et al.: Retinal blood flow changes in patients with insulin-dependent diabetes mellitus and no diabetic retinopathy. *Am J Physiol* 1996, 270:R61–R70
17. Krolewski AS, Warram JH, Rand LI, et al.: Risk of proliferative diabetic retinopathy in juvenile-onset type I diabetes: a 40-yr follow-up study. *Diabetes Care* 1984, 9:443–452.
18. Klein R, Klein BE, Moss SE, et al.: The Wisconsin epidemiologic study of diabetic retinopathy. II. Prevalence and risk of diabetic retinopathy when age at diagnosis is less than 30 years. *Arch Ophthalmol* 1984, 102:520–536.
19. Klein R, Moss SE, Klein BE, et al.: 1987. New management concepts for timely diagnosis of diabetic retinopathy treatable by photocoagulation. *Diabetes Care* 1987, 10:633–638.
20. American Academy of Pediatrics: Screening for retinopathy in the pediatric patient with type I diabetes mellitus. *Pediatrics* 1998, 101:313–314.

21. Klein, BE, Moss SE, Klein R: Effect of pregnancy on progression of diabetic retinopathy. *Diabetes Care* 1990, 13:34–40.

22. The Early Treatment Diabetic Retinopathy Study Research Group: Grading diabetic retinopathy from stereoscopic color fundus photographs: an extension of the modified Airlie House classification. ETDRS report number 10. *Ophthalmology* 1991, 98:786–806.

23. The Early Treatment Diabetic Retinopathy Study Research Group: Early photocoagulation for diabetic retinopathy. ETDRS report number 9. *Ophthalmology* 1991, 98:766–785.

24. The Diabetic Retinopathy Study Research Group: Photocoagulation treatment of proliferative diabetic retinopathy. Clinical application of Diabetic Retinopathy Study (DRS) findings, DRS Report Number 8. *Ophthalmology* 1981, 88:583–600.

25. The Diabetic Retinopathy Study Research Group: Indications for photocoagulation treatment of diabetic retinopathy: Diabetic Retinopathy Study Report no. 14. *Int Ophthalmol Clin* 1987, 27:239–253.

26. The Early Treatment Diabetic Retinopathy Study Research Group: Photocoagulation for diabetic macular edema. Early Treatment Diabetic Retinopathy Study report number 1. *Arch Ophthalmol* 1985, 103:1796–1806.

27. Cavallerano J: Diabetic retinopathy. *Clinical Eye and Vision Care* 1990, 2:4–14.

28. Ferris F: Early photocoagulation in patients with either type 1 or type 2 diabetes. *Trans Am Ophthalmol Soc* 1996, 94:505–537.

29. The Diabetes Control and Complications Trial Research Group: The effect of intensive diabetes treatment on the progression of diabetic retinopathy in insulin-dependent diabetes mellitus: the Diabetes Control and Complications Trial. *Arch Ophthalmol* 1995, 113:36–51.

30. The Diabetic Retinopathy Vitrectomy Study Research Group: Early vitrectomy for severe proliferative diabetic retinopathy in eyes with useful vision. Clinical application of results of a randomized trial: Diabetic Retinopathy Vitrectomy Study Report 4. *Ophthalmology* 1988, 95:1321–1334.

31. Michaelson IC: The mode of development of the vascular system of the retina, with some observations on its significance for certain retinal diseases. *Trans Ophthalmol Soc UK* 1948, 68:137–180.

32. Aiello LP, Northrup JM, Keyt BA: Hypoxic regulation of vascular endothelial growth factor in retinal cells. *Arch Ophthalmol* 1995, 113:1538–1544.

33. Aiello LP, Avery RL, Arrigg PG, et al.: Vascular endothelial growth factor in ocular fluid of patients with diabetic retinopathy and other retinal disorders [see comments]. *N Engl J Med* 1994, 331:1480–1487.

34. Aiello LP, Pierce EA, Foley ED, et al.: Suppression of retinal neovascularization in vivo by inhibition of vascular endothelial growth factor (VEGF) using soluble VEGF-receptor chimeric proteins. *Proc Natl Acad Sci USA* 1995, 92:10457–10461.

35. Adamis AP, Shima DT, Tolentino MJ, et al.: Inhibition of vascular endothelial growth factor prevents retinal ischemia-associated iris neovascularization in a nonhuman primate. *Arch Ophthalmol* 1996, 114:66–71.

36. Robinson GS, Pierce EA, Rook SL, et al.: Oligodeoxynucleotides inhibit retinal neovascularization in a murine model of proliferative retinopathy. *Proc Natl Acad Sci USA* 1996, 93:4851–4856.

37. Smith LE, Wesolowski E, McLellan A, et al.: Oxygen-induced retinopathy in the mouse. *Invest Ophthalmol Vis Sci* 1994, 35:101–111.

38. Aiello LP: Vascular endothelial growth factor. 20th-century mechanisms, 21st-century therapies. *Invest Ophthalmol Vis Sci* 1997, 38:1647–1652.

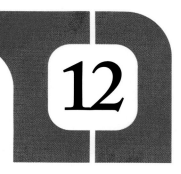

DIABETES AND THE KIDNEY

Robert C. Stanton

Diabetic nephropathy is a serious public health concern because it has become the major cause of end-stage renal disease in the United States (see Fig. 12-1). It is characterized primarily by the clinical presentation of microalbuminuria, which slowly progresses to frank proteinuria, followed by a gradual decline in glomerular filtration rate, eventually leading to renal failure. Nodular sclerosis of the mesangium in the glomerular tuft is the characteristic pathologic change seen in diabetic nephropathy. A minority of patients with diabetes mellitus develop renal failure, but the number of cases of diabetic nephropathy is increasing every year, mostly because of the aging of patients with type 2 diabetes mellitus. Success in prolonging the lives of patients with both type 1 and type 2 diabetes mellitus has led to an increase in the numbers of patients with complications of the disease. In the past 15 years, much has been learned about the possible causes of diabetic nephropathy. This understanding has led to the development and use of specific therapies that have been effective in slowing the progression to renal failure. Although effective, these therapies are not cures. Thus, there is an ongoing effort to further identify 1) the

factors predisposing to renal failure; 2) the causes of diabetic nephropathy; and 3) the factors that lead to progression to renal failure. This chapter presents an overview of the demographics, diagnosis, and natural history as well as current ideas about the pathogenesis underlying the development and progression of diabetic nephropathy. An understanding of these mechanisms has provided specific directions for the development of new, effective treatments that hold promise for the development of new clinically applicable therapies in the next 5 to 10 years. This chapter does not differentiate between the nephropathy of type 1 diabetes mellitus and the nephropathy of type 2 diabetes mellitus because recent evidence suggests that both pathogenesis and therapy for diabetic nephropathy in type 1 and type 2 diabetes mellitus are similar. Although there are clear differences in susceptibility to diabetic nephropathy, and there are some differences in the approach to screening and therapy, it is believed that there are more similarities than differences. A recent review by Ruggenenti and Remuzzi provides more information on diabetic nephropathy in patients with type 2 diabetes mellitus[1].

Demographics and Incidence

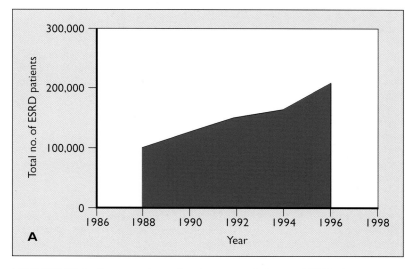

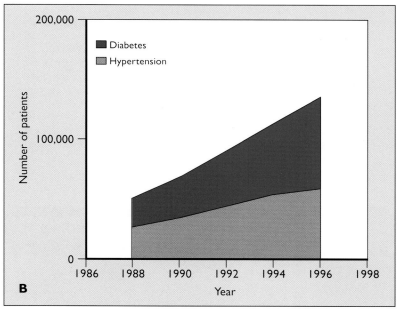

FIGURE 12-1. Demographics of end-stage renal disease (ESRD). Diabetic nephropathy occurs in about 20% to 40% of patients with type 1 diabetes mellitus and 10% to 15% of patients with type 2 diabetes mellitus. It is a significant cause of morbidity in these patients; the appearance of nephropathy leads to both a significant decrease in life expectancy and a significant increase in hospitalizations and medical care costs. **A** and **B**, The major causes of ESRD in the United States are diabetes, hypertension, and glomerulonephritis, and since the late 1980s, diabetes has become the leading cause [2]. The 1998 report of

the U.S. Renal Data System shows that over the past 10 years the percentage of patients with ESRD has increased from 24% to 37%. This figure also shows that the rate of increase in ESRD due to diabetes is greater than the increase for other causes.

PREVALENCE AND INCIDENCE OF END-STAGE RENAL DISEASE BY CAUSE

Cause	Prevalence	Incidence
Diabetes Mellitus	92,211	30,933
Hypertension	69,538	18,844
Glomerulonephritis	50,378	7,882

FIGURE 12-2. Prevalence and incidence of end-stage renal disease by top three causes in 1996 [2]. Prevalence—number of patients with endstage renal disease on December 31, 1996; incidence—number of patients starting in end-stage renal disease in all of 1996.

Diabetic Nephropathy Diagnosis

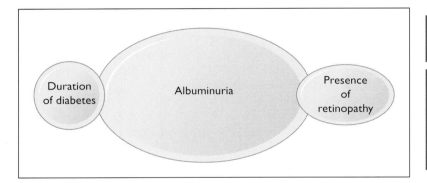

FIGURE 12-3. Diagnosis of diabetic nephropathy. The hallmark of the diagnosis of diabetic nephropathy is albuminuria. Microalbuminuria is the earliest detectable clinical sign of diabetic nephropathy. Typically, microalbuminuria progresses to frank proteinuria over a period of years. The rate of progression is based on a number of factors, which are discussed later in this chapter. In addition to microalbuminuria, patients with early diabetic nephropathy have increased glomerular filtration rates, and their kidneys undergo hypertrophy. Thus, increased creatinine clearance and increased kidney size are additional signs of early diabetic nephropathy. There are clear associations between diabetic nephropathy and two other diagnostically important factors: 1) the duration of diabetes and 2) pre-existing retinopathy. It is unusual for diabetic nephropathy to appear in patients who have had diabetes for less than 5 years. Most patients (as many as 90%) with diabetic nephropathy also have retinopathy [3]. Thus, either short duration of diabetes or no evidence of retinopathy in a patient with evidence of renal dysfunction should lead the clinician to consider other renal diseases.

REASONS TO CONSIDER OTHER RENAL DISEASES IN PATIENTS WITH DIABETES MELLITUS

Absence of albuminuria

Diabetes mellitus present for less than 5 years

Rapidly increasing serum creatinine

Presence of active urinary sediment

FIGURE 12-4. Reasons to consider other renal diseases in patients with diabetes mellitus. 1) If there is no albuminuria/proteinuria, then the patient does not have diabetic nephropathy. Less definite, but still important, considerations in the diagnosis of diabetic nephropathy are listed in Figure 12-4. 2) Worsening renal function in a patient with less than 5 years of diabetes mellitus should prompt the physician to consider other causes of renal failure. 3) Typically, the decrease in glomerular filtration rate occurs over years. If a patient has a decreasing creatinine clearance or increasing serum creatinine that occurs over weeks to months, other renal diseases should be considered. 4) The presence of an active urinary sediment (ie, the presence of such elements as red blood cells, white blood cells, and red blood cell casts) should lead the physician to consider other renal diseases. Although most patients with diabetic nephropathy have a relatively inactive urinary sediment, as many as 25% to 30% of patients with diabetic nephropathy may have hematuria and even red blood cell casts [4]. The finding of an active sediment, therefore, should alert the physician to consider other causes, but by itself it may not be a reason to strongly pursue evidence for other renal diseases.

MICROALBUMINURIA AND MACROALBUMINURIA

Definition of Microalbuminuria
  <30 mg/24 hours or >20 µg/min
  Albumin/creatinine ratio of >30 mg/g
Definition of frank albuminuria or macroalbuminuria
  > 300 mg/24 hours or >200 µg/min
Common causes of transient increases in albuminuria
  Exercise
  Pregnancy
  Poor glycemic control
  Congestive heart failure
  Hypertension
  Urinary tract infection

FIGURE 12-5. Detection of microalbuminuria. Microalbuminuria is the hallmark of early diabetic nephropathy, so all diabetic patients should be routinely screened for the presence of microalbuminuria. Although a timed urine collection is a very effective way to determine albumin excretion accurately, it is neither convenient nor cost-effective. Recent studies have shown that the albumin/creatinine ratio, obtained by measuring a spot urine sample for albumin and creatinine, is a highly accurate method for screening and following patients with diabetes mellitus [5]. The dipsticks used for the determination of protein in the urine are not sensitive enough to measure protein excretion less than 300 mg per 24 hours, however, so direct laboratory measurement of albumin is required to detect microalbuminuria. A spot measurement of albumin alone is affected by the urine volume, but normalizing to the amount of creatinine in the urine eliminates this concern. As shown, a value of 30 mg/g is suggestive of the presence of microalbuminuria. A number of studies have shown that the albumin/creatinine ratio is a highly accurate and effective test for the detection and following of patients with diabetes mellitus.

In determining the presence of microalbuminuria, causes of transient increases in albuminuria must be considered. Macroalbuminuria reflects progressive diabetic nephropathy. Increased attention to treatment (see fig. 12-21) should be given. Thus, repeat measurements of albumin excretion are recommended before labeling a patient with a diagnosis of early diabetic nephropathy.

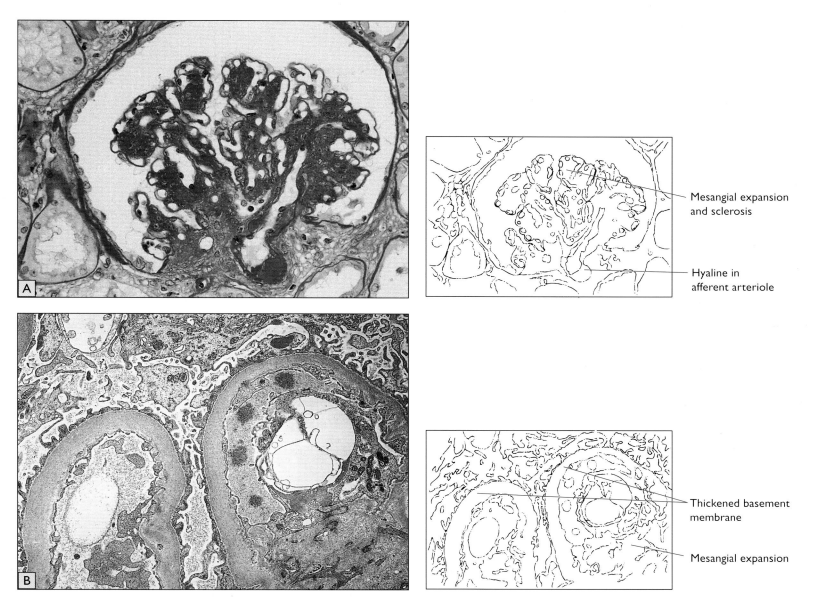

FIGURE 12-6. (*see* Color Plate) Pathology of diabetic nephropathy. Typical changes of diabetic nephropathy are seen in the light micrograph (**A**) and in the electron micrograph (**B**) [6]. *Panel A* shows nodular sclerosis, mesangial expansion, and hyaline deposition in the afferent arteriole. *Panel B* shows two capillary loops. The capillary loop on the right shows basement membrane thickening and mesangial expansion. Although these changes are typical of diabetic nephropathy, they are not pathognomonic. Two other diseases also must be considered in a patient with these renal biopsy findings: light chain deposition disease and amyloid. It is possible to differentiate among these diseases by specific stains and history. (*Courtesy of* Dr. Helmut Rennke, Boston, MA.)

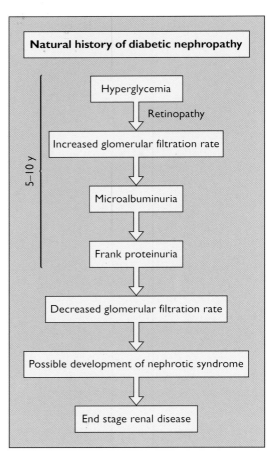

Natural history of diabetic nephropathy

5–10 y

Hyperglycemia

→ Retinopathy

Increased glomerular filtration rate

Microalbuminuria

Frank proteinuria

Decreased glomerular filtration rate

Possible development of nephrotic syndrome

End stage renal disease

FIGURE 12-7. Natural history of diabetic nephropathy. If a patient with diabetes mellitus develops microalbuminuria, the progression to renal failure tends to be inexorable unless specific interventions are done. Figure 12-7 shows the likely progression in an idealized patient. As previously noted, the presence of microalbuminuria is the first easy and reliably detectable evidence of renal failure. A patient who is going to develop renal failure usually has detectable retinopathy and will show evidence of renal failure 5 to 10 years after the diagnosis of diabetes mellitus. Interestingly, if the patient has not developed proteinuria after 15 to 20 years of diabetes, the likelihood of the development of renal disease with progression to renal failure is greatly reduced [7]. The reasons for progression are multifactorial. The ensuing figures discuss both the possible causes of the development of diabetic nephropathy and the reasons for the progression of diabetic nephropathy.

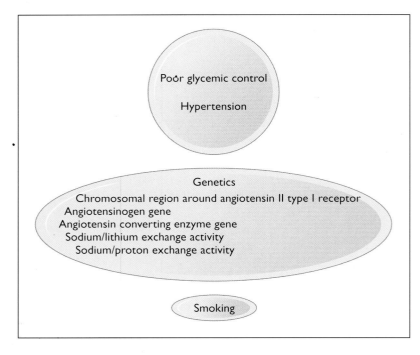

Poor glycemic control

Hypertension

Genetics

Chromosomal region around angiotensin II type I receptor
Angiotensinogen gene
Angiotensin converting enzyme gene
Sodium/lithium exchange activity
Sodium/proton exchange activity

Smoking

FIGURE 12-8. Risk factors for development of diabetic nephropathy. Poor glycemic control and hypertension have been shown to increase the likelihood of developing diabetic nephropathy [8]. Both of these factors are independently correlated with the development of diabetic nephropathy. Patients with poor glycemic control also are more likely to have hypertension than are patients with good glycemic control [8]. In addition, there has been a concerted effort to detect specific genes that predispose patients to the development of diabetic nephropathy. The existence of such genes is supported by a number of findings. A family history of diabetic nephropathy increases the likelihood of developing nephropathy [9]. In addition, certain genetically similar groups are more susceptible to nephropathy than are other groups. For example, members of the Pima Indian tribe in Arizona have a high rate of development of type 2 diabetes, and above age 45 more than 60% have developed nephropathy, a percentage that is much higher than the average [10]. Specific genes listed in this figure have been suggested to be associated with the development of nephropathy. Smoking, probably because of its deleterious effects on vascular endothelial cells, also has been shown to increase the likelihood of developing diabetic nephropathy in patients with both type 1 and type 2 diabetes mellitus [11].

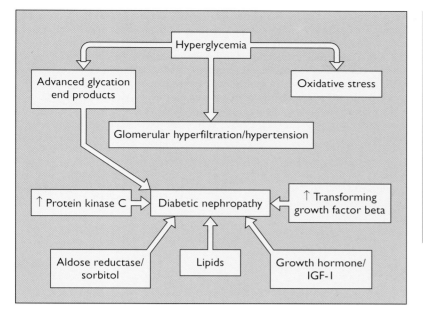

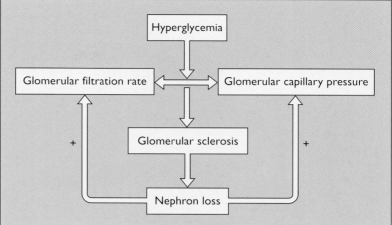

FIGURE 12-9. Suggested mechanisms underlying the development and progression of diabetic nephropathy. A number of mechanisms have been proposed to be responsible for the development of diabetic nephropathy. None of these are mutually exclusive, and it is likely that interactions of among many of these factors contribute to diabetic nephropathy. An understanding of these mechanisms is essential so that appropriate therapies may be produced to prevent both the development and progression of diabetic nephropathy. A number of existing therapies, as well as treatments currently in development or in clinical trials, are based on altering one or more of the mechanisms shown in this figure. The ensuing figures provide a brief review of each of these mechanisms.

FIGURE 12-10. Glomerular hyperfiltration. Glomerular hyperfiltration is a hallmark of diabetic nephropathy. Glomerular filtration rates (GFR) of 150 mL/min and greater are seen in early diabetic nephropathy. Zatz and coworkers were the first to show that intervention directed at decreasing hyperfiltration significantly slowed the progression of diabetic nephropathy in rats [12]. The hypothesis is that the increased GFR is associated with increased pressure in the glomerular capillary tuft. This glomerular hypertension then leads to glomerular sclerosis and loss of functioning nephrons. Although the total glomerular filtration rate eventually decreases when enough nephrons undergo sclerosis, the hypothesis suggests that the filtration and, thus, the pressure in the remaining functioning glomeruli will be high because the filtered load delivered to the kidney is the same as it was when there were more functioning glomeruli. Much research supports this general hypothesis. More importantly, efforts to use interventions that lead specifically to a reduction in glomerular capillary pressure are now mainstays of treatment for diabetic nephropathy (eg, angiotensin-converting enzyme [ACE] inhibitors and low protein diets). An extension of this hypothesis was recently suggested by Brenner and colleagues, who proposed that one predisposing factor for the progression of renal disease and possibly for the development of diabetic nephropathy is the number of glomeruli one is born with [13]. That is, the presence of fewer glomeruli would lead to relative glomerular hyperfiltration/hypertension, which would slowly lead to renal failure. This hypothesis is still controversial.

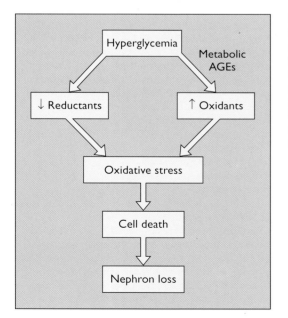

FIGURE 12-11. Oxidative stress. Many studies in both humans and animals have determined that patients with diabetes have evidence of increased oxidant stress [14]. Intracellular oxidants can increase as a result of intracellular production of oxidants or by exposure to extracellular oxidants. The cell carefully regulates the level of intracellular oxidants by a series of enzymes that reduce the oxidants. Defects in the actions of these enzymes also would contribute to an excessive level of intracellular oxidants. Hyperglycemia alone can increase the level of intracellular oxidants. Increased oxidants can cause defects in a number of intracellular events and cause cell death. In addition, increased oxidants lead to increased activity of protein kinase C (PKC), thus linking two pathophysiologic mechanisms. A number of studies currently underway are aimed at determining whether antioxidants such as vitamin E have a therapeutic role in the treatment of diabetic nephropathy.

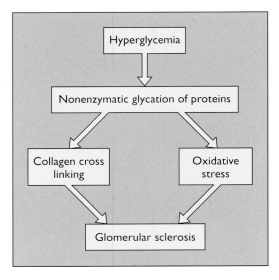

FIGURE 12-12. Advanced glycation end products. Advanced glycation end products (AGEs) are proteins that have reacted nonenzymatically with glucose. Although they exist normally, the number of AGEs increases significantly in patients with diabetic nephropathy. AGEs have been implicated in the development of complications of diabetes [15]. In particular, AGE production leads to increased oxidant stress. AGEs also can cause collagen cross-linking and, by binding to specific receptors, can lead to intracellular increases in oxidants. Administration of AGEs to animals can cause a number of changes that are seen in animals with diabetes, including glomerular sclerosis [16]. Accumulation of AGEs parallels the severity of diabetic nephropathy [17]. A number of trials currently are underway using an inhibitor of the formation of AGEs, aminoguanidine, to determine whether this drug can help patients with established nephropathy and also help prevent diabetic nephropathy.

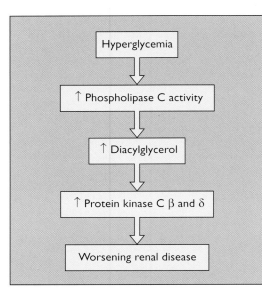

FIGURE 12-13. Protein kinase C. Protein kinase C (PKC) is a serine/threonine kinase that has been shown to play important roles in normal cell growth, in cancerous cell growth, and in a number of other intracellular processes. Work by King and associates has shown that hyperglycemia leads to activation of PKC [18]. More detailed work has demonstrated that specific isoforms of protein kinase C are specifically activated by hyperglycemia. The prevention of PKC activation may reduce mesangial expansion and prevent the progression of renal disease. The deleterious effects of PKC on the kidney may be the result of stimulation of the production of the cytokine transforming growth factor β (see Fig. 12-14). In particular, PKC β has been suggested to play an important pathophysiologic role in the development of vascular, retinal, and other complications of diabetes mellitus. Ishii and colleagues showed in diabetic rats that an inhibitor that specifically blocks PKC greatly reduced the increase in renal transforming growth factor β and also reduced the increase in other proteins associated with sclerosis [19]. This suggests that PKC inhibitors may play an important role in future treatments for diabetic nephropathy.

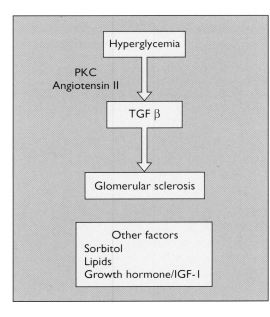

FIGURE 12-14. Transforming growth factor β. Transforming growth factor β (TGFβ) is a cytokine that can stimulate some cells to grow and inhibit the growth of other cells. Ziyadeh and colleagues have provided a strong body of work that supports the hypothesis that TGFβ is an important mediator of the lesions seen in diabetic nephropathy [20]. The suggestion that TGFβ plays a role in the pathogenesis of diabetic nephropathy is supported by the following evidence: 1) patients with diabetic nephropathy have increased levels of TGFβ; 2) TGFβ can cause glomerular sclerosis in animal models of diabetic nephropathy; and 3) neutralizing antibodies to TGFβ have prevented the development of diabetic nephropathy in an animal model. An interesting speculation is that increased activity of protein kinase C (PKC) leads to increased expression of TGFβ. Thus, hyperglycemia could be the initiating point that leads to increased oxidative stress, which leads to increased activity of PKC, which leads to increased expression of TGFβ. In addition, hyperglycemia leads to the production of AGEs. Thus, all of these mechanisms, separately and together, contribute to the development and progression of diabetic nephropathy.

Other factors have been implicated as well. Aldose reductase activity and the production of sorbitol have been implicated in diabetic nephropathy. Sorbitol is produced by the reduction of glucose by aldose reductase. Sorbitol is osmotically active, and, thus, increased sorbitol may lead to cell swelling and cell death. In addition, the action of aldose reductase leads to the loss of intracellular antioxidants, thereby increasing oxidative stress. Although increased aldose reductase activity appears to play a significant role in the pathogenesis of diabetic neuropathy, it remains to be shown whether it plays an important role in diabetic nephropathy. Epidemiologic studies have implicated increased lipids as possible mediators. Although it seems clear that increased lipids are associated with progression of diabetic nephropathy, the mechanism underlying this association has not been well defined. The important association of worsening vascular disease with increased lipids may be the mechanism by which lipids contribute to the progression of diabetic nephropathy. Lastly, a growing body of research suggests that growth hormone/IGF-1 may play an important role in the pathogenesis of diabetic nephropathy. A recent study showed a strong positive correlation between urinary levels of growth hormone and IGF-1 with the development of microalbuminuria and increased kidney size in patients with type 1 diabetes mellitus [20].

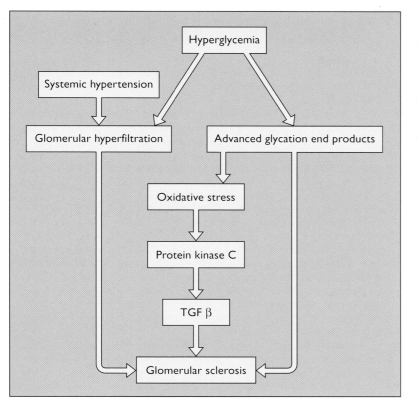

FIGURE 12-15. Possible connections between various mechanisms that may contribute to diabetic nephropathy. This model suggests that controlling the blood sugar is of paramount importance. Research from the Diabetes Control and Complications Trial (DCCT) strongly supports this idea [21]. Nevertheless, after there is evidence of diabetic nephropathy, many of these mechanisms may occur independent (to some extent) of the current blood glucose control. For example, if nephron loss has occurred, then glomerular hyperfiltration/hypertension will continue even in the presence of tight control of blood sugar. Other mechanisms shown in the figure also may become somewhat autonomous after initial damage to the glomerulus is accomplished. Thus, tight control of the blood sugar as well as other interventions that block mechanisms shown in this figure probably are needed to prevent the progression of diabetic nephropathy.

FIGURE 12-16. The efficacy in humans of various treatments for diabetic nephropathy, listed according to mechanism. As previously noted, a combined therapeutic approach probably is the most beneficial.

TREATMENT FOR DIABETIC NEPHROPATHY

Mechanism	Treatment	Efficacy in humans
Hyperglycemia	Tight control of blood sugar	Proven
Systemic hypertension	Antihypertensives agents	Proven
Glomerular hypertension	ACE inhibitors	Proven
	Calcium channel blockers	
	Low protein diet	
Lipids/cholesterol	Lipid-lowering agents	Important adjunctive therapy
Advanced glycation end products	Aminoguanidine	In trials
Oxidative stress	Antioxidants (eg, Vitamin E)	In trials
Increased protein kinase C	PKC inhibitors	Unknown
TGF β	?Antibodies to TGF β	Unknown
	PKC inhibitors	
Increased aldose reductase/sorbitol	Aldose reductase inhibitors (eg, Tolrestat)	Questionable
Growth hormone/IGF-1	No obvious therapy	Unknown

Treatment and Prevention

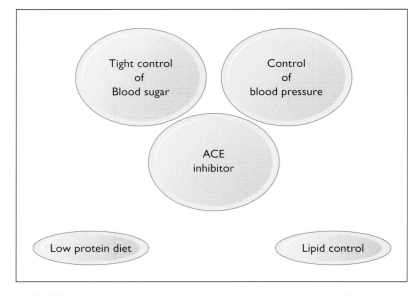

FIGURE 12-17. Treatment and prevention of diabetic nephropathy. The mainstay of prevention is tight control of the blood sugar and control of hypertension. The DCCT clearly showed that control of the blood sugar is very beneficial in preventing both the onset and the progression of diabetic nephropathy [21]. This is entirely consistent with the information presented in Figures 12-10 through 12-15 suggesting that hyperglycemia can be the predominant mechanism that leads to the activation of the other proposed mechanisms. In addition, many studies have clearly indicated that hypertension both predisposes to and worsens diabetic nephropathy [22]. Thus, before microalbuminuria has developed, all

patients should be urged to monitor blood sugars closely and to control blood pressure. The current recommendation is to aim for a blood pressure lower than 135/85 [22].

When microalbuminuria develops, the principal therapies are those shown here. In addition to tight control of the blood glucose and control of hypertension, all patients should be taking an angiotensin-converting enzyme inhibitor (ACE I). The ACE I drugs, although not a cure, have been clearly shown to slow the progression of diabetic nephropathy. These drugs reduce the levels of angiotensin II. A reduction in angiotensin II leads to a decrease in glomerular filtration and a decrease in glomerular pressure. In addition to its vasoactive properties, angiotensin II is also a growth factor. Thus, it has been proposed that ACE I drugs also work by inhibiting the growth-promoting effects of angiotensin II [23]. A new class of drugs, the angiotensin II receptor blockers (eg, Valsartan and Losartan), recently have become available. Studies are ongoing as to whether these drugs are as effective as ACE I in slowing the progression of diabetic nephropathy, but the general consensus is that they are as effective as ACE I. The angiotensin II receptor blocker drugs are especially useful in patients who develop a cough while taking ACE I. In addition, for unclear reasons, the hyperkalemia that can occur in patients taking ACE I is much less common in patients taking angiotensin II receptor blockers.

Other recommended treatments are adherence to a low-protein diet and control of lipids. A low-protein diet probably acts similarly to ACE I by decreasing intraglomerular pressure. In practical terms, it is somewhat difficult to achieve a low enough intake of protein, because the diet is rather bland. Nevertheless, it is recommended that diet counseling be done for both blood sugar control and low protein intake so that the patients do not ingest a high-protein diet that could potentially accelerate progression of renal disease. When patients are nearing end-stage renal disease, it is important for protein intake to be liberalized, because at this point there is little benefit to a low-protein diet and the risk of malnutrition is significant.

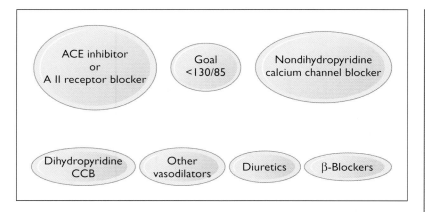

FIGURE 12-18. Antihypertensive agents. In addition to diet modifications and ACE I drugs, other antihypertensive agents play important roles in the treatment of hypertension in diabetic nephropathy. Of particular interest are the calcium channel blockers. Specifically, the nondihydropyridine calcium channel blockers (eg, diltiazem and verapamil) offer benefits in both reducing blood pressure and slowing the progression of renal disease that are similar to those provided by ACE I drugs [24]. Dihydropyridine calcium channel blockers (eg, nifedipine and amlodipine) also are useful in treating hypertension, but, alone, they do not offer the same effects on the slowing of progression of renal disease that is observed with the ACE I drugs and the nondihydropyridines. Various combinations of antihypertensive agents also have been evaluated and may offer further benefits. A combination of nondihydropyridine and ACE I may be more effective than either drug alone in slowing the progression of diabetic nephropathy [25].

Other antihypertensive agents also can be used in patients with diabetic nephropathy, such as diuretics, -blockers and vasodilators, but used alone they do not have the same effects on diabetic nephropathy as do ACE I and nondihydropyridines.

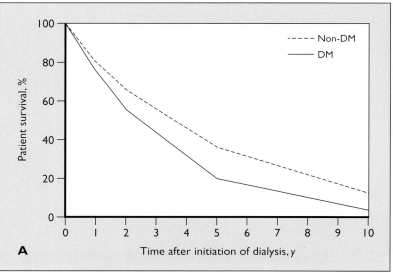

FIGURE 12-19. Survival estimates for patients on dialysis. As noted in Figure 12-1, diabetic nephropathy is the leading cause of end-stage renal disease (ESRD) in the United States. In addition, the rate of increase in ESRD resulting from diabetes is significantly greater than that for the other leading causes of renal failure. Most of this increase reflects an aging population in which type 2 diabetes mellitus is prevalent. A recent review covers the general issues of ESRD in the diabetic population [26]. Probably because of the many comorbid conditions that are present in diabetic patients, diabetic patients on dialysis (**A**) or posttransplantation

(Continued on next page)

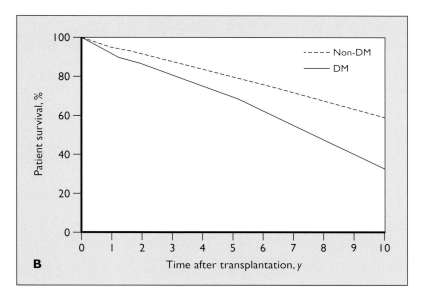

FIGURE 12-19. (*Continued*) (**B**) have a lower survival than do nondiabetic ESRD patients [26]. It is not clear whether the mode of dialysis has any effects, positive or negative, on morbidity or mortality, although most ESRD diabetic patients are treated by hemodialysis [26]. The decision to use hemodialysis versus peritoneal dialysis should be made on consideration of such factors as lifestyle, overall health of the patient, and comorbid conditions (*eg*, vision impairment). The use of peritoneal dialysis may simplify or complicate glucose management. Because peritoneal dialysate contains varying concentrations of glucose (1.5%. 2.5%, and 4.25%), glucose control can be significantly affected when dialysate exchanges occur. This problem is minimized by injecting insulin directly into the dialysate solution. This insulin delivery method can be used not only to counteract the effects of the acute exposure to the high glucose concentrations but also as a way to provide a constant level of insulin that may help in maintaining a reasonably stable blood glucose throughout the day. This method of insulin delivery is effective for overall blood glucose maintenance only for patients who do fluid exchanges during the day. Many patients prefer to do peritoneal dialysis by repeated nighttime exchanges using a machine that cycles the fluid in and out of the abdomen. During the day these patients have no fluid exchanges. The insulin injected in each bag at night is dosed to maintain a steady glucose concentration through the night, and the patient follows a standard schedule of subcutaneous injections throughout the day. DM— diabetes mellitus. (*Data from* U. S. Renal Data System [28].)

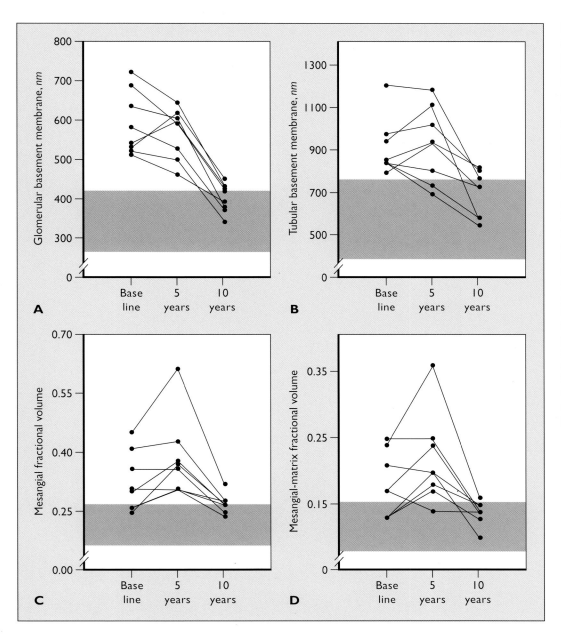

FIGURE 12-20. Kidney and pancreas transplantation. Kidney or kidney/pancreas transplantation generally is believed to be the preferred therapy for ESRD patients. Survival rates after transplantation are higher than those for patients who remain on dialysis (see Fig. 12-19). Diabetic nephropathy recurs in most kidney transplant recipients, however, although it usually is many years before diabetic nephropathy is severe enough to cause loss of the transplant (**A** through **D**). Loss of the transplant because of the recurrence of diabetic nephropathy is rare, therefore.

Pancreas transplantation usually is done only in conjunction with a kidney transplant. It has been believed that because blood glucose levels can be controlled with insulin, pancreas transplantation offers too many risks as compared to benefits. The biggest risks relate to immunosuppression and the increased risk of life-threatening infections. In addition, there has been little evidence showing that early pancreas transplant would affect the progression of diabetic nephropathy. An intriguing study by Fioretto and coworkers shows, however, that pancreas transplant alone can cause actual reversal in the lesions of diabetic nephropathy that become evident only after 5 years of normoglycemia [27]. This intriguing finding may increase interest in pancreas transplant as a way to prevent the development of diabetic nephropathy. (*From* Fioretto *et al.* [27]; with permission.)

JOSLIN DIABETES CENTER SCREENING AND TREATMENT RECOMMENDATIONS FOR MICRO- AND MACROPROTEINURIA

Screening:

Screen for microalbuminuria by checking for albumin/creatinine ratio (A/C):

Annually in patients 10-65 years of age

As clinically indicated in patients > 65 years of age.

Continue use of routine urinalysis as clinically indicated.

Treatment:

If A/C ratio < 20 μg/mg (30 mg/24 h)

Recheck in 1 year

If A/C ratio 20-300 μg/mg (30–300 mg/24 h)

Confirm presence of microalbuminuria with at least 2 positive collections of 3 done within 3–6 mo. In the process rule out confounding factors that cause false positive results, eg urinary tract infection, pregnancy, excessive exercise.

Once confirmed:

Initiate/modify use of ACE inhibitor. Consider use for type 2 diabetes. If side effects to ACE inhibitor occur, consider angiotensin II receptor antagonist treatment.

Initiate/modify hypertension treatment with a goal blood pressure under 130/85mm Hg or MAP < 90

Encourage home blood pressure monitoring.

Refer to diabetes education.

Refer to registered dietician for dietary management.

Strive to improve glycemic control with an optimal goal HbA1c < 8% or as otherwise clinically indicated.

Monitor serum creatinine and potassium, and treat appropriately.

Repeat A/C ratio testing at least every 12 mo. Consider testing more often when changes in medication are made.

If A/C ratio > 300 μg/mg (> 300 mg/24 h) or overt proteinuria

Follow all guidelines as stated for A/C ratio 20–300 μg/mg

Consider a consultation with nephrology team when:

A/C ratio is > 300 μg/mg

Rapid rise in creatinine (eg, 0.8 to 1.4 in 12 mo); presence of hematuria, or sudden increase in proteinuria

Questioning etiology of nephropathy

For refinement of treatment program to prevent further decline in renal function.

Refer to renal team for collaborative care when:

Creatinine is elevated (> 1.8 women, > 2.0 in men)

Problems with ACE inhibitors, difficulties in management of hypertension or hyperkalemia

FIGURE 12-21. Screening and treatment recommendations for proteinuria. The current recommendations for treatment for proteinuria at the Joslin Diabetes Center in Boston, Massachusetts are based on the level of proteinuria. The physicians at the Joslin Diabetes Center believe that a collaborative model of care is best for the patient with diabetes. Thus, patients with early diabetic nephropathy are cared for primarily by an endocrinologist in consultation with a nephrologist. When patients near end-stage renal disease, much of the care of the patient transfers to the nephrologist, but the other caregivers (eg, endocrinologist, ophthalmologist, dietitian) continue to work collaboratively to care for the patient.

References

1. Ruggenenti P, Remuzzi G: Nephropathy of type-2 diabetes mellitus. *J Am Soc Nephrol* 1998, 9:2157–2169.

2. Agodoa LY: U.S. Renal Data System, USRDS 1998 Annual Data Report. In *NIH, National Institute of Diabetes and Digestive and Kidney Diseases,* 1998:23–36

3. Stephenson JM, Fuller JH, Viberti GC, *et al.*: EURODIAB IDDM complications study group. Blood pressure, retinopathy, and urinary albumin excretion in IDDM. *Diabetologia* 1995, 38:599–603.

4. Chihara J, Takebayashi S, Takashi T, *et al.*: Glomerulonephritis in diabetic patients and its effect on the prognosis. *Nephron* 1986, 43:45–49.

5. Warram JH, Krowleski AS: Use of the albumin/creatinine ratio in patient care and clinical studies. In *The Kidney and Hypertension in Diabetes Mellitus.* Edited by Mogensen CE. London: Kluwer Academic Publishers, 1998: 85–96

6. Tisher CC, Hostetter TH: Diabetic nephropathy. In *Renal Pathology*, edn 2. Edited by Tisher CC, Brenner BM. Philadelphia: JB Lippincott; 1994:1387–1412.

7. Parving HH, Hommel E, Mathiesen E, *et al.*: Prevalence of microalbuminuria, arterial hypertension, retinopathy, and neuropathy in patients with insulin dependent diabetes. *Br Med J* 1988, 296:156–160.

8. Krolewski AS, Fogarty DG, Warram JH: Hypertension and nephropathy in diabetes mellitus: what is inherited and what is acquired? *Diab Res Clin Practice* 1998, 39(suppl):S1–S14.

9. Quinn M, Angelico MC, Warram JH, *et al.*: Familial factors determine the development of diabetic nephropathy in patients with IDDM. *Diabetologia* 1996, 39:940–945.

10. Nelson RG, Newman JM, Knowler WC, *et al.*: Incidence of end stage renal disease in Type 2 (non-insulin dependent) diabetes mellitus in Pima Indians. *Diabetologia* 1988, 31:730–736.

11. Biesenbach G, Grafinger P, Janko O, *et al.*: Influence of cigarette-smoking on the progression of clinical diabetic nephropathy in type 2 diabetic patients. *Clin Nephrol* 1997, 48:146–150.

12. Zatz R, Rentz DB, Meyer TW, *et al.*: Prevention of diabetic glomerulopathy by pharmacological amelioration of glomerular capillary hypertension. *J Clin Invest* 1986, 77:1925–1930.

13. Brenner B, Mackenzie HS: Nephron mass as risk factor for the progression of renal disease. Kidney Int 1997, 63(suppl) :S124–S127.

14. Giugliano D, Ceriello A, Paolissa G: Oxidative stress and diabetic vascular complications. *Diabetes Care* 1996, 19:257–267.

15. Bierhaus A, Hofmann MA, Ziegler R, *et al.*: AGEs and their interaction with AGE-receptors in vascular disease and diabetes mellitus. I. The AGE concept. *Cardiovasc Res* 1998, 37:586–600.

16. Vlassara H, Striker LJ, Teichberg S, *et al.*: Advanced glycation end products induce glomerular sclerosis and albuminuria in normal rats. *Proc Natl Acad Sci U S A* 1994, 91:11704–11708.

17. Makita Z, Radoff S, Rayfield EJ, *et al.*: Advanced glycation end products in patients with diabetic nephropathy. *N Engl J Med* 1991, 325:836–842.

18. Koya D, King GL: Protein kinase C activation and the development of diabetic complications. *Diabetes* 1998, 47:859–866.

19. Ishii H, Jirousek MR, Koya D, *et al.*: Ameliorations of vascular dysfunctions in diabetic rats by an oral PKC beta inhibitor. *Science* 1996, 272:728–731.

20. Hoffman BB, Sharma K, Ziyadeh FN: Potential role of TGF-β in diabetic nephropathy. *Min Electrol Metab* 1998, 24:190–196.

21. The Diabetes Control and Complications Trial Research Group: The effect of intensive treatment of diabetes on the development and progression of long-term complications in insulin-dependent diabetes mellitus. *N Engl J Med* 1993, 329:977–986.

22. Bakris GL: Progression of diabetic nephropathy. A focus on arterial pressure level and methods of reduction. *Diab Res Clin Prac* 1998,39(Suppl):S35–S42.

23. Wolf G, Ziyadeh FN: The role of angiotensin II in diabetic nephropathy: emphasis on nonhemodynamic mechanisms. *Am J Kidney Dis* 1997, 29:153–163.

24. Slataper R, Vicknair N, Sadler R, *et al.*: Comparative effects of different antihypertensive treatments on progression of diabetic renal disease. *Arch Int Med* 1993, 153:973–979.

25. Bakris GL, Weir MR, DeQuattro V, *et al.*: Effects of an ACE inhibitor/ calcium antagonist combination on proteinuria in diabetic nephropathy. *Kidney Int* 1998, 54:1283–1289.

26. Williams ME: The diabetic patient with end stage renal disease. In *Therapy in Nephrology and Hypertension.* Edited by Brady HR, Wilcox CS. Philadelphia: WB Saunders; 1999:249–255.

27. Fioretto P, Steffes MW, Sutherland DER, *et al.*: Reversal of lesions of diabetic nephropathy after pancreas transplantation. *N Engl J Med* 1998, 339:69–75.

28. U. S. Renal Data System: *USRDS 1996 Annual Data Report.* Bethesda, MD: The National Institutes of Health, National Institute of Diabetes and Digestive and Kidney Diseases. April 1996.

DIABETIC NEUROPATHIES

Aaron Vinik

Diabetic neuropathy is not a single entity but rather a number of different syndromes, each with a range of clinical and subclinical manifestations. According to the San Antonio Conference [1], the main groups of neurologic disturbance in diabetes mellitus include subclinical neuropathy determined by abnormalities in electrodiagnostic and quantitative sensory testing, diffuse clinical neuropathy with distal symmetric sensorimotor and autonomic syndromes, and focal syndromes. There is reason to add proximal neuropathy as a separate entity based on the nature of the pathology and response to treatment. However, we have found it more appropriate to classify neuropathy into different clinical syndromes based on their pathogenesis because this is what ultimately determines the choice of treatment. We classify neuropathies into somatic and autonomic. There are two types of autonomic neuropathy, focal and diffuse. The focal neuropathies are mononeuritis and entrapment syndromes. The diffuse neuropathies are proximal neuropathies and large- and small-fiber distal symmetric polyneuropathies.

Estimates of the prevalence of diabetic neuropathy range from 10% to 90% of the diabetic population, depending on the criteria used to define neuropathy [1–6]. Neurologic complications occur equally in patients with type 1 and type 2 diabetes mellitus, as well as various forms of acquired diabetes.

In this pictorial overview, clinical presentations and therapeutic approaches to common forms of neuropathy are presented and discussed, including distal symmetric, proximal motor, and autonomic neuropathies. Also provided are algorithms for recognition and management of common pain and entrapment syndromes. A global approach is used for recognition of syndromes requiring specialized treatments based on our improved understanding of their etiopathogenesis.

Pathogenesis

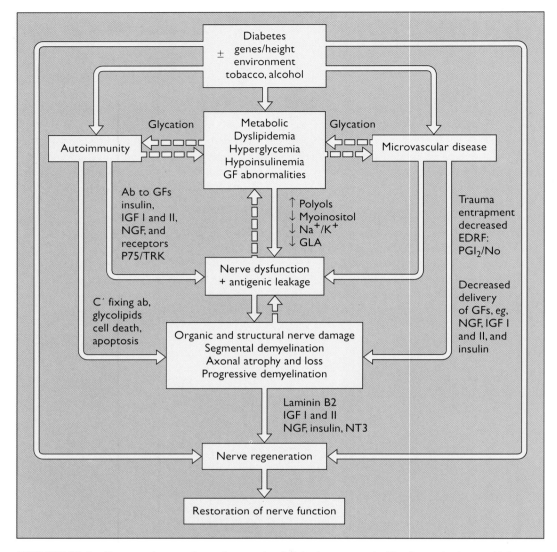

Diabetes
± genes/height
environment
tobacco, alcohol

Glycation

Glycation

Autoimmunity

Metabolic
Dyslipidemia
Hyperglycemia
Hypoinsulinemia
GF abnormalities

Microvascular disease

Ab to GFs
insulin,
IGF I and II,
NGF, and
receptors
P75/TRK

↑ Polyols
↓ Myoinositol
↓ Na$^+$/K$^+$
↓ GLA

Trauma
entrapment
decreased
EDRF:
PGI$_2$/No

Nerve dysfunction
+ antigenic leakage

C´ fixing ab,
glycolipids
cell death,
apoptosis

Decreased
delivery
of GFs, eg,
NGF, IGF I
and II, and
insulin

Organic and structural nerve damage
Segmental demyelination
Axonal atrophy and loss
Progressive demyelination

Laminin B2
IGF I and II
NGF, insulin, NT3

Nerve regeneration

Restoration of nerve function

FIGURE 13-1. Current view on the pathogenesis of diabetic neuropathy. The figure depicts multiple causes, as discussed above, including metabolic, vascular, autoimmune, and neurohormonal growth factor deficiency. Although there is increasing evidence that the pathogenesis of diabetic neuropathy comprises several mechanisms, the prevailing theory implicates persistent hyperglycemia as the primary factor within the metabolic hypothesis [7,8]. Persistent hyperglycemia increases polyol pathway activity with accumulation of sorbitol and fructose in nerves, damaging them by an as yet unknown mechanism. This is accompanied by decreased myoinositol uptake and inhibition of the sodium-potassium ion adenosine triphosphatase pathway, resulting in sodium retention, edema, myelin swelling, axoglial disjunction and nerve degeneration. Deficiency of dihomo γ linoleic acid (GLA) as well as N acetyl L carnitine also have been implicated [9]. Metabolic factors cannot account for all forms of neuropathy nor for the heterogeneity of the clinical syndromes. In a subpopulation of patients with neuropathy, immune mechanisms may be responsible for the

clinical syndrome, especially in patients with the proximal variety of neuropathy and those with a more marked motor component to their neuropathy. Our data support the hypothesis that circulating antineuronal antibodies are present in diabetic serum, at least in some patients. The circulating autoantibodies directed against motor and sensory nerve structures have been detected by indirect immunofluorescence, and antibody and complement deposits in various components of sural nerves have been shown [10–12].

Microvascular insufficiency has been proposed by a number of investigators as a possible cause of diabetic neuropathy [13–15]. The interest in microvascular derangement in patients with diabetic neuropathy has arisen from studies, suggesting that absolute or relative ischemia may exist in the nerves of patients with diabetes owing to altered function of the endoneurial or epineurial blood vessels, or both. Histopathologic studies show the presence of different degrees of endoneurial and epineurial microvasculopathy, mainly thickening of blood vessel wall or occlusion [16,17]. A number of functional disturbances have also been demonstrated in the microvasculature of the nerves of patients with diabetes. Studies have demonstrated decreased neural blood flow, increased vascular resistance, decreased oxygen pressure and altered vascular permeability characteristics such as a loss of the anionic charge barrier and decreased charge selectivity [18-20]. It also has been shown that abnormalities of cutaneous blood flow correlate with neuropathy [21].

Apart from the metabolic, immunologic and vascular factors involved in the pathogenesis of neuropathy, data exist to support a role for growth factor deficiency. Many of the neuronal changes characteristic of diabetic neuropathy are similar to those observed following either removal of target-derived growth factors by axotomy or depletion of endogenous growth factors by experimental induction of growth factor autoimmunity. Because neuronal growth factors can promote the survival, maintenance, and regeneration of neurons subject to the noxious effects of diabetes, the success of patients with diabetes in maintaining normal nerve morphology and function may ultimately depend on the expression and efficacy of these factors [9]. Ab— antibody; EDRF—endothelium-derived relaxing factor; GF—growth factor; IGF—insulin-like growth factor; NGF—neuronal growth factor; NO—nitric oxide; NT3—neurotropin 3; PGI$_2$—prostaglandin I$_2$.

Mononeuropathy and Entrapment

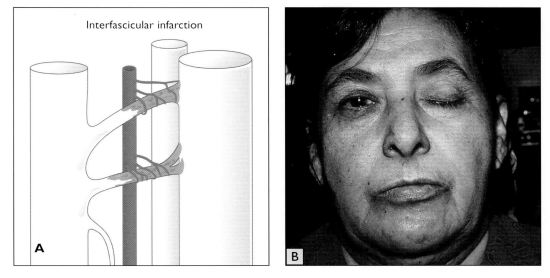

Interfascicular infarction

A

B

Medial and lateral plantar entrapments decrease sensation in the inside and outside of the foot, respectively. The entrapment neuropathies are highly prevalent in the diabetic population and should be actively sought in every patient with signs and symptoms of neuropathy because the treatment may be surgical [23].

Carpal tunnel syndrome occurs twice as frequently in a diabetic population compared with a normal healthy population. Its increased prevalence in patients with diabetes may be related to repeated undetected trauma, metabolic changes, or accumulation of fluid or edema within the confined space of the carpal tunnel [22]. If recognized, the diagnosis can be confirmed by an electrophysiologic study, and therapy is simple with surgical release. The unaware physician seldom realizes that symptoms may spread to the whole hand or arm in carpal tunnel syndrome, and the signs may extend beyond those subserved by the entrapped nerve. Thus, the very nature of the trouble goes unrecognized, and an opportunity for successful therapeutic intervention often is missed. The mainstays of nonsurgical treatment are avoidance of the use of the wrist, placement of a wrist splint in a neutral position for day and night use, and anti-inflammatory medications. Surgical treatment consists of sectioning the volar carpal ligament. The decision to proceed with surgery should be based on several considerations, including severity of symptoms, appearance of motor weakness. and failure of nonsurgical treatment.

FIGURE 13-2. Focal neuropathies: mononeuritis and entrapment syndromes. Mononeuropathies are due to vasculitis and subsequent ischemia or infarction of nerves (A) [22]. Mononeuropathies heal spontaneously, usually within 6 to 8 weeks. The isolated peripheral nerve lesions involve particularlyu lnar, median. radial, femoral, and lateral cutaneous nerves of the thigh. In mononeuropathies in which weakness is a prominent feature, such asperoneal palsy, physical therapy may be necessary to maintain good muscle tone and prevent contractures.

The common mononeuropathies (B) involve cranial nerves 3, 4, 6 and 7; and thoracic and peripheral nerves including peroneal, sural, sciatic, femoral, ulnar, and median. Their onset is acute and associated with pain and their course is self-limiting, resolving over a period of 6 weeks. The common mononeuropathies must be distinguished from entrapment syndromes, which start slowly, progress, and persist without intervention. Common entrapments involve the median nerve with impaired sensation in the first three fingers and a positive Tinel sign. Ulnar entrapment decreases sensory perception in the little and ring fingers.

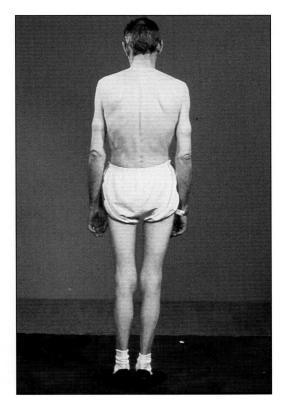

FIGURE 13-3. Proximal motor neuropathy can be identified clinically based on proximal muscle weakness and muscle wasting. This neuropathy may be symmetric or asymmetric in distribution and is sometimes associated with pain in the lateral aspect of the thighs [24,25]. The condition is readily recognizable clinically. Prevailing weakness of the iliopsoas, obturator, and adductor muscles is observed together with relative preservation of the gluteus maximus and minimus, and hamstrings [24,25]. Those affected have great difficulty rising out of a chair unaided and often climb up their bodies. Heel or toe standing is surprisingly good. In the classic form of diabetic amyotrophy, axonal loss is the predominant process, and the condition coexists with distal sensory polyneuropathy [10]. Electrophysiologic evaluation reveals lumbosacral plexopathy [11]. In contrast, if demyelination predominates and the motor deficit affects proximal and distal muscle groups, the diagnosis of chronic inflammatory demyelinating polyneuropathy should be considered [11,12]. It is important to divide proximal syndromes into these two subcategories because the CIDP variant responds dramatically to intervention [12], whereas amyotrophy runs its own course over months to years. Until more evidence is available, we consider them to be separate syndromes. Another frequently seen focal syndrome is multifocal, predominantly sensory neuropathy, which easily can be identified based on clinical evaluation. (*From* Chia *et al.* [26]; with permission.)

Distal Neuropathy

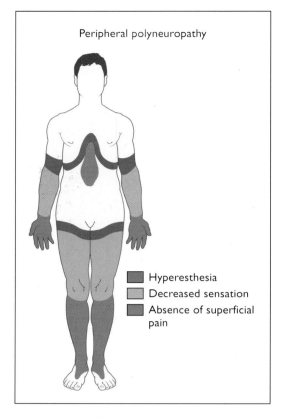

Peripheral polyneuropathy

■ Hyperesthesia
□ Decreased sensation
■ Absence of superficial pain

FIGURE 13-4. Peripheral polyneuropathy. The spectra of clinical neuropathic syndromes described in patients with diabetes mellitus include dysfunction of almost every segment of the somatic peripheral and autonomic nervous systems [22]. Each syndrome can be distinguished by its pathophysiologic, therapeutic, and prognostic features. Initial neurologic evaluation should be directed toward detection of the specific part of the nervous system affected by diabetes. Diabetes may damage small fibers, large fibers, or both. Small nerve fiber dysfunction usually, but not always, occurs early and often is present before objective signs or electrophysiologic evidence of nerve damage is found [27–29]. Small nerve fiber dysfunction is manifested first in the lower limbs by pain and hyperalgesia. Loss of thermal sensitivity follows, with reduced light touch and pinprick sensation. Large fiber neuropathies may involve sensory or motor nerves, or both. The neuropathies are manifested by reduced vibration (often the first objective evidence of neuropathy) and position sense, weakness, muscle wasting, and depressed tendon reflexes. Most patients with distal sensory polyneuropathy have a mixed variety, with both large and small nerve fiber involvement. In the case of distal sensory polyneuropathy, a "glove and stocking" distribution of sensory loss is almost universal [22]. Early in the course of the neuropathic process, multifocal sensory loss may also be found.

Diabetic peripheral symmetric polyneuropathy is thought to be a dying-back disorder, with prevailing effects on the axons and consequent demyelination. There is an early functional phase in which metabolic abnormalities are responsible for the clinical symptoms and signs. Later structural changes occur in the nerves so that treatment strategies have been to arrest or slow the rate of progression. When neuronal cell death occurs, little can be done to induce recovery. Clearly, all attempts at treating neuropathy should be oriented toward the reversible phase of the disorder.

Components of Cutaneous Nerve

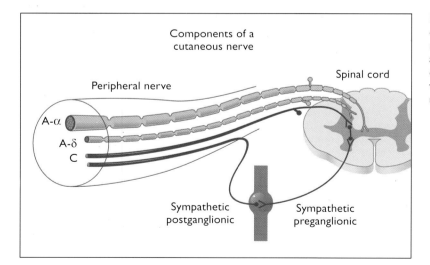

Components of a cutaneous nerve

Spinal cord

Peripheral nerve

A-α
A-δ
C

Sympathetic postganglionic
Sympathetic preganglionic

FIGURE 13-5. Cutaneous nerve components. Peripheral nerves are comprised of several different types of nerve fibers, each with their own function. The large myelinated α fibers conduct rapidly and subserve motor power and proprioception and coordination. The thinner yet myelinated A-δ fibers subserve cold thermal detection and deep-seated pain. The thin unmyelinated fibers are responsible for warm detection threshold, heat pain, part of touch sensation, and sympathetic nerve supply to the skin.

Large Fiber Neuropathy

CLINICAL PRESENTATION AND MANAGEMENT OF LARGE FIBER NEUROPATHY

Presentation
Impaired vibration perception
Pain of A-δ type: deep-seated, gnawing
Ataxia
Wasting of small muscles, intrinsic minus feet with hammer toes
Weakness
Increased blood flow, the hot foot
  Risk: Charcot neuroarthropathy
Management
  Proper shoes
  Orthotics
  Tendon lengthening
  Foot reconstruction

FIGURE 13-6. Clinical presentation and management of large fiber neuropathy.

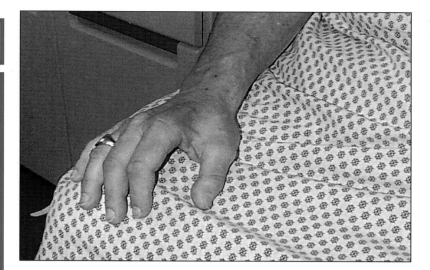

FIGURE 13-7. Wasting of the small muscle of the hand in large fiber neuropathies. This must not be mistaken for ulnar entrapment, which is amenable to treatment. In large fiber neuropathies all peripheral nerves are affected equally and the sensory disturbance is of the "glove and stocking" variety not confined to the nerve distribution. In ulnar entrapment the sensory loss involves the ring and little fingers.

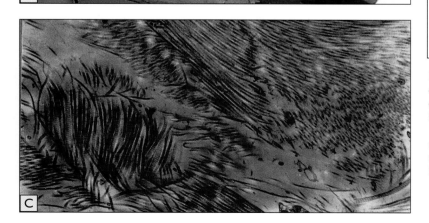

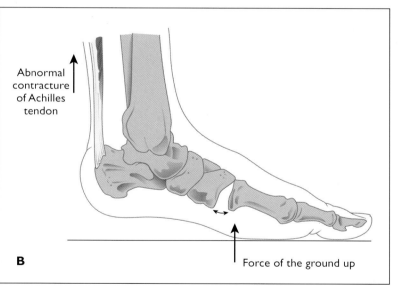

FIGURE 13-8. In large fiber neuropathies there is wasting of the small muscles of the feet: intrinsic minus feet as well as talipes equinovarus owing to shortening of the Achilles tendon **A**, Measurement of the angle of the ankle in full flexion. Using a goniometer the flexion should be at least 90 degrees. **B**, Greater than 100 degrees indicates tendo-achilles shortening, with its impact on increasing midfoot pressure and breakdown of Lisfranc's joint in the midfoot. **C**, Electron micrograph of disrupted collagen fibers in the Achilles tendon in a patient with large nerve neuropathy.

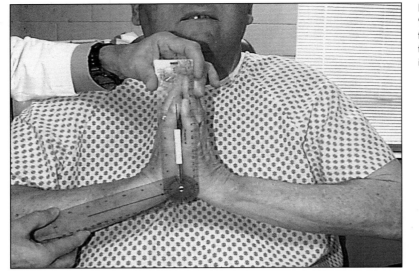

FIGURE 13-9. The patient is unable to extend his hands at the wrist to beyond 90 degrees, as shown using the goniometer. Note the separation of the small fingers creating a diamond-shaped open space indicative of cheiroarthropathy. These features accompany large fiber neuropathies as well as entrapment syndromes. This is not universal and the two conditions may well have different causes.

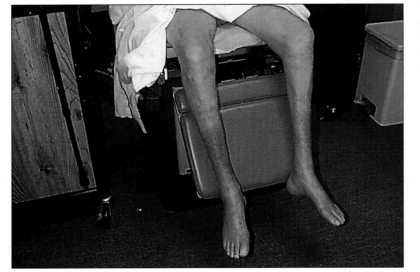

FIGURE 13-10. The patient shows a combination of severe muscle wasting of the lower limbs resembling that seen in Charcot-Marie-Tooth disease, the equinus of the feet owing to shortening of the Achilles tendon and wasting of the proximal muscles of the thigh owing to a combination of a proximal neuropathy and a distal large fiber neuropathy.

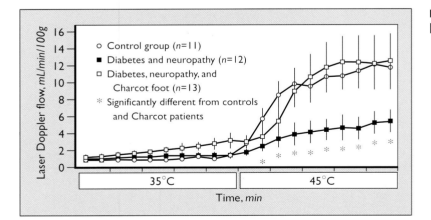

FIGURE 13-11. Neurovascular dysfunction in neuropathy. (*From* Shapiro *et al.* [30]; with permission.)

C-Fiber Dysfunction in Small Fiber Neuropathy

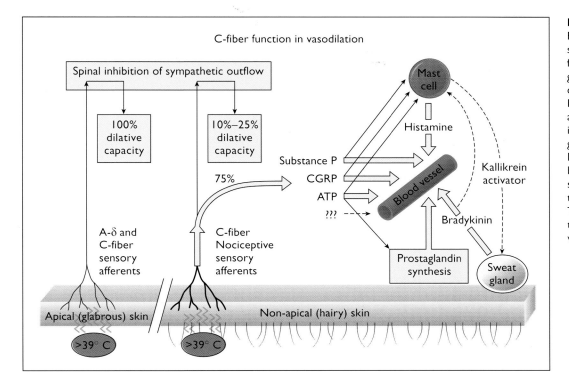

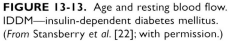

FIGURE 13-12. Vasodilation and C-fiber function. Factors controlling vasodilation in glabrous skin such as that found on the pads and soles hairy skin found on the dorsum of the feet and hands. In glabrous skin, vasodilation is for the most part a consequence of relaxation of the sympathetic tone. In hairy skin, C fibers are essential for vasodilation, a process mediated by a variety of neurotransmitters including the neuropeptides, substance P, and calcitonin gene-related peptide (CGRP) as well as bradykinin. Defective trophic support for skin with reduced levels of neuronal growth factor result in decreased substance P and CGRP, thereby impairing the ability to dilate in response to noxious stimuli and heat. Thus nutrient delivery is compromised and susceptibility to ulceration. (*From* Burnstock and Ralvic [31]; with permission.)

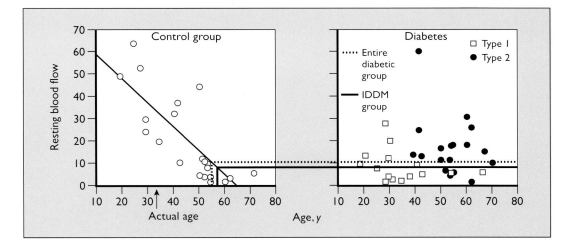

FIGURE 13-13. Age and resting blood flow. IDDM—insulin-dependent diabetes mellitus. (*From* Stansberry et al. [22]; with permission.)

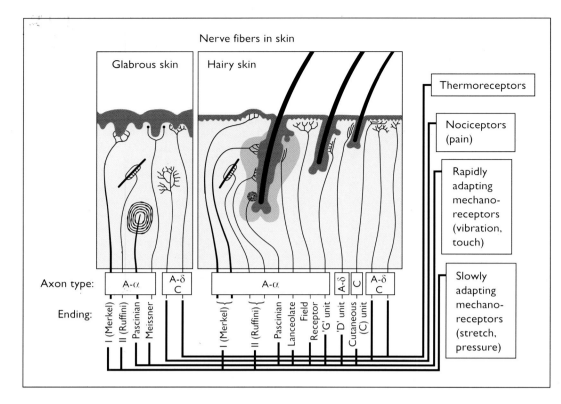

Nerve fibers in skin

| Glabrous skin | Hairy skin |

Axon type:

Ending:

Thermoreceptors

Nociceptors (pain)

Rapidly adapting mechano-receptors (vibration, touch)

Slowly adapting mechano-receptors (stretch, pressure)

FIGURE 13-14. Different nerve fibers in skin and their different roles in sensory perception and mechanoreceptor function. C-fiber type pain generally is described as throbbing, shooting, stabbing, sharp, hot, burning, and tender. Touch is misinterpreted as pain, *ie*, allodynia, and patients cannot bear contact with bedclothes or other objects. In contrast, A-δ pain often is described as cramping, gnawing, aching, heavy, splitting, tiring and exhausting, sickening, fearful, and punishing and cruel. A patient may say, "I have toothache in my foot," "there is a dog gnawing at the bones of my feet," or "my feet feel as if they are encased in concrete." These pains derive from different fibers and have a different mechanism of production. The scheme is based on this information, which proves helpful in the management of patients with neuropathic pain.

Pain disappears when a loss of C-fibers occurs, and the loss heralds the phase of hypoalgesia, and hypesthesia, with impairment of warm thermal perception and insensitivity to heat pain. These symptoms are particularly dangerous and are the forerunners of repeated minor injury and subsequent loss of toes and feet.

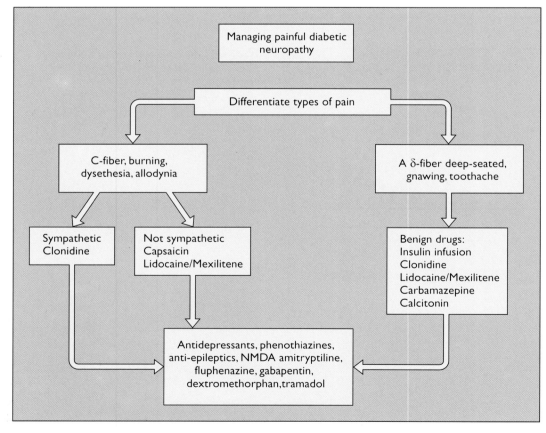

Managing painful diabetic neuropathy

Differentiate types of pain

C-fiber, burning, dysethesia, allodynia

A δ-fiber deep-seated, gnawing, toothache

Sympathetic Clonidine

Not sympathetic Capsaicin Lidocaine/Mexilitene

Benign drugs: Insulin infusion Clonidine Lidocaine/Mexilitene Carbamazepine Calcitonin

Antidepressants, phenothiazines, anti-epileptics, NMDA amitryptiline, fluphenazine, gabapentin, dextromethorphan, tramadol

FIGURE 13-15. Managing painful diabetic neuropathy.

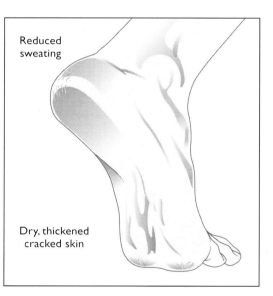

Reduced sweating

Dry, thickened cracked skin

FIGURE 13-16. Clinical presentation of small fiber neuropathy. This signs of this disorder include pain (C-fiber type, burning and superficial), late hypoalgesia, hypoesthesia impaired warm thermal perception decreased sweating, and impaired cutaneous blood flow (the cold foot). The risks are foot ulcers, gangrene, and amputations.

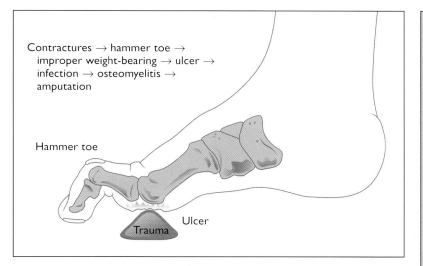

Contractures → hammer toe → improper weight-bearing → ulcer → infection → osteomyelitis → amputation

Hammer toe

Ulcer

Trauma

FIGURE 13-17. Management of small fiber neuropathies. In the United States, 65,000 amputations are performed each year. Half of these are attributable to diabetes and small fiber neuropathy is implicated in 87% of cases. The combination of decreased pain perception with decreased warm thermal perception and the resulting hammer toe deformity that follows intrinsic minus feet leads to blisters on the top of the knuckles of the toes or ulcers over the heads of the metatarsals. These high-pressure points are easily recognized by forced gate analysis (F) scans of the feet. With correct shoes, padded socks and orthotics, the likelihood of amputation can be reduced by half. Patients should be instructed to protect their feet with padded socks, wear shoes that have adequate support, regularly inspect their feet and shoes, be careful of exposure to heat, and to use emollient creams for sympathetic dysfunction.

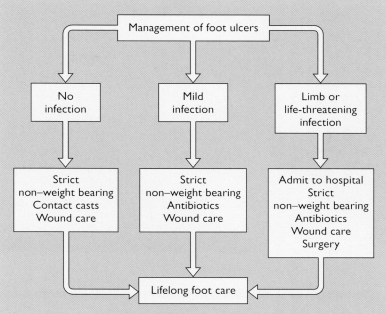

FIGURE 13-18. Management of foot ulcers.

Neuroarthropathy

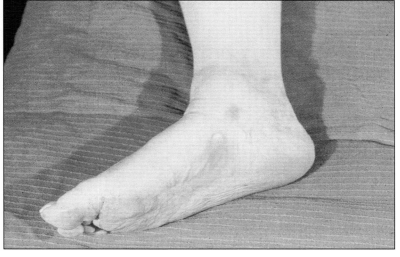

FIGURE 13-19. (*see* Color Plate) The hot foot of Charcot neuroarthropathy showing the end result of large fiber neuropathy. Note the red inflamed foot that is easily mistaken for infection and the collapse of the midfoot.

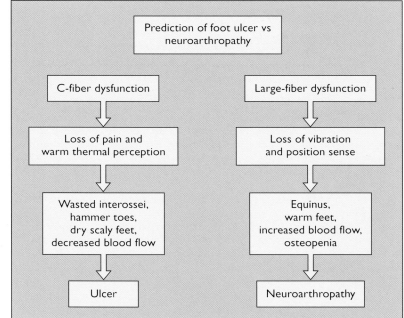

FIGURE 13-20. Prediction of foot ulcers vs. neuroarthropathy.

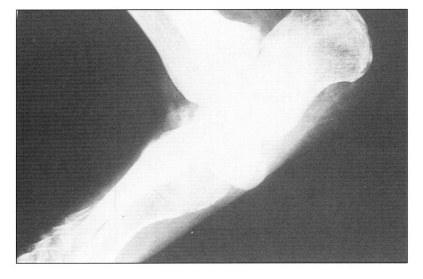

FIGURE 13-21. Radiograph of the foot shown in Figure 14-19. Note the rarefaction and osteopenia of the calcaneus with collapse of the midfoot and loss of architecture of the foot. These results of large fiber neuropathy and increased blood flow could have been prevented if recognized early.

Autonomic Neuropathy

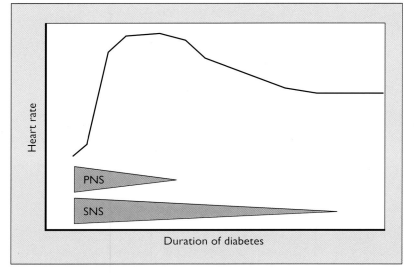

FIGURE 13-22. Model of the effects of autonomic neuropathy on heart rate. The rule in diabetic neuropathy is that the longest fibers are affected early and more severely. In the autonomic nervous system the longest fibers are those in the vagus (parasympathetic nervous system) nerves. Thus, the earliest observations in people with autonomic neuropathy of the cardiovascular system is an increase in heart rate.

Later as the short efferent fibers of the sympathetic nervous system (SNS) become involved the heart rate slows down, but not to normal. It is indeed a denervated heart. With loss of the afferent fibers there also is loss of pain perception, accounting for the high incidence of painless myocardial infarctions in patients with diabetic neuropathy. (*From* Ewing [33]; with permission.)

FIGURE 13-23. RR intervals and effects of cardiac autonomic dysfunction. The most sensitive indicator of cardiac autonomic neuropathy is the loss of the normal sinus arrhythmia with breathing. This loss can be measured on an electrocardiogram as loss of the change in the RR interval with deep breathing at 6 breaths per minute and reflects almost entirely damage to the parasympathetic nervous system. With more sophisticated approaches computerized spectral analysis of the ECG tracing allows one to infer the status of the sympathetic nervous system as well. Late in the course of cardiac autonomic neuropathy the advent of *orthostasis* (a decrease in blood pressure of > 30 mm Hg when arising from a lying position) reflects sympathetic nerve damage. Peripheral measures of autonomic function are described in Figures 13-11–13-13 on blood flow in the diabetic foot.

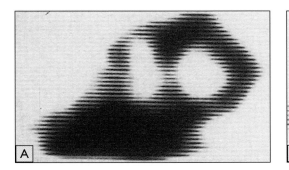
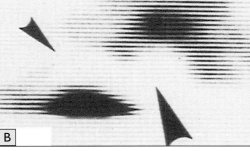
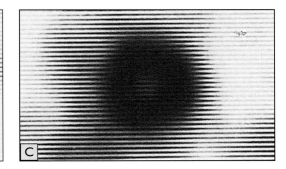

FIGURE 13-24. Segmental loss of sympathetic nerve fibers in the heart, demonstrable using meta-iodobenzylguanidine **B**. The multiple gated acquisition (MUGA) and thallium scans shown in panels **A** and **C** do not demonstrate ventricular wall defects. It is now thought that this imbalance in the sympathetic nerve supply of the myocardium is what leads to the irritable foci leading to arrhythmia and possible accounting for the sudden death in diabetic patients with autonomic neuropathy. This mechanism also is thought to operate in people who have had a myocardial infarction and may be the reason for the effectiveness of β blockade in reducing mortality in patients who have had a myocardial infarction. (*From* Kahn [34]; with permission.)

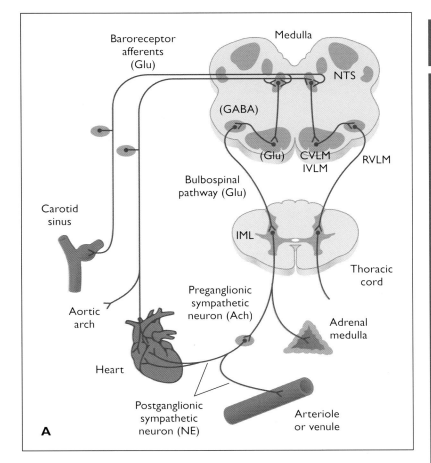

B. ORGANIZATION OF THE AUTONOMIC NERVOUS SYSTEM OF THE HEART

Eye
  Abnormal pupillary reaction, with night blindness
Cardiovascular
  Sudden death, silent myocardial infarction
  Orthostasis
  Impaired peripheral vascular reflexes
Respiratory
  Failure of hypoxia-induced respiration
Gut
  Gustatory sweating
  Gastroparesis
  Diarrhea
  Constipation
  Loss of anal sphincter tone and incontinence
Metabolic
  Hypoglycemia unawareness
  Hypoglycemia unresponsiveness
  Hypoglycemia-associated autonomic failure
Genitourinary
  Overflow incontinence
Sexual
  Males, erectile dysfunction
  Females, decreased vaginal lubrication

FIGURE 13-25. Schematic outline of the organization of the autonomic nervous system of the heart (**A**). Note that diabetes affects the afferent and efferent components of the sympathetic and parasympathetic nervous s stems and has diffuse effects throughout the body (**B**). CVLM and IVLM—paraventricular nuclei of vasomotor center; GABA—γ-aminobutyric acid; IML—intermediolateral nucleus; NTS—solitary tract nucleus; RVLM—motor nucleus of vagus.

Gastropathy

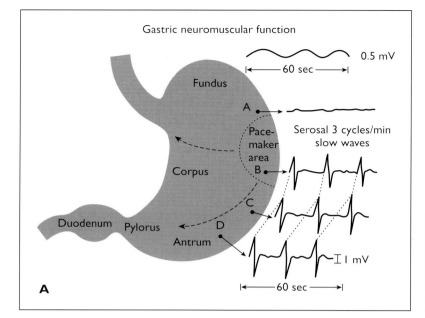

Gastric neuromuscular function

0.5 mV

|← 60 sec →|

Fundus

A →

Pace-maker area

Serosal 3 cycles/min slow waves

B →

Corpus

C →

Duodenum Pylorus D

Antrum

⊥1 mV

|← 60 sec →|

A

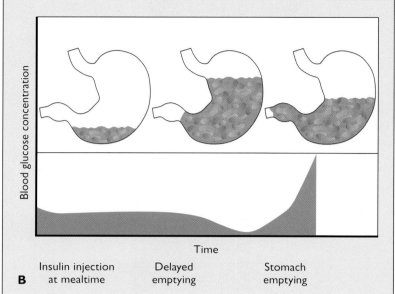

Blood glucose concentration

Time

Insulin injection at mealtime   Delayed emptying   Stomach emptying

B

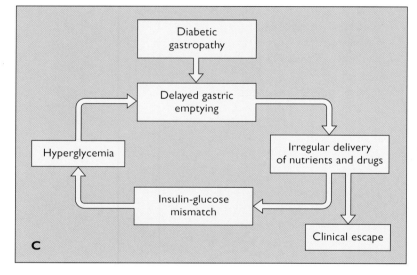

Diabetic gastropathy

↓

Delayed gastric emptying

Hyperglycemia   Irregular delivery of nutrients and drugs

Insulin-glucose mismatch

Clinical escape

C

FIGURE 13-26. Gastropathy. **A** and **B,** Gastric neuromuscular function. The stomach is a complex neuromuscular organ. It has a pacemaker that discharges rhythmic electrical impulses that initiate propulsive contractions. It is sensitive to volume, viscosity, osmolarity, caloric density, and the nature of the fuel within.

Functional disturbances may occur such as arrhythmias, tachygastria and brady-gastria, pylorospasm, and hypomotility. Organic lesions include gastroparesis. Antral dilation and obstruction, inflammation, ulceration, and bezoar formation. Gastric dysfunction should be suspected in patients with Type I and Type II diabetes; who have had diabetes for over 120 years; who display evidence of distal symmetric polyneuropathy and autonomic neuropathy; observations of brittle diabetes in patients with previously well-controlled symptoms; and symptoms of early satiety, bloating, and a succussion splash. Anorexia, nausea, vomiting, and dyspepsia are nonspecific and herald other conditions.

C, Clinical presentation of gastropathy. Many more people with gastropathy present with brittle diabetes than do those who present with gastric symptoms. In fact, it has been shown that many of the gastrointestinal symptoms of gastropathy can be nonspecific and do not reflect an abnormality in gastric emptying. The most fertile soil for discovery of those with gastric dysfunction are patients with "difficult to control diabetes." The stomach can be regarded as the coarse regulator of blood glucose concentrations, releasing fuel to the small bowel at its own predetermined rate. Any dysfunction in the bowel therefore would result in a mismatch of fuel delivery and either endogenous or exogenous insulin, thereby creating the apparent pattern of insulin resistance or brittle diabetes. Of interest is that the irregular pattern of delivery applies to drugs used in the treatment of diabetes and may confound the problem. Similar concern applies to other drugs that may fail to reach their absorptive site in the small bowel leading to clinical escape from the condition being treated. Overzealous adjustment of the insulin dose may result because the real cause may be easily overlooked.

FIGURE 13-27. Normal electrogastrogram. An electrogastrogram obtained in a normal patient showing the predominant frequency of 3 to 6 cpm.

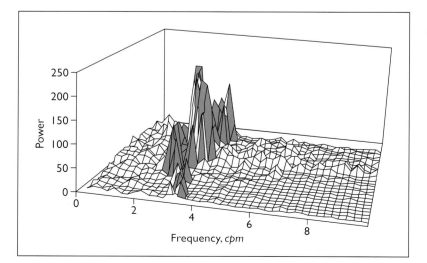

Power

250
200
150
100
50
0

0   2   4   6   8

Frequency, cpm

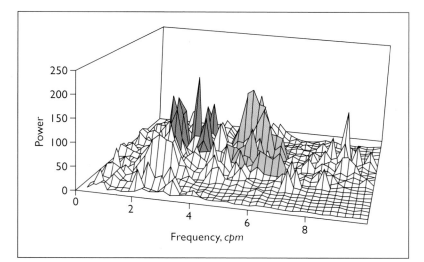

FIGURE 13-28. Hyperglycemia-induced tachygastrias. Note two peaks of activity, one at the usual frequency of 3 to 6 cpm and the major peak at over 6 cpm. Thus, hyperglycemia *per se* can markedly affect gastric function and many have made the costly error of carrying out gastric-emptying studies when the blood glucose is over 400 mg/dL. Not only does this induce tachygastria but it may inhibit the interdigestive myoelectric complex and thus give the erroneous impression of gastroparesis. Doing a gastric-emptying study when the blood glucose is elevated is a costly way to discover the blood glucose level.

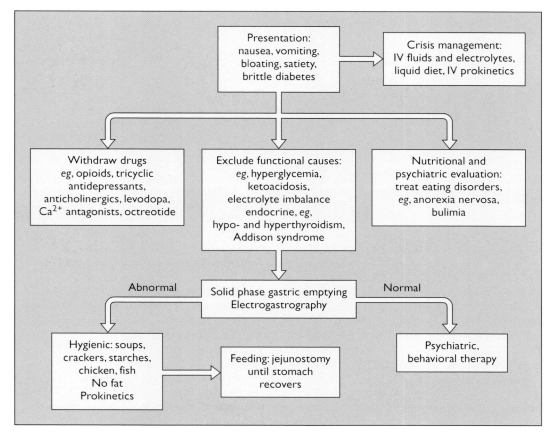

FIGURE 13-29. Algorithm for the management of gastropathy in patients with diabetes.

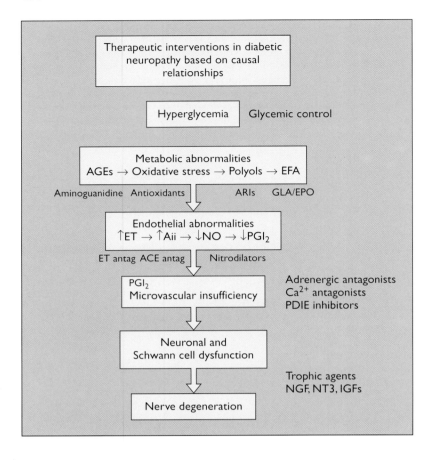

FIGURE 13-30. Specific interventions in diabetic neuropathy designed to target the major defect. Many of these intervention already have been tested in animal models and currently are in phase 2 and 3 clinical trials in the United States. Some of these interventions are further along and may well be in clinic trials shortly. ACE—angiotensin-converting enzyme; AGEs—advanced glycation endproduct; Antag—antagonists; ARIs—aldose-reductose inhibitors; Ca^{2+}—calcium ion; EFA—essential fatty acid; ET—endothelin; GLA/EPγ—gamma linolenic acid; IGF—insulin-like growth factor; NGF—neuronal growth factor; NO—nitric oxide; NT3—neurotropin 3; PDIE—phosphodiesterase; PGI_2—prostaglandin I_2.

References

1. American Diabetes Association, American Academy of *Neurology*: Consensus statement: report and recommendations of the San Antonio Conference on Diabetic Neuropathy. *Diabetes Care* 1988, 11:592–597.

2. Vinik AI. Mitchell BD. Leichter SB, *et al.*: Epidemiology of the complications of diabetes. In *Diabetes: Clinical Science and Practice* Edited by Leslie RDG, Robbins DC. Cambridge: Cambridge University Press, 1995:15,221.

3. Kjiturnan M, Welborn T, McCann V, *et al.*: Prevalence of diabetic complications in relation to risk factors. *Diabetes* 1986, 35:1332–1339.

4. Young MJ, Boulton AJ, MacLeod AF, *et al.*: A multicenter study of the prevalence of diabetic neuropathy in the United Kingdom hospital clinic population. *Diabetologia* 1993, 36:150–154.

5. Feldman JN, Hirsch SR, Bever BS, *et al.*: Prevalence of diabetic nephropathy at time of time of treatment for diabetic retinopathy. In *Diabetic Renal-Retinal Syndrome.* Edited by Friedman L'Esperance FA. London: Grune & Stratton, ; 1982:9.

6. Dyck PJ, Kratz KM, Karnes MS. *et al.*: The prevalence by staged severity of various types of diabetic neuropathy, retinopathy, and nephropathy in a population based cohort: The Rochester Diabetic Neuropathy Study. *Neurology* 1993); 43:817–824.

7. Brownlee M: Advanced products of nonenzymatic glycosylation and the pathogenesis of diabetic complications. In *Diabetes Mellitus. Theory and Practice* Edited by Rifkin H, Porte D. New York: Elsevier, 1990:279.

8. Diabetes Control and Complications Trial Research Group: Effect of intensive diabetes treatment on nerve conduction in the Diabetes Control and Complications Trial. *Ann Neurol* 1995 38(6):869–80.

9. Vinik AI, Newlon PG, Lauterio TJ, *et al.*: Nerve survival and regeneration in diabetes. *Diabetes Rev* 1995, 3:139–157. by Riflin H, Porte D. New York, Amsterdam, London: Elsevier, 1990:279.

10. Said G, Goulon-Gorcau C, Lacroix C, Moulonguet A: Nerve biopsy findings in different patterns of proximal diabetic neuropathy. *Ann Neurol* 1994, 35:559–569.

11. Krendel DA, Costigan DA, Hopkins LC: Successful treatment of neuropathies in patients with diabetes mellitus. *Arch Neurol* 1995, 52:1053–1061.

12. Vinik AL, Milicevic Z, Colen LB, *et al.*: Histopathological and electro-physiologic heterogeneity in patients with proximal diabetic neuropathy (PDN) [abstract]. *Diabetes* 1996, 769:209A.

13. Malik RA, Tesfaye S. Thompson SD, *et al.*: Transperineurial capillary abnormalities in the sural nerve of patients with diabetic neuropathy. *Microvasc Res* 1994, 48:236–245.

14. Dyck P, Hansen S, Karnes J: Capillary number and percentage closed in human diabetic sural nerve. *Proc Natl Acad Sci* USA 1985, 82:2513–2517.

15. Low P, Lagerlund T, McManis : Nerve blood flow and oxygen delivery in normal. diabetic. and ischemic neuropathy. *Int Rev Neurobiol* 1989, 33 1:355–438.

16. Yasuda H, Dyck P: Abnormalities of endoneurial microvessels and sural nerve pathology in diabetic neuropathy. *Newurology* 1987, 37:20–28.

17. Malik RA, Veves A, Masson EA, *et al.*: Endoneurial capillary abnormalities in human diabetic neuropathy. *J Neurol Neurosurg Psychiatry* 1992, 55:557–561.

18. Tuck RR, Schinelzer JD, Low PA: Endoneurial blood flow and oxygen tension in the sciatic nerves of rats ,with experimental diabetic neuropathy. *Brain* 1984, 107:935–950.

19. Newrick PG, Wilson AJ, Jakubowski J, *et al.*: Sural nerve oxygen tension in diabetes. *Brit Med J* 1986, 293:1053–1054.

20. Zachodne DW, Ho LT. Normal blood flow but lower oxygen tension in diabetes of' young rats: microenvironment and the influence of sympathectomy. *Can J Physiol Pharmacol* 1992, 70:651–659.

21. Hotta N, Koh N, Sakakibara F, *et al.*: Effect of proplionyl-L-carnitine on motor nerve conduction, autonomic cardiac function, and nerve blood flow in rats with streptozotocin-induced diabetes: comparison with an aldose reductase inhibitor. *Diabetes* 1992, 41:587–591.

22. Vinik AI, Holland MT, LeBeau JM, et al.: Diabetic neuropathies. *Diabetes Care* 1992, 15:1926–1975.

23. Dawson DM. Entrapment neuropathies of the upper extremities. *N Engl J Med* 1993, 329:2013[?]–218.

24. Leedman PJ, Davis S, Harrison LS: Diabetic amyotrophy. Reassessment of the clinical spectrum. *Aust NZ J Med* 1988, 18:768–773.

25. Barohn RJ, Salienk Z, Warmolts JR, Mendell JR: The Bruns Garland syndrome (diabetic amyotrophy). *Arch Neurol* 1991, 48:1130–1135.

26. Chia L, Fernandez A, Lacroix C: Contribution of nerve biopsy findings to the diagnosis of disabling neuropathy in the elderly. A retrospective review of 100 consecutive patients. *Brain* 1996, 119:1091–1098.

27. Hanson PH, Schumaker P. Debugne Tf 1, Clerin M. Evaluation of somatic and autonomic small fibers neuropathy in diabetes. *Am J Phys Med Rehabil* 1992, 71:44–47.

28. Dyck PJ: Small-fiber neuropathy determination. *Muscle Nerve* 1988, 11:998–999.

29. Jarnal GA, Hansen S, Weir AI, Ballantyne JP: The neurophysiologic investigation of small fiber neuropathies. *Muscle Nerve* 1987, 10:537–545.

30. Shapiro SA, Vinik AJ, et al.: Normal blood flow response and vasomotion in the diabetic. Charcot foot. *J Diab Complications* 1998, 12:147–153.

31. Burnstock G, Ralevic: New insights into the local regulation of blood flow by perivascular nerves and endothelium. *British J Plastic Surg* 1994, 47(8):527–543.

32. Stansberry KB, Vinik AJ, et al.: Impairment of peripheral blood flow responses in diabetes resembles an enhanced aging effect. *Diab Care* 1997, 20:1711–1716.

33. Ewing J, Campbell IW, Clarke BF, et al.: Heart rate changes in diabetes mellitus. *Lancet* 1981, 1:183–186.

34. Kahn J, Ida B, Vinik A: Stress and cardiovascular function in diabetes. *Diabetes Care* 1985, 12:3–5.

Secondary Forms of Diabetes

Veronica M. Catanese

Primary forms of diabetes mellitus include type 1, or insulin-dependent diabetes mellitus, and type 2, or non–insulin-dependent diabetes mellitus. Secondary forms of diabetes and glucose intolerance may occur in association with a variety of disorders of both endocrinologic and nonendocrinologic origin [1].

Most endocrine diseases associated with glucose intolerance produce the metabolic abnormality through excessive production of insulin counterregulatory hormones, such as growth hormone, glucocorticoids, glucagon, and catecholamines. These hormones affect both glucose production (through glycogenolysis and gluconeogenesis) and glucose utilization (through insulin secretion and insulin action) to varying degrees. In these diseases, the secondary diabetes is usually reversible with successful treatment of the underlying disorder, and the risk for ketoacidosis is low.

Nonendocrine conditions associated with abnormal glucose tolerance may be grouped into three major categories: diseases affecting pancreatic function (pancreatoprivic); drug-induced glucose intolerance; and complex genetic syndromes that affect multiple aspects of hepatic, renal, and musculoskeletal function. Pancreatitis, pancreatectomy, and hemochromatosis are the main components of the pancreatoprivic group. As expected, these conditions are associated with variable amounts of insulin deficiency and at least the potential for ketoacidosis. Pharmacologic agents can alter glucose tolerance by affecting insulin secretion, insulin action, or both. Genetic syndromes producing diabetes have multiple mechanisms, but in most cases, the exact cause still remains poorly understood.

Microangiopathic complications of diabetes are uncommon in patients with glucose intolerance secondary to diseases of hormonal overproduction. This is because these diseases rarely persist in an untreated state for many years. Retinal, renal, and neurologic sequelae do occur, however, in patients whose disease has lasted a decade or more. Because duration of hyperglycemia is a critical factor in the development of microvascular complications, it is not surprising that patients with long-standing pancreatitis, exocrine, and endocrine pancreatic dysfunction secondary to pancreatic reductive surgery, hemochromatosis, and genetic syndromes that include glucose intolerance are at risk for the development of classic diabetic complications.

Therapy for all types of secondary diabetes should center on correction of the underlying disturbance when possible. If this cannot be accomplished or until this is accomplished, treatment should reflect an understanding of the pathophysiologic basis of the diabetes. If insulin secretion is impaired (for example, in patients with pheochromocytoma), then exogenous insulin therapy should be instituted promptly until the underlying source of the problem has been eliminated. Patients with preserved insulin secretion should be treated with diet or oral hypoglycemic agents given as single drugs or in combination. In these cases, insulin should also be used if necessary to achieve glycemic goals. In all cases, little evidence suggests a correlation between the need for insulin therapy during a period of secondary diabetes and the risk for permanently altered glucose tolerance after successful treatment of the underlying primary disease.

FIGURE 14-1. Secondary forms of diabetes mellitus.

SECONDARY FORMS OF DIABETES

Endocrine Diseases
  Changes in balance of insulin counter-regulatory hormones disrupt glucose homeostasis
Nonendocrine Conditions
  Pancreatic functional defects
  Drug-induced glucose intolerance
  Genetic syndromes

Abnormal Glucose Homeostasis Secondary to Endocrinologic Disorders: Acromagaly

ACUTE AND DELAYED EFFECTS OF SUPRAPHYSIOLOGIC GROWTH HORMONE ON CARBOHYDRATE METABOLISM

Metabolic Variable	Short-Term GH Administration	Chronic GH Excess
Glucose uptake	↑	↓
Glucose utilization	↑	↓

FIGURE 14-2. Acute and delayed effects of supraphysiologic growth hormone (GH) on carbohydrate metabolism. Intravenous administration of GH produces insulinomimetic effects during the first 4 hours after infusion. Glucose uptake and glucose utilization by insulin-sensitive tissues are increased, and plasma glucose and free fatty acid levels decrease. These effects may result from a rapid, direct effect of GH on insulin secretion, GH-mediated increase in hepatic production of insulin-like growth factor-I, or GH-induced activation of some of the early steps in insulin receptor intracellular signaling pathways [2]. The delayed effects of GH administration, however, counter insulin action. Glucose uptake and use by insulin-sensitive tissues are impaired, resulting in hyperinsulinism and varying patterns of glucose tolerance. Free fatty acid levels increase only with concomitant fasting; this supports the concept that excess GH does not promote significant lipolysis in the presence of adequate insulin.

A. RESPONSES TO ORAL GLUCOSE TOLERANCE TESTING IN ACROMEGALY

Abnormal OGTT	Normal OGTT
↑ Glucose	→ Glucose
↑ Insulin	↑ Insulin
↑ Glucose	→ Glucose
↓ Insulin	→ Insulin

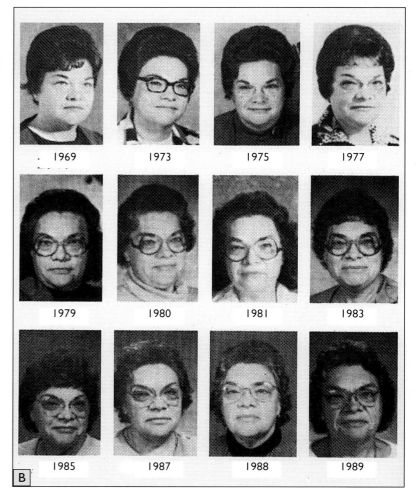

FIGURE 14-3. Spectrum of response to oral glucose tolerance testing in acromegaly. The prevalence of glucose intolerance in patients with acromegaly is approximately 60%; the spectrum of abnormalities in glucose homeostasis in such patients is shown in **A**. Most acromegalic patients with abnormal results on oral glucose tolerance tests (OGTTs) have normal fasting plasma glucose levels but impaired handling of a glucose load associated with elevated basal or stimulated insulin levels. A small subset have low basal insulin levels and profoundly impaired insulin responses to glucose loading and clinically manifest severe hyperglycemia. It is not clear whether these patients represent a distinct subgroup with coincident insulin-dependent diabetes or B-cell desensitization as a consequence of prolonged hyperglycemia. Acromegalic patients with normal glucose tolerance, however, often exhibit insulin resistance as defined by elevated plasma insulin levels under basal or glucose-stimulated conditions. In these patients, glucose uptake in skeletal muscle and nonoxidative glucose metabolism are impaired in the postabsorptive state [3]. Therefore, oral glucose tolerance testing underestimates the prevalence of insulin resistance in patients with acromegaly. It is not clear, however, that progression from hyperinsulinemic euglycemia to a more severe defect manifested by hyperglycemia occurs with progressive acromegaly, such as that seen in the patient photographed over time in **B**. (*From* Thorner, et al. [3a]; with permission.)

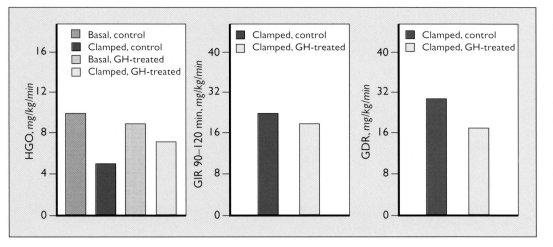

FIGURE 14-4. Growth hormone (GH)–induced hepatic and peripheral insulin resistance. Continuous administration of recombinant human GH to normal rats reduces insulin-mediated suppression of hepatic glucose output (HGO) and produces significant decreases in steady-state glucose infusion rate (GIR) and glucose disposal rate (GDR) during hyperinsulinemic glucose clamping. Similar results have been obtained in normal humans studied under conditions of continuous GH infusion [4]. In both rats and humans, fasting plasma glucose and insulin levels during GH treatment did not differ from those in controls, providing an experimental correlate of patients with acromegaly who have evidence of impaired insulin action in the postabsorptive state. The mechanisms responsible for this insulin resistance, however, remain unclear. Impairment of early events in insulin signal transduction in liver and muscle is a likely contributing factor. Insulin receptor substrate (IRS)-1 and IRS-2 tyrosine phosphorylation and association of these substrates with phosphatidylinositol 3-kinase are reduced in the livers and muscle of rats receiving long-term GH therapy [6]. It is not known whether troglitazone, which alleviates the GH-induced alterations in HGO, GIR, and GDR [4], affects the changes in IRS-1 and IRS-2 phosphorylation and phosphatidylinositol 3-kinase association or activity observed in liver or muscle of GH-treated rats. (*Adapted from* Sugimoto *et al.* [5].)

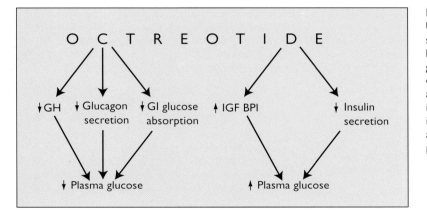

FIGURE 14-5. Effects of octreotide on glucose homeostasis in acromegaly. Unlike other effective treatment options for acromegaly, octreotide (the synthetic, long-acting somatostatin analogue) has complex effects on several hormonal factors that affect carbohydrate metabolism. In addition to inhibiting growth hormone (GH) and insulin-like growth factor-I (IGF-I) hypersecretion, octreotide inhibits insulin and glucagon secretion, delays gastrointestinal glucose absorption, and increases production of insulin-antagonistic IGF BP1 [7]. The interplay of these pharmacologic effects may lead to concomitant improvement in glucose tolerance with control of the GH hypersecretion; however, it may also cause worsened glucose tolerance upon institution of octreotide therapy, particularly if GH secretory profiles remain abnormal [8]. BP1—binding protein 1.

Cushing Syndrome

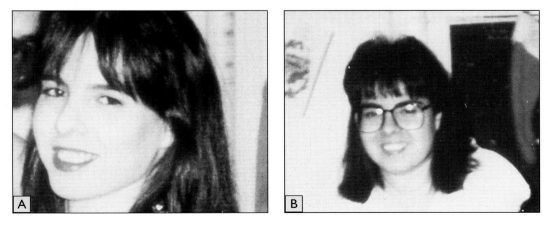

FIGURE 14-6. Cushing syndrome is a common endocrine cause of secondary glucose intolerance and diabetes. Abnormal glucose homeostasis may result from exogenous daily or alternate-day administration of glucocorticoids or as a consequence of chronic endogenous excess of glucocorticoids due to pituitary hypersecretion of adrenocorticotropic hormone (ACTH), paraneoplastic production of ACTH by tumor cells, or autonomous adrenal cortical hyperfunction. The latter affected this patient, photographed before (**A**) and after (**B**) presentation with phenotypic Cushing syndrome. The patient was found to have an adrenal cortical adenoma.

Although fasting hyperglycemia occurs in approximately 5% of patients with Cushing syndrome, insulin resistance with basal or stimulated hyperinsulinemia occurs in up to 90% of patients. Patients with Cushing syndrome may present in a hyperosmolar, nonketotic state [1]. This presentation is extremely unusual in patients with acromegaly, who otherwise display a spectrum of abnormal glucose and insulin profiles similar to those of patients with Cushing syndrome. (*Courtesy of* Jaishree Jagirdar, Department of Pathology, New York University School of Medicine.)

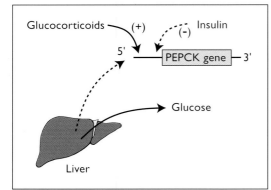

FIGURE 14-7. Glucocorticoid excess promotes hepatic glucose production. Several key enzymes controlling the production and utilization of metabolic fuels are directly regulated by glucocorticoids at the level of gene transcription. Phosphoenolpyruvate carboxykinase (PEPCK), a critical enzyme in gluconeogenesis, is positively regulated by glucocorticoids [9]. Transgenic mice overexpressing PEPCK, in fact, exhibit impaired glucose tolerance [10]. In addition, exposure of pregnant rats during late gestation to glucocorticoid excess permanently increases hepatic expression of PEPCK and glucocorticoid receptor and causes glucose intolerance in adult offspring [11]. Under normal physiologic conditions, however, insulin regulates PEPCK even more potently and dominantly in a negative manner [12]. Thus, repelete insulin prevents the enhanced gluconeogenesis that would be caused by glucocorticoid excess. In the presence of insulin deficiency or impaired insulin action, however, the stimulatory effects of glucocorticoids on glucose production become apparent. Because patients with Cushing syndrome almost always have insulin resistance, the stage is set for glucocorticoid-enhanced gluconeogenesis, which contributes to glucose intolerance.

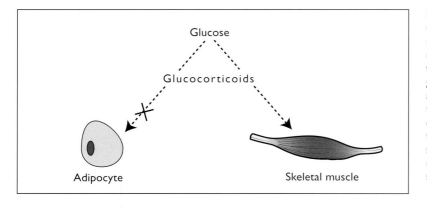

FIGURE 14-8. Glucocorticoid excess diminishes peripheral glucose utilization. Glucocorticoids induce resistance to insulin-stimulated glucose uptake in rat adipocytes [13]. This effect may be at least partly mediated by direct glucocorticoid-mediated inhibition of insulin-induced protein kinase C translocation from cytosol to plasma membrane. Glucocorticoids also inhibit activation of glucose transport in rat skeletal muscle by insulin, insulin-like growth factor-I, and hypoxia [14]. In rat soleus muscle, this effect is associated with preservation of total content of GLUT4 glucose transporters but also reduced translocation of GLUT4 transporter units to the plasma membrane [15]. In addition to these effects on GLUT4 subcellular trafficking, glucocorticoids affect early steps in insulin receptor signaling in skeletal muscle and in the liver [16]. As a result, both basal and insulin-stimulated glucose uptake and utilization are subject to modulation by excess glucocorticoids.

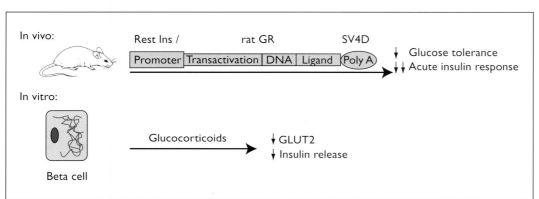

FIGURE 14-9. Glucocorticoids inhibit insulin secretion from pancreatic beta cells. Insulin resistance has long been a recognized consequence of glucocorticoid excess. Effects of glucocorticoids on insulin secretion in vivo and in vitro, however, have only recently been described. Transgenic mice overexpressing the glucocorticoid receptor under the control of the insulin promoter have increased glucocorticoid sensitivity that is restricted to pancreatic beta cells [17]. These animals have normal fasting and postabsorptive blood glucose levels but also have a markedly reduced insulin response and impaired glucose tolerance during intravenous glucose loading. This in vivo evidence suggesting a diabetogenic effect of glucocorticoids on pancreatic beta cells is supported by in vitro evidence for dexamethasone-induced, posttranslational degradation of beta cell GLUT2 glucose transporters [18] and by dexamethasone-induced inhibition of exocytotic insulin release from rodent islets in culture [19]. Diminished glucose utilization in Cushing syndrome may therefore be a composite result of deficient insulin secretion and impaired insulin action.

Glucagonoma

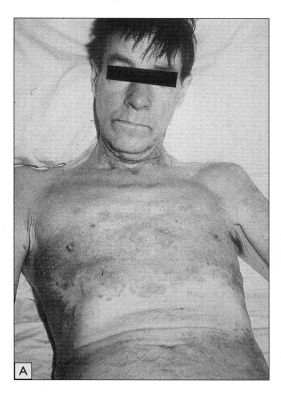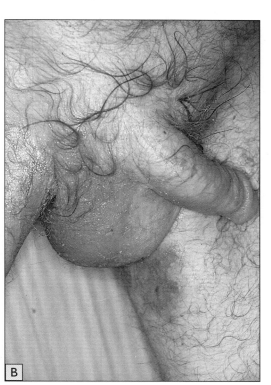

FIGURE 14-10. (*see* Color Plate) Glucose intolerance in the "glucagonoma syndrome." Although hyperglucagonemia may be associated with a variety of secretory islet-cell tumors and is rarely associated with multiple endocrine neoplasia type I (MEN I), the characteristic glucagonoma syndrome is most frequently seen in patients with clinically malignant, glucagon-producing tumors of pancreatic alpha cells. Central to the classic glucagonoma syndrome is necrolytic migratory erythema—the pathognomonic erythematous rash involving the perineum, extremities, trunk, or perioral region. This rash may be reproduced by infusion of glucagon into normal individuals and can be alleviated by infusion of parenteral amino acids, despite continued hyperglucagonemia. Thus, it is likely that amino acid deficiency produced by glucagon-induced muscle proteolysis is responsible for the rash. The incidence of glucose intolerance in patients with glucagonoma approaches 100%, with metabolic defects ranging from mild to very severe. Despite the excess production of glucagon and its potent effects on glycogenolysis and gluconeogenesis, ketoacidosis is rare. This probably reflects the stimulatory effect of glucagon on insulin secretion and the importance of the relative concentrations of both insulin and glucagon to hepatic glucose production and ketogenesis. In addition, functional heterogeneity of the various circulating species of immunoreactive glucagon may titrate glucagon's biological effects. (*Courtesy of* Dr. C.R. Kahn, Joslin Diabetes Center.)

ished glucose utilization. Insulin resistance has not been described clinically in patients with glucagonoma. Glucagon is a potent stimulus of epinephrine release; thus, alpha-adrenergic receptor–mediated inhibition of insulin secretion may diminish glucose disposal in patients with glucagonoma syndrome. Excess glucagon also has direct, paracrine, stimulatory effects on beta cell insulin secretion. Beta cells in the nontumoral endocrine pancreatic tissue of patients with glucagonoma have reduced immunoreactive insulin content and have ultrastructural features suggestive of accelerated insulin synthesis and secretion.

A, A beta cell from a control human pancreas, with moderate amounts of rough endoplasmic reticulum, a small Golgi apparatus, and numerous mature granules with crystal-like cores. **B,** A beta cell from a glucagonoma-associated pancreas. This cell contains several elongated rough endoplasmic reticulum cisternae, stacks of Golgi with adjacent progranules (*arrows*), and fewer secretory granules, which primarily contain immature rounded cores. It is therefore possible that the balance of multiple effects of hyperglucagonemia on insulin secretion may determine the degree of impairment in glucose utilization rate. (*From* from Bani *et al.* [20]; with permission.)

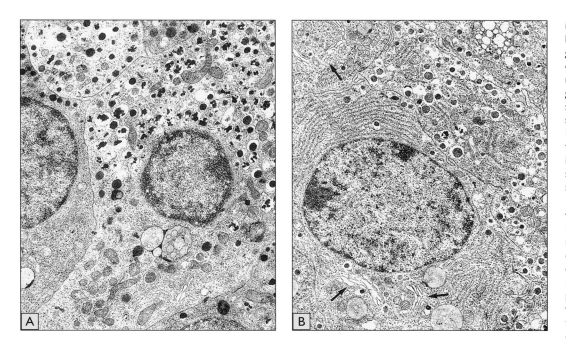

FIGURE 14-11. Effects of endogenous hyperglucagonemia on pancreatic beta cells. It is unlikely that an increased glucose production rate alone could produce glucose intolerance in the absence of an absolute or relative decrease in glucose disposal rate. Decreased insulin secretion or insulin resistance could result in dimin-

Pheochromocytoma

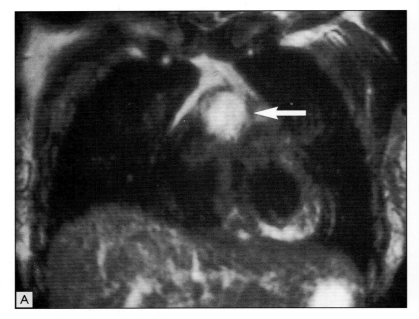

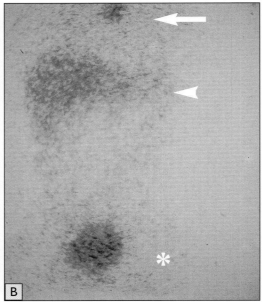

FIGURE 14-12. Glucose intolerance is a prominent feature in pheochromocytoma. Continuous or intermittent overproduction of the insulin counterregulatory hormones epinephrine or norepinephrine by pheochromocytomas results in glucose intolerance in up to 75% of patients. Ninety percent of tumors are located within the adrenal medulla, but tumors may occur in several other sites, including along the abdominal aorta, in the organ of Zuckerkandl, in the urinary bladder, or in the mediastinum. As an adjunct to biochemical diagnosis, the tumor may be localized before surgery by many techniques, including computed tomography and magnetic resonance imaging. Multiple tumor foci, as well as metastatic sites, are best visualized by 131I-labeled metaiodobenzylguanidine (MIBG) scanning. This nuclear medicine technique is accurate in 80% to 95% of pheochromocytomas, but its specificity is reduced by its capacity to detect neuroblastomas, medullary carcinomas of the thyroid, and carcinoid tumors [21]. In this figure, mediastinal metastases in a patient with a previously resected adrenal medullary pheochromocytoma are demonstrated by magnetic resonance imaging (**A**, *arrow*) and by 131I-MIBG (**B**; *arrow* points to the pheochromocytoma, *arrowhead* to the liver, *asterisk* to the bladder). (*Courtesy of* Dr. Elissa Kramer, Division of Nuclear Medicine, Department of Radiology, New York University School of Medicine.)

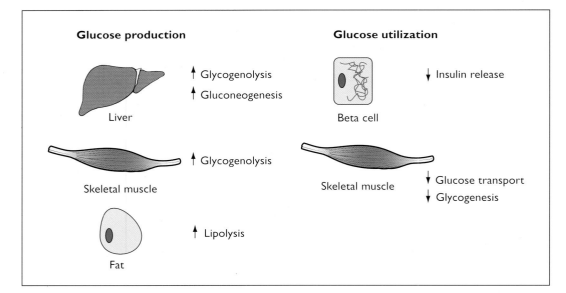

FIGURE 14-13. Excess catecholamines affect both glucose production and glucose utilization. Under pathologic conditions, the effects of catecholamines on glucose disposal are more profound than the effects on glucose production. Epinephrine directly interferes with exocytosis of insulin from pancreatic beta cells [22] and does so at a step distal to the membrane depolarization-induced increase in intracellular calcium [23]. Catecholamines also impair insulin sensitivity, particularly in skeletal muscle [24], by inhibiting both insulin-stimulated glucose transport [25] and insulin-mediated muscle glycogenesis [26]. Catecholamines, especially epinephrine, increase net glucose production rate by directly affecting liver glycogenolysis and gluconeogenesis, muscle glycogenolysis, and fat lipolysis. The effects of catecholamines on pancreatic insulin secretion are mediated mainly through alpha-adrenergic receptors, whereas the effects on insulin target tissues are mediated primarily through beta-adrenergic receptor activation. Glucose tolerance in patients with pheochromocytoma is often restored by administration of alpha-adrenergic blockers, such as phentolamine; this supports the notion that the effects of excess catecholamines on glucose utilization outweigh the effects on glucose production.

Thyrotoxicosis

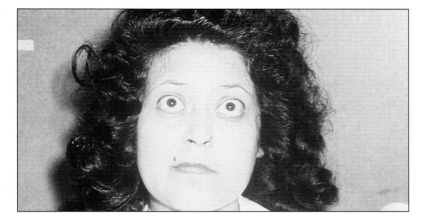

FIGURE 14-14. Glucose production and glucose utilization are altered in the thyrotoxic state. Hyperthyroidism of any cause, including thyrotoxic Graves disease—as manifested by this patient—alters glucose homeostasis. Thyroid hormones directly affect the activity of several glycometabolic enzymes, such as hepatic [27] and muscle [28] glycogen synthase, and also impair insulin-mediated suppression of hepatic glycogenolysis and gluconeogenesis [29]. In addition to their direct effects on glucose production, thyroid hormones in excess may also impair glucose-induced growth hormone suppression [30]; this adds another factor favoring the development of glucose intolerance. Glucose disposal, particularly in adipocytes, also is affected by thyrotoxicosis. Insulin-stimulated glucose transport is minimally increased [31], and this effect is associated with an increase in appearance of GLUT4 glucose transporters in the plasma membrane of adipocytes [32]. More important, hyperthyroidism increases basal rates of lipolysis, augments the maximal response of lipolysis to norepinephrine stimulation, and blunts the sensitivity of norepinephrine-stimulated lipolysis to suppression by insulin [31]. Clinically, these effects on glucose tolerance and insulin sensitivity appear more pronounced in obese than nonobese hyperthyroid women [33], perhaps because the decrease in nonoxidative glucose metabolism caused by hyperthyroidism cannot be adequately compensated for in the presence of the impaired oxidative glucose metabolism of obesity [34]. (*Courtesy of* Dr. Herbert Samuels, Departments of Medicine and Pharmacology, New York University School of Medicine.)

Hyperprolactinemia

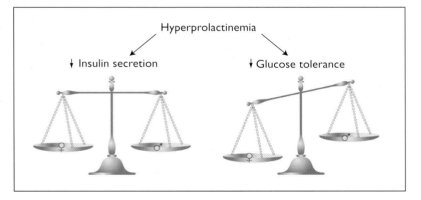

FIGURE 14-15. Sexual dimorphism of the diabetogenic effects of hyperprolactinemia. Moderate chronic hyperprolactinemia is associated with reduced thresholds for basal and glucose-induced insulin release [35] and pancreatic beta cell proliferation [36], mediated largely by altered expression of glucokinase, hexokinase, and GLUT2 glucose transporter in islet cells [37]. However, prolactin also affects insulin resistance in extramammary tissue and glucose tolerance [38]. Studies in hyperprolactinemic, pituitary-grafted mice [39] and rats [40], however, suggest that prolactin's effects on hepatic insulin action, unlike its sex-neutral effects on insulin secretion, may require estrogen for full expression. The molecular basis for prolactin's effects on insulin action in the presence and absence of estrogen has not been elucidated, and well-controlled studies testing this hypothesis in hyperprolactinemic men and women have not yet been performed.

Pancreatoprivic Diabetes:
Pancreatectomy and Chronic Pancreatitis

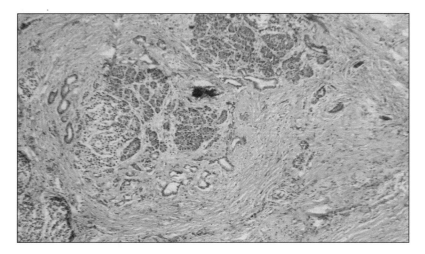

FIGURE 14-16. (*see* Color Plate) Reductions in pancreatitic functional mass impair glucose tolerance by affecting multihormonal islet-cell activity. Pancreatic exocrine and endocrine deficiency develop predictably with removal or destruction of more than 75% of pancreatic tissue. Glucose intolerance after pancreatectomy,

fibrocalcific or "J-type" tropical diabetes, and chronic pancreatitis, particularly as a result of alcoholism, share several features that distinguish them from other types of primary and secondary diabetes. Endocrine secretion from all islet-cell types is reduced, resulting not only in insulin deficiency under basal or stimulated conditions, but also diminished pancreatic glucagon, somatostatin, and pancreatic polypeptide secretion. Despite preserved secretion of glucagon-like substances of duodenal origin in patients who have not undergone pancreatoduodenectomy, reduced levels of pancreatic glucagon account for the relative resistance of these patients to ketoacidosis under conditions of insulin deficiency. In addition, iatrogenic hypoglycemia is common, and the response to spontaneous or induced hypoglycemia is delayed compared to that observed in both insulin-dependent and non–insulin-dependent diabetics. Although carbohydrate intolerance in these patients is usually attributed to reduced insulin secretion, insulin deficiency alone may not be the only factor responsible for secondary diabetes under these conditions. Hepatic resistance to insulin, accompanied by loss of sensitivity to insulin-induced hepatic glucose suppression, is a prominent feature of canine chronic pancreatitis. Deficiency of pancreatic polypeptide has been implicated as a factor in this resistance. Infusion of bovine pancreatic polypeptide improves glucose tolerance and restores suppression of hepatic glucose output by insulin in pancreatic polypeptide–deficient animals [41] and patients with chronic pancreatitis [42]. Hemotoxylin and eosin stain (*Courtesy of* Dr. Howard Mizrachi, Department of Pathology, New York University School of Medicine.)

Hemochromatosis

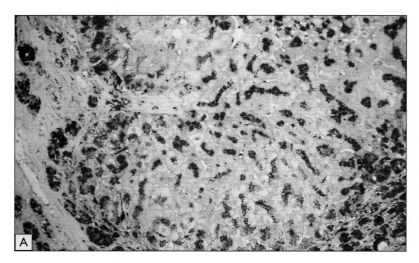

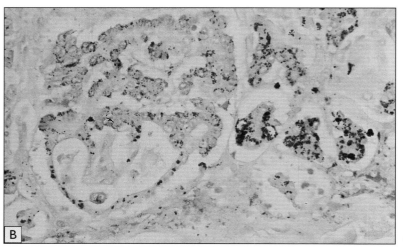

FIGURE 14-17. (*see* Color Plate) Hemochromatosis, whether hereditary or secondary to iron overload, is associated with abnormal glucose tolerance. Clinical diabetes or impaired glucose tolerance occurs in 75% to 90% of patients with primary hemochromatosis and in up to 65% of patients with hemochromatosis as a consequence of hemolytic anemia, multiple transfusion, or iron ingestion. Although the presence of cirrhosis increases the likelihood of abnormal glucose metabolism, hepatic iron content (shown by Prussian blue staining in **A**), serum ferritin levels, or extent of liver damage correlate poorly with the presence of impaired glucose homeostasis. A positive family history of diabetes may be the best predictor of glucose intolerance, at least among

patients with hereditary hemochromatosis [43]. Hepatic insulin resistance clearly plays an important role in patients with both varieties of hemochromatosis [44, 45]. Defective first-phase insulin secretion, however, is also observed, even in the absence of significant degrees of islet iron deposition, such as that shown in **B**. Taken together, these physiologic abnormalities resemble those seen during the natural history of non–insulin-dependent diabetes. The relative importance of genetic factors versus iron overload in the pathophysiology of diabetes secondary to hemochromatosis, however, is not yet clear. (*Courtesy of* Dr. Howard Mizrachi, Department of Pathology, New York University School of Medicine).

Pharmacologic Effects on Glucose Homeostasis

DRUGS CAUSING DIABETES

Drugs That Affect Insulin Secretion

Anticonvulsant	Cations	Hormones	Antihelminthics
Phenytoin	Barium	Somatostatin	Pentamidine
Diuretics	Cadmium	Pesticides	Antineoplastics
Thiazides	Lithium	DDT	L-Asparaginase
Furosemide	Potassium	Fluoride	Mithramycin
Ethacrynic acid	Zinc	Pyriminil (Vacor)	

Drugs that affect insulin action

Hormones
 Growth hormone

Drugs that affect both insulin secretion and insulin action

Hormones/Hormone Antagonists	Antihypertensive	Blocking agents	Psychopharmacologic agents
Glucagon	Clonidine	β-Adrenergic blockers	Benzodiazepines
Glucocorticoids	Diazoxide	Calcium-channel blockers	Ethanol
Octreotide	Prazosin	Histaminergic blockers	Opiates
Adrenergic compounds			Phenothiazines
Epinephrine			
Norepinephrine			

FIGURE 14-18. Drug-induced diabetes. The list of pharmacologic agents that can induce diabetes is long. Individual drugs may affect glucose homeostasis by interfering with insulin secretion, insulin action, or both. Whether its effect is primarily on insulin secretion or insulin action, a drug itself may mediate the effect directly, or indirectly through hormones or cations critical to the mechanisms that control insulin release or biological effect. Glucohomeostatic effects of supraphysiologic levels of growth hormone, glucocorticoids, and catecholamines best illustrate the direct and indirect consequences of "pharmacologically" altered insulin action. As the links between altered insulin sensitivity and altered insulin secretion tighten, it becomes more and more difficult to assign an effect to a drug solely on the basis of insulin action. Clinically, these agents may uncover previously silent insulin secretory defects or insulin resistance and consequently induce glucose intolerance in a previously undiagnosed patient or worsen the diabetic state when administered to patients with antecedent diabetes mellitus. (*From* Argetsinger and Carter-Su [2]; with permission.)

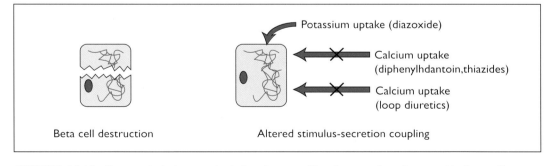

Potassium uptake (diazoxide)
Calcium uptake (diphenylhdantoin, thiazides)
Calcium uptake (loop diuretics)
Beta cell destruction
Altered stimulus-secretion coupling

FIGURE 14-19. Prototypical pharmacologic impairment of insulin secretion: direct and indirect effects. Insulin secretion by pancreatic beta cells may be impaired directly by destruction of the beta cells themselves or by interference with the normal mechanism of stimulated insulin secretion. Pentamidine, a widely used anti-helminthic agent active against *Pneumocystis carinii*, produces beta cell–selective necrosis and irreversibly reduces beta cell responses to glucose and nonglucose secretagogues after initially causing cytolytic release of insulin [46]. In contrast, diphenylhydantoin, at therapeutic blood levels, reversibly reduces both first and second phases of insulin release by inhibiting calcium inflow into the beta cell through voltage-dependent Ca^{2+} channels [47]. Unlike diphenylhydantoin, thiazide diuretics were thought to adversely affect insulin secretion and promote glucose intolerance indirectly through production of hypokalemia [48] in a manner similar to that proposed for primary hyperaldosteronism. Although prevention or correction of hypokalemia does alleviate thiazide-induced glucose intolerance, direct effects of thiazides themselves on the beta cell secretory recently have been described. Unlike the structurally related compound diazoxide, thiazides do not hyperpolarize beta cells by opening the adenosine triphosphate–sensitive potassium channels closed by the sulfonylureas [49]. Instead, they, like diphenylhydantoin, may affect stimulus-secretion coupling in the beta cell by inhibiting calcium uptake [50]. Similarly, the loop diuretics, thought to share with the thiazides an indirect effect on beta cell secretion mediated through hypokalemia, also directly affect insulin secretion by inhibiting chloride pump function in the beta cell membrane [51].

Genetic Syndromes Associated with Impaired Glucose Tolerance

GENETIC SYNDROMES ASSOCIATED WITH IMPAIRED GLUCOSE TOLERANCE

Acute intermittent porphyria

Alström syndrome (obesity, deafness, retinitis pigmentosa)

Ataxia-telangiectasia

Cockayne syndrome

Cystic fibrosis

Friedreich ataxia (spinocerebellar ataxia)

Glycogen storage disease type I

Herrmann syndrome (photomyoclonus, nerve deafness, nephropathy, cerebral dysfunction)

Huntington chorea

Isolated growth hormone deficiency

Klinefelter syndrome

Laurence-Moon-Biedl syndrome

Leprechaunism

Lipoatrophic diabetes

Machado disease (ataxia, nystagmus, dysarthria, depressed tendon reflexes, distal muscle atrophy)

Myotonic dystrophy

Panhypopituitary dwarfism

Prader-Willi syndrome

Trisomy 21

Turner syndrome

Werner syndrome

Wolfram syndrome (hereditary optic atrophy, visual loss, neurosensory deafness)

FIGURE 14-20. The list of genetic syndromes that include glucose intolerance as part of their profile is extensive and growing. Among members of this list, relatively "pure" defects in insulin secretion are represented by diseases such as cystic fibrosis; leprechaunism, on the other hand, may be regarded as a prototypical syndrome of insulin resistance. It is clear, however, that multiple pathophysiologic mechanisms that affect both glucose production and glucose utilization coalesce, in most cases, to produce the full-blown syndromes and the glucose intolerance that characterize them. It is likely that advances in the molecular genetics and molecular pathophysiology of these syndromes will shed light not only on the dysregulated glucose handling in these syndromes, but also on mechanisms of altered glucose homeostasis common both to secondary and primary forms of diabetes.

References

1. Catanese VM, Kahn DR: Secondary forms of diabetes. In: *Principles and Practice of Endocrinology and Metabolism*. Edited by Becker KL, Bremner WJ, Hung W, Kahn CR, *et al.* Philadelphia: J.B. Lippincott; 1995:1220–1228.

2. Argetsinger L, Carter-Su C: Mechanism of signaling by growth hormone receptor. *Physiol Rev* 1996, 76:1089–1107.

3. Foss MC, Saad MJ, Paccola GM, *et al.*: Peripheral glucose metabolism in acromegaly. *J Clin Endocrinol Metab* 1991, 72:1048–1053.

3a. Thorner MO, Vance ML, Laws ER, et al.: The Anterior Pituitary. In *Williams Textbook of Endocrinology*, edn. 9. Edited by Wilson JD, Foster DW, Kronenberg HM, Larsen PR. Philadelphia, WB Saunders, 1998: 296.

4. Orskov L, Schmitz O, Jorgensen JOL, *et al.*: Influence of growth hormone on glucose-induced glucose uptake in normal men as assessed by the hyperglycemic clamp technique. *J Clin Endocrinol Metab* 1989, 68:276–282.

5. Sugimoto M, Takeda N, Nakashima K, *et al.*: Effects of troglitazone on hepatic and peripheral insulin resistance induced by growth hormone excess in rats. *Metabolism* 1998, 47:783–787.

6. Thirone ACP, Carvalho CRO, Brenelli SL, *et al.*: Effect of chronic growth hormone treatment on insulin signal transduction in rat tissues. *Mol Cell Endocrinol* 1997, 130:33–42.

7. Ezzat S, Ren SG, Braunstein GD, *et al.*: Octreotide stimulates insulin-like growth factor-binding protein-1: a potential pituitary-independent mechanism for drug action. *J Clin Endocrinol Metab* 1992, 75:1459–1463.

8. Koop BL, Harris AG, Ezzat S: Effect of octreotide on glucose tolerance in acromegaly. *Eur J Endocrinol* 1994, 130:581–586.

9. Imai E, Stromstedt PE, Quinn PG, *et al.*: Characterization of a complex glucocorticoid response unit in the phosphoenolpyruvate carboxykinase gene. *Mol Cell Biol* 1990, 10:4712–4719.

10. Valera A, Pujol A, Pelegrin M, *et al.*: Transgenic mice overexpressing phosphoenolpyruvate carboxykinase develop non-insulin-dependent diabetes. *Proc Natl Acad Sci U S A* 1994, 91:9151–9154.

11. Nyirenda MJ, Lindsay RS, Kenyon CJ, *et al.*: Glucocorticoid exposure in late gestation permanently programs rat hepatic phosphoenolpyruvate carboxykinase and glucocorticoid receptor expression and causes glucose intolerance in adult offspring. *J Clin Invest* 1998, 101:2174–2181.

12. O'Brien RM, Granner DK: Regulation of gene expression by insulin. *Biochem J* 1991, 278:609–619.

13. Ishizuka T, Nagashima T, Kajita K, *et al.*: Effect of glucocorticoid receptor antagonist RU 38486 on acute glucocorticoid-induced insulin resistance in rat adipocytes. *Metabolism* 1997, 46:997–1002.

14. Weinstein SP, Paquin T, Pritsker A, *et al.*: Glucocorticoid-induced insulin resistance: dexamethasone inhibits the activation of glucose transport in rat skeletal muscle by both insulin- and non-insulin-related stimuli. *Diabetes* 1995, 44:441–445.

15. Dimitriadis G, Leighton B, Parry-Billings M, *et al.*: Effects of glucocorticoid excess on the sensitivity of glucose transport and metabolism to insulin in rat skeletal muscle. *Biochem J* 1997, 321:707–712.

16. Saad MJA, Folli F, Kahn JA, *et al.*: Modulation of insulin receptor, insulin receptor substrate-1, and phosphatidylinositol 3-kinase in liver and muscle of dexamethasone-treated rats. *J Clin Invest* 1993, 92:2065–2072.

17. Delaunay F, Khan A, Cintra A, *et al.*: Pancreatic beta cells are important targets for the diabetogenic effects of glucocorticoids. *J Clin Invest* 1997, 100:2094–2098.

18. Gremlich S, Roduit R, Thorens B: Dexamethasone induces posttranslational degradation of GLUT2 and inhibition of insulin secretion in isolated pancreatic beta cells. *J Biol Chem* 1997, 272:3216–3222.

19. Lambillotte C, Gilon P, Henquin JC: Direct glucocorticoid inhibition of insulin secretion. *J Clin Invest* 1997, 99:414–423.

20. Bani D, Biliotti G, Sacchi TB: Morphological changes in the human endocrine pancreas induced by chronic excess of endogenous glucagon. *Virchows Archiv B Cell Pathol* 1991, 60:199–206.

21. Keiser HR: Pheochromocytoma and other diseases of the sympathetic nervous system. In: *Principles and Practice of Endocrinology and Metabolism*. Edited by Becker KL, Bremner WJ, Hung W, *et al.* Philadelphia: J.B. Lippincott; 1995:762–770.

22. Lehr S, Herbst M, Kampermann J, *et al.*: Adrenaline inhibits depolarization-induced increases in capacitance in the presence of elevated intracellular calcium concentration in insulin secreting cells. *FEBS Lett* 1997, 415:1–5.

23. Renstrom E, Ding WG, Bokvist K, *et al.*: Neurotransmitter-induced inhibition of exocytosis in insulin-secreting beta cells by activation of calcineurin. *Neuron* 1996, 17:513–522.

24. Capaldo B, Napoli R, Di Marino L, *et al.*: Epinephrine directly antagonizes insulin-mediated activation of glucose uptake and inhibition of free fatty acid release in forearm tissues. *Metab Clin Exp* 1992, 41:1146–1149.

25. Laakso M, Edelman SV, Brechtel G, *et al.*: Effects of epinephrine on insulin-mediated glucose uptake in whole body and leg muscle in humans: role of blood flow. *Am J Physiol* 1992, 263:E199–204.

26. Raz I, Katz A, Spencer MK: Epinephrine inhibits insulin-mediated glycogenesis but enhances glycolysis in human skeletal muscle. *Am J Physiol* 1991, 260:E430–435.

27. Malbon CC, Campbell R: Thyroid hormones regulate hepatic glycogen synthase. *Endocrinology* 1984, 115:681–686.

28. Dimitriadis GD, Leighton B, Vlachonikolis IG, *et al.*: Effects of hyperthyroidism on the sensitivity of glycolysis and glycogen synthesis to insulin in the soleus muscle of the rat. *Biochem J* 1988, 253:87–92.

29. Holness MJ, Sugden MC: Hepatic carbon flux after re-feeding: hyperthyroidism blocks glycogen synthesis and the suppression of glucose output obse

30. Tosi F, Moghetti P, Castello R, *et al.*: Early changes in plasma glucagon and growth hormone response to oral glucose in experimental hyperthyroidism. *Metabolism* 1996, 45:1029–1033.

31. Fryer LG, Holness MJ, Sugden MC: Selective modification of insulin action in adipose tissue by hyperthyroidism. *J Endocrinol* 1997, 154:513–522.

32. Matthei S, Trost B, Hamann A, *et al.*: Effect of in vivo thyroid hormone status on insulin signalling and GLUT1 and GLUT4 glucose transport systems in rat adipocytes. *J Endocrinol* 1995, 144:347–357.

33. Gonzalo MA, Grant C, Moreno I, *et al.*: Glucose tolerance, insulin secretion, insulin sensitivity and glucose effectiveness in normal and overweight hyperthyroid women. *Clin Endocrinol* 1996, 45:689–697.

34. Bonadonna RC, DeFronzo RA: Glucose metabolism in obesity and type II diabetes. In: *Obesity*. Edited by Bjorntorp P, Brodoff BN. Philadelphia: J.B. Lippincott; 1992:474–501.

35. Sorenson RL, Brejle TC, Hegre OD, *et al.*: Prolactin (in vitro) decreases the glucose stimulation threshold, enhances insulin secretion, and increases dye coupling among islet B cells. *Endocrinology* 1987, 121:1447–1453.

36. Brejle TC, Parsons JA, Sorenson RL: Regulation of islet beta-cell proliferation by prolactin in rat islets. *Endocrinology* 1994, 43:263–273.

37. Weinhaus AJ, Stout LE, Sorenson RL: Glucokinase, hexokinase, glucose transporter 2, and glucose metabolism in islets during pregnancy and prolactin-treated islets in v̌itro: mechanisms for long term up-regulation of islets. *Endocrinology* 1996, 137:1640–1649.

38. Wade GN, Schneider JE: Metabolic fuels and reproduction in female mammals. *Neurosci Biobehav Rev* 1992, 16:235–272.

39. Matsuda M, Mori T: Effect of estrogen on hyperprolactinemia-induced glucose intolerance in SHN mice. *Proc Soc Exp Biol Med* 1996, 212:243–247.

40. Reis FM, Reis AM, Coimbra CC: Effects of hyperprolactinaemia on glucose tolerance and insulin release in male and female rats. *J Endocrinol* 1997, 153:423–428.

41. Sun YS, Brunicardi FC, Druck P, *et al.*: Reversal of abnormal glucose metabolism in chronic pancreatitis by administration of pancreatic polypeptide. *Am J Surg* 1986, 151:130–140.

42. Brunicardi FC, Chaiken RL, Ryan AS, *et al.*: Pancreatic polypeptide administration improves abnormal glucose metabolism in patients with chronic pancreatitis. *J Clin Endocrinol Metab* 1996, 81:3566–3572.

43. Hramiak IM, Finegood DT, Adams PC: Factors affecting glucose tolerance in hereditary hemochromatosis I. *Clin Invest Med* 1997, 20:110–118.

44. Stremmel W, Niederau C, Berger M, *et al.*: Abnormalities in estrogen, androgen, and insulin metabolism in hereditary hemochromatosis. *Ann N Y Acad Sci* 1988, 526:209–223.

45. Merkel PA, Simonson DC, Amiel SA, *et al.*: Insulin resistance and hyperinsulinemia in patients with thalassemia major treated by hypertransfusion. *N Engl J Med* 1988, 318:809–814.

46. Shen M, Orwoll ES, Conte JE Jr, *et al.*: Pentamidine-induced pancreatic beta-cell dysfunction. *Am J Med* 1989, 86:726–728.

47. Siegel EG, Janjic D, Wollheim CB: Phenytoin inhibition of insulin release. Studies on the involvement of Ca^{2+} fluxes in rat pancreatic islets. *Diabetes* 1982, 31:265–269.

48. Helderman JH, Elahi D, Andersen DK, *et al.*: Prevention of the glucose intolerance of thiazide diuretics by maintenance of body potassium. *Diabetes* 1983, 32:106–111.

49. Tucker SJ, Gribble FM, Zhao C, *et al.*: Truncation of Kir6.2 produces ATP-sensitive K^+ channels in the absence of the sulphonylurea receptor. *Nature* 1997, 387:179–183.

50. Sandstrom PE: Inhibition by hydrochlorothiazide of insulin release and calcium influx in mouse pancreatic beta cells. *Br J Pharmacol* 1993, 110:1359–1362.

51. Sandstrom PE: Bumetanide reduces insulin release by a direct effect on the pancreatic beta cells. *Eur J Pharmacol* 1990, 187:377–383.

Obesity

Eleftheria Maratos-Flier

Obesity, generally defined as weight exceeding 20% of ideal body weight or a body mass index (BMI) greater than 30, is a complex problem. In the United States, the prevalence of clinically significant obesity is more than 25%. Obesity is associated with excess mortality because of the elevated risk for such diseases as diabetes, hypertension, lipid disorders, and coronary artery disease and increased rates of endometrial and colonic carcinoma. Despite the magnitude of the problem, the cause of obesity is poorly understood and effective weight loss is difficult to achieve.

Recent work in mouse models has increased our understanding of the molecular mechanisms that may lead to obesity. The identification of leptin has provided insight into peripheral signals important in mediating eating behavior. Leptin, the product of the obese gene, is predominantly expressed in white adipose tissue and signals information about peripheral energy stores to the central nervous system. In ob/ob mice, a premature stop codon prevents transcription of the mature leptin peptide and leads to a severe obesity syndrome. Leptin interacts with two leptin receptor variants, the long form and the short form. Severe obesity is seen in db/db mice, which do not make the long form of the leptin receptor, are leptin resistant, and have high circulating leptin levels. In ob/ob animals, exogenous leptin leads to weight reduction, restoration of fertility, and correction of abnormal physiologic measures, including hyperglycemia and hyperinsulinemia and hypercortisolemia. Leptin administration also reduces hypothalamic neuropeptide Y messenger RNA (mRNA).

Attention has recently focused on a number of neuropeptides that are known to affect feeding behavior in mice. For example, ablation of the melanocortin-4 receptor leads to rodent obesity and has brought to the fore the importance of the melanocortin pathway. Similarly, ablation of melanin concentrating hormone (MCH) leads to a model of rodent leanness, indicating the MCH is a significant contributor to feeding.

The findings of single gene defects in rodents focused attention on certain peptides and receptors and led to a search for single gene defects in humans. Thus far, humans with obesity secondary to leptin deficiency, leptin receptor deficiency, preproopiomelanocortin abnormalities, melanocortin-4 receptor abnormalities, prohormone convertase-1 abnormalities, and abnormalities of peroxisome proliferator-activated receptor-gamma have been identified.

The neuropeptides regulating body weight and eating probably interact at several levels in the central nervous system; however, the anatomic and functional basis for this interaction has not been defined. In addition, the molecular basis by which signals from the lateral hypothalamus might be integrated into systems involved in weight regulation has only recently been explored.

Prevalence of Obesity

PREVALENCE OF OBESITY IN THE US POPULATION

Preobesity: BMI 25.0–25.9

Constant rate over last 3–4 decades, prevalence has remained constant at 32%

Obesity: BMI>30

Prevalence is increasing

~13% in 1960

~23% in 1994

More than half the adult US population has a BMI that exceeds the healthy range.

FIGURE 15-1. In the United States, the prevalence of obesity has increased during the past four decades. In some populations, such as non-Hispanic white men 50 to 59 years of age, the prevalence of overweight and obesity (body mass index [BMI] greater than 25) is 72.9%. The prevalence in non-Hispanic black women of the same age is 78.1% [1].

Obesity and the Risk for Other Diseases

DISEASES FOR WHICH OBESITY IS A RISK FACTOR

Diabetes
Cardiovascular disease
Hypertension
Sleep apnea
Endometrial cancer
Breast cancer
Colon cancer
Gallbladder disease

FIGURE 15-2. Obesity increases the risk for many diseases [2].

EXAMPLES OF INCREASED RISK RELATED TO OBESITY

Relative risk in persons 20–44 years of age:
Diabetes—3.8
Hypertension—5.6
Hypercholesterolemia—2.1

FIGURE 15-3. Obesity is associated with a substantially increased risk for diabetes and cardiovascular disease, even in young persons.

OBESITY AND TYPE 2 DIABETES

80% to 90 % of people with non–insulin-dependent diabetes are obese.

Weight loss (as little as 10–20 pounds) can be single, adequate treatment.

Most people (>90%) cannot lose weight successfully.

Patients with non–insulin-dependent diabetes are at risk for usual complications, including cardiovascular disease, retinopathy, neuropathy, and nephropathy.

FIGURE 15-4. Non–insulin-dependent diabetes typically occurs in obese persons and has a significant component of insulin resistance. Even modest weight loss can lead to normalization of glucose control or to improved control with any given dose of oral medication. However, successful weight loss is unusual.

REGIONAL FAT DEPOSITS

Visceral Tissue	Subcutaneous
Mesenteric	Superficial
Omental	Deep
Retroperitoneal	
Perirenal	

FIGURE 15-5. Visceral fat deposits include mesenteric, omental, retroperitoneal, and perirenal deposits. According to location, fat deposits have different metabolic characteristics and thus pose different levels of risk for the complications of obesity. Central fat can be assessed by computed tomography, but a fairly good estimate can also be obtained by determining the waist-to-hip ratio. The abdominal circumference halfway between the lower rib and the iliac crest is compared to the circumference at the level of the greater trochanter [3]. Consideration of the waist-to-hip ratio augments evaluation of the risks of obesity. Data from a study by Goodpaster *et al.* [4] indicate that in men, for any given body mass index, increased waist-to-hip ratio confers additional risk. This increase is also seen in women. (see Fig. 15-39 for relative risk.)

Role of Molecular Mechanisms

REQUIREMENT FOR STABLE WEIGHT

Calories in:	Calories out:
Can only equal what one eats	Basal metabolic rate
	Thermogenesis
	Activity

FIGURE 15-6. Stable weight requires a match between calories consumed and calories expended. Fat-free mass is a major determinant of resting energy expenditure [5]. Weight gain leads to an increase in both fat and fat-free mass; thus, the basal metabolic rate of obese persons is higher than that of lean persons of the same height [6]. Obesity results from chronic excess of calories ingested over calories expended. Calories expended include the resting metabolic rate, the thermic effect of food, the thermic effect of exercise, and adaptive thermogenesis. Body fat is not significantly influenced by resting energy expenditure or the thermic effect of food [7], but changes in energy expenditure resulting from physical activity influence weight and body composition [8].

VIEWS OF ENERGY HOMEOSTASIS

Very old view
  Obesity is the result of excess calories and sloth voluntary
  overeating and laziness indicate moral fault.

Old view
  Obesity is the result of excess calories, but some lucky people can
  eat more because they have "faster metabolism."

New view
  Obesity is the result of interactions between factors that regulate
  appetite and total energy expenditure.

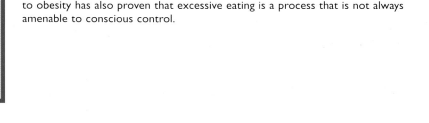

FIGURE 15-7. For many years, obesity was considered to be the consequence of a moral fault. Eating was considered a process entirely under voluntary control, and decreased energy expenditure was ascribed to sloth. Over time, various studies revealed that thermogenesis varied among people and that when placed diets consisting of equal calories, people might gain, maintain, or even lose weight. The discovery of leptin in 1994 revolutionized understanding of the pathophysiologic basis of obesity. It is now clear that multiple factors regulate appetite and total energy expenditure. The demonstration that single gene defects can lead to obesity has also proven that excessive eating is a process that is not always amenable to conscious control.

HYPOTHALAMIC ORGANIZATION

Lateral hypothalamus—eatring center (1951)

  Stimulates eating behavior

  Triggers feeding

  Ablative lesions cause aphagia, adipsia, and weight loss

Medial hypothalamus—satiety center (1940)

  Inhibits eating behavior

  Electrical stimulation of ventromedial hypothalamus inhibits eating

  Ablative lesions (surgical and goldthioglucose) cause hyperphagia
  and obesity

FIGURE 15-8. The role of the hypothalamus in the regulation of eating behavior was initially defined decades ago in studies of electrical stimulation and anatomical lesions. The role of the lateral hypothalamus in mediating eating was first considered in 1951 [9]. Experimental hypothalamic lesions of the ventromedial hypothalamus were reported to produce obesity in 1940 [10].

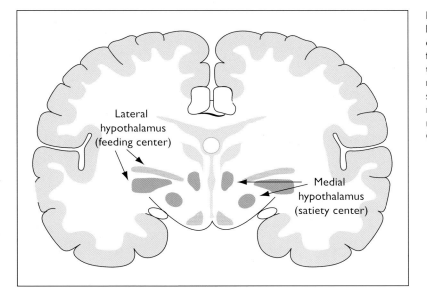

FIGURE 15-9. The hypothalamic areas implicated in eating behavior. The lateral hypothalamus is green (the lighter green area indicates the zona incerta). Melanin concentrating hormone [11] and orexin [12] localize to this area and stimulate feeding. The medial hypothalamus (ventral medial and dorsal medial) is red, and the paraventricular nucleus is yellow. The arcuate nucleus, in which cell bodies making neuropeptide Y, preproopiomelanocortin (the precursor to melanocyte-stimulating hormone), agouti-related peptide, and cocaine- and amphetamine-regulated transcript [CART] are localized, is pink. Neuropeptide Y and agouti-related peptide stimulate eating, and melanocyte-stimulating hormone and CART inhibit eating.

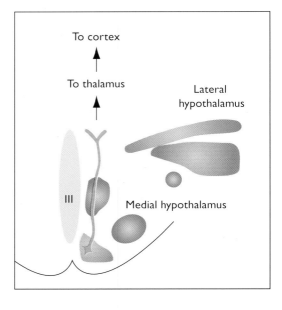

FIGURE 15-10. Neuropeptide Y (NPY) is made in neurons in the arcuate nucleus. The role of NPY in eating is attributed to direct projections of NPY to the paraventricular nucleus [13]. Repetitive injection of NPY into the hypothalamus induces hyperphagia and obesity [14]. Neuropeptide Y also alters energy metabolism. After repetitive injections of NPY, brown-fat thermogenic activity is decreased and white-fat lipoprotein lipase activity is decreased [15]. This finding suggests that the neuropeptides regulating appetite may have multiple roles.

One action of leptin is the suppression of neuropeptide Y (NPY) synthesis in the arcuate nucleus. This peptide appears to function as an important central regulator in eating behavior. Injection of NPY into rat lateral ventricles leads to a marked increase in eating; NPY-treated animals eat six- to ten-fold more than control animals over the ensuing 24-hour period. Repetitive injections over a several-day period cause weight gain. Neuropeptide Y also suppresses energy expenditure through actions on the sympathetic nervous system. Although NPY is diffusely expressed, it is the NPY-synthesizing neurons in the arcuate nucleus that project to paraventricular nucleus and the dorsal medial hypothalamus that is responsible for mediating eating behavior. In the ob/ob mouse, messenger RNA (mRNA) levels in the arcuate nucleus are two- to three-fold higher than mRNA levels in control mice; peptide levels are also increased in the ob/ob mouse. Similar results are seen in the Zucker fatty rat.

Both central intracerebroventricular and peripheral leptin treatment of ob/ob animals reduced NPY messages in the arcuate nucleus, suggesting that NPY is a leptin target. In normal animals, peripheral administration of leptin significantly inhibits the increase in the arcuate NPY mRNA levels seen with starvation. Although NPY may normally mediate eating behavior, NPY knockout mice lacking NPY in all tissues have no demonstrable changes in eating behavior. Cross-breeding of the NPY knockout mice with ob/ob mice revealed that the double-knockout offspring mice had an attenuated obesity phenotype. These data indicate that NPY is an important but not exclusive regulator of eating behavior and energy expenditure.

Role of Monogenic Mechanisms

MONOGENIC CAUSES OF RODENT OBESITY

Spontaneous
  Leptin deficiency (ob/ob)
  Absence of long form of leptin receptor (db/db)
  Ectopic agouti expression (Ay mouse)
  Fat (fa/fa)
  Tub
Engineered
  Serotonin 2C-receptor knockout
  Melanocortin-4 receptor knockout
  AgRP overexpression
  NPY 1 and NPY 5 receptor knockouts
  CRH overexpression
  B-3 receptor knockout
  Bombesin B-3 receptor knockout
  Glut-4 overexpression in fat

FIGURE 15-11. The identification of spontaneously occurring monogenic causes of obesity provided significant clues to understanding regulation of body weight. Identification of the fat hormone leptin [16] provided a mechanism by which fat can signal the status of peripheral energy stores to the brain [17]. Leptin is also important in regulating physiologic responses to fasting [18]. Analysis of other models of obesity, such as the Ay mouse, provided significant insight into pathways that are important in regulating body weight. Engineered models have been important in confirming the importance of the pathways and in identifying the roles of different peptides. AgRP—agouti-related peptide; CRH—corticotropin-releasing hormone; NPY—neuropeptide Y.

MONOGENIC CAUSES OF HUMAN OBESITY

Leptin deficiency	Mutations
Leptin receptor deficiency	PC-1 mutations
POMC gene mutations	PPARg2 mutations
Melanocortin-4 receptor mutations	

FIGURE 15-12. Monogenic obesity also occurs in humans. Key peptides identified in mice led to the pursuit of patients with similar defects. These studies were done in patients with morbid obesity of very early onset. In many cases (such as leptin deficiency, leptin receptor deficiency, melanocortin receptor abnormalities, and PC-1 mutations), the human phenotype is similar to the rodent phenotype. Some mutations, however, such as POMC gene mutations and PPARg2 mutations, have been described only in humans.

MONOGENIC CAUSES OF RODENT LEANNESS

Uncoupling protein overexpression in white adipose and brown adipose tissue

Glut-4 gene ablation

Dopamine D₁ receptor knockout

Melanin concentrating hormone knockout

Protein kinase A knockout

Hepatic leptin overexpression

Mahogany mutation

FIGURE 15-13. Most monogenic causes of rodent leanness have been specifically engineered lesions. The mechanism by which some of these manipulations cause leanness is understood, as in the case of hepatic leptin overexpression and melanin concentrating hormone deficiency [19]. In other cases, however, such as protein kinase A knockout, the mechanism of leanness is not understood. Of note, ablation of the *NPY* gene in rodents did not cause leanness or any change in the eating phenotype [20]. However, absence of neuropeptide Y led to an attenuation of the obesity seen in the Lep^ob/Lep^ob mouse [21].

MONOGENIC CAUSES OF HUMAN LEANNESS

None

FIGURE 15-14. Monogenic causes of human leanness have not been identified because the pursuit of such mutations would be complicated. Setting criteria for screening appropriate families would be difficult because weights, although reduced, might still be in the normal range.

PEPTIDES THAT REGULATE EATING

Increase Feeding	Decrease Feeding
Neuropeptide Y	Leptin
Melanin concentrating hormone	α-Melanocyte-stimulating hormone
Agouti related peptide	Glucagon-like peptide-1
Galanin	Neurotensin
Orexin A and B (?)	Corticotrophin-releasing hormone
Dynorphin	Urocortin
B-Endorphin	CART
	Bombesin
	Cholecystokinin
	Enterostatin

FIGURE 15-15. Partial listing of peptides that regulate eating. Several peptides are known to stimulate eating, and more are known to suppress eating. In addition, eating is regulated by monoamines (not discussed here).

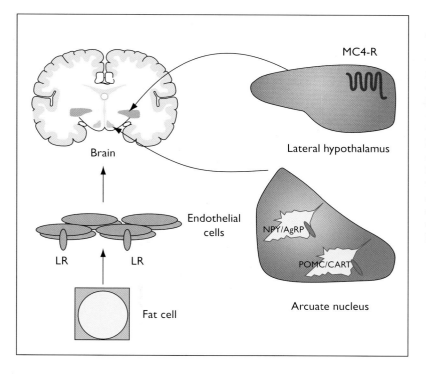

FIGURE 15-16. The relationship among peptides involved in the regulation of eating is complex. This figure summarizes some of the known interactions. Leptin is synthesized by adipocytes and released into the circulation. Leptin transport across the blood–brain barrier is mediated by the short form of the leptin receptor (LR). In the brain, leptin targets long-form receptors [22] in both the arcuate and the dorsal medial hypothalamus (not shown). In the arcuate hypothalamus, leptin regulates cell bodies that co-express agouti-related peptide (AgRP) and neuropeptide Y (NPY) (peptides that stimulate eating) and cells that co-express preproopiomelanocortin (POMC, the melanocyte-stimulating hormone precursor) and cocaine- and amphetamine-regulated transcript (CART) (peptides that inhibit eating). Cells from the arcuate project to several areas, including the lateral hypothalamus [23], where the melanocortin-4 receptor [24], which responds to POMC and AgRP, is expressed. This receptor may be present on neurons expressing orexin or melanin concentrating hormone (MCH), although this localization has not yet been confirmed. This figure provides an overview of sites where single gene lesions that lead to human obesity have been described.

FEATURES OF CONGENITAL LEPTIN DEFICIENCY

1. Homozygous frame shift mutation of leptin gene to synthesis of an unsecreted truncated lyk species
2. Normal birthweight, early severe obesity

   Patient I: 82 kg, age 8

   Patient 2: 30 kg, age 2
3. HPA axis normal, normal glycemic control, slightly elevated TSH level
4. Parents of both patients are heterozygotes

FIGURE 15-17. Leptin deficiency causes of the syndrome of obesity seen in ob/ob mice. These mice develop early obesity associated with hyperphagia and insulin resistance. Leptin deficiency has been described in two related children. Both had normal birthweight but were markedly obese during infancy. The hypothalamus-pituitary-adrenal (HPA) axis was normal in these children, although the thyroid-stimulating hormone (TSH) level was slightly elevated. In both children, glycemic control was normal; this finding differs from the severe insulin resistance seen in mice. Both sets of parents were of normal weight. Analysis of the leptin gene revealed that parents were heterozygotes and that the children were homozygous for a frame-shift mutation that led to synthesis of a truncated, unsecreted species [25].

CLINICAL FEATURES OF HUMAN LEPTIN RECEPTOR MUTATION*

Age, y	Sex	Weight, kg	BMI	Genotype	Leptin level, mg/mL
12	Male	37	16	wt/wt	5.6
13	Female	159	71.5	m/m	670
16	Male	87	30	wt/m	212
17	Female	102	34	wt/wt	88
19	Female	166	65.5	m/m	600
19	Female	133	52.5	?	526
22	Female	76	27.5	m/wt	240
24	Female	67.8	26.5	m/wt	294

Additional features: growth delay; no overnight burst of growth hormone; poor response of growth hormone to stimulation tests; low IgF levels; low TSH; sustained TSH response to thyroid-releasing hormone; hypothalamus-pituitary-adrenal axis grossly normal.

FIGURE 15-18. Leptin receptor deficiency has been described in a large family [26]. The proband presented with significant obesity and hypogonadotrophic hypogonadism. Affected homozygotes have 100-fold increased leptin levels (BMIs) in excess of fat content. Affected heterozygotes had BMIs in the preobese or minimally obese range and leptin levels of approximately 200 mg/mL. TSH—thyroid-stimulating hormone level.

THE STRANGE LINK BETWEEN EATING AND PIGMENTATION

Agouti

Melanocortin-4 receptor

Melanocyte stimulating hormone

Agouti-related peptide

Melanin-concentrating hormone

FIGURE 15-19. Peptides involved in regulating eating behavior and pigmentation. The intriguing connection between pigmentation and eating was first suggested by the finding that spontaneously mutant yellow mice (Ay), known as agouti mice, were also markedly obese. Agouti (normally expressed in the skin) acts on melanocytes as a paracrine factor to inhibit the conversion of phycomelanin (yellow) to eumelanin (black). Most mice are brown because of variable mixtures of these two pigments. Ay mice express agouti in all tissues and in an unregulated form. These findings suggested that melanocortin receptors have a role in mediating eating behavior.

Agouti protein is expressed in the skin and regulates skin coloration acting through the melanocortin 1 receptor, where it inhibits the action of melanocyte-stimulating hormone; when expressed ubiquitously, it leads to yellow pigmentation (inhibiting melanocortin 1 receptor) and obesity by inhibiting centrally expressed melanocortin 4 receptors. These receptors are expressed in the central nervous system; when activated by melanocyte-stimulating hormone, they mediate inhibition of eating behavior [27]. Melanin concentrating hormone regulates skin pigmentation in fish, where it is made in the pituitary and released into the circulation and acts on melanophores (cells containing pigment granules) to cause granule aggregation and skin darkening. It has no known role on pigmentation in mammals, but in mammals it is made in the lateral hypothalamus; it stimulates eating behavior through a still-unidentified receptor. A potential endogenous antagonist ligand for the hypothalamic melanocortin receptors is agouti-related protein, a recently cloned homologue of agouti. This protein is expressed in the arcuate nucleus of the hypothalamus, and its messenger RNA is upregulated in both ob/ob and db/db mice. Agouti-related protein appears to inhibit the melanocortin receptor in a manner similar to that of agouti.

THE AY MOUSE

Homozygous lethal

Heterozygote is obese, macrosomic, insulin resistant

Heterozygote has mustard yellow color

Syndrome results from ectopic expression of agouti in all organs

  Why is the mouse yellow?

  Why is the mouse obese?

FIGURE 15-20. The Ay mouse, in which normal agouti protein is expressed ectopically, is yellow and obese [28] .

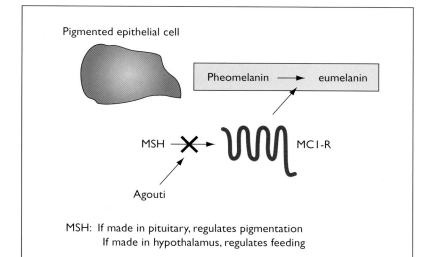

MSH: If made in pituitary, regulates pigmentation
      If made in hypothalamus, regulates feeding

FIGURE 15-21. Agouti protein is normally expressed in hair follicles in the skin and regulates pigmentation of skin and fur. Agouti protein expressed peripherally inhibits the melanocortin-1 receptor (MC1-R) and prevents the melanocyte-stimulating hormone (MSH)–mediated conversion of yellow pigment to black pigment [29].

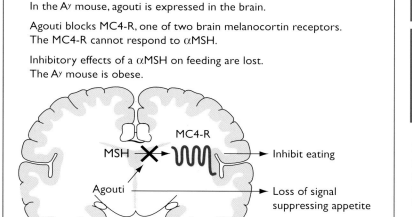

In the A^y mouse, agouti is expressed in the brain.

Agouti blocks MC4-R, one of two brain melanocortin receptors. The MC4-R cannot respond to αMSH.

Inhibitory effects of a αMSH on feeding are lost. The A^y mouse is obese.

FIGURE 15-22. Agouti (Ay) protein expressed centrally acts on the melanocortin-4 receptor (MC4-R) [30] and inhibits melanocyte-stimulating hormone (MSH)–mediated inhibition of eating. The obesity syndrome could be mimicked by genetically engineering a mouse that lacked MC4-R [31]; this capability demonstrates the importance of this receptor.

EXPRESSION OF AGOUTI AND AGRP

Agouti is not expressed in brain of normal animals.

A related peptide AgRP is expressed in the brain.

AgRP is found exclusively in arcuate neurons, which are leptin responsive and co-express neuropeptide Y.

FIGURE 15-23. Because agouti is not normally expressed in the central nervous system, the finding of the agouti effect on centrally expressed melanocortin receptors led to a search for agouti-like peptides in the central nervous system. Agouti-related peptide (AgRP) [32,33] is expressed in the arcuate nucleus and is one of the central nervous system peptides regulating the melanocortin-4 receptor (MC4-R). In addition, attention has focused on alpha-melanocyte-stimulating hormone (MSH), a product of preproopiomelanocortin in the arcuate, and on the role of alpha-MSH in the regulation of eating by acting as an agonist on MC4-R.

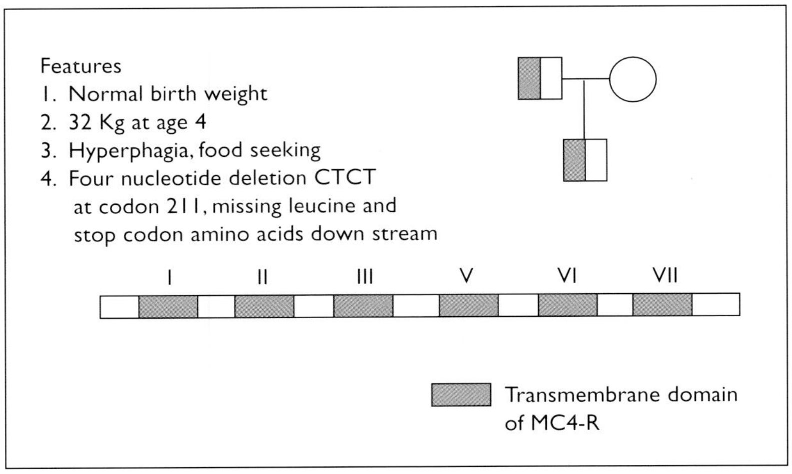
Features
1. Normal birth weight
2. 32 Kg at age 4
3. Hyperphagia, food seeking
4. Four nucleotide deletion CTCT
at codon 211, missing leucine and
stop codon amino acids down stream
I
II
III
V
VI
VII
Transmembrane domain
of MC4-R

FIGURE 15-24. A cohort of severely obese children was screened for mutations in melanocortin-4 receptor (MC4-R) by using direct nucleotide sequencing [34]. One patient was heterozygous for a 4–base pair deletion at codon 211 of the MC4-R. This mutation resulted in a stop codon in the region encoding for the fifth transmembrane domain. Residues at the fifth and sixth transmembrane domain are important for MC4-R signaling so this mutation results in a nonfunctional receptor. The proband's mother is normal weight, but the father is obese (body mass index, 41). The same mutation was identified in the father.

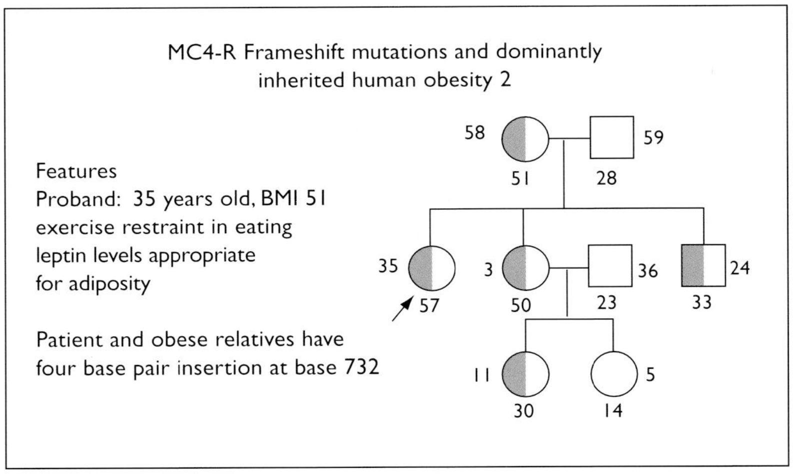
MC4-R Frameshift mutations and dominantly
inherited human obesity 2
Features
Proband: 35 years old, BMI 51
exercise restraint in eating
leptin levels appropriate
for adiposity
Patient and obese relatives have
four base pair insertion at base 732
58
51
59
28
35
57
3
50
36
23
24
33
11
30
5
14

FIGURE 15-25. A French population was screened by selecting persons with a history of obesity in infancy and highest lifetime body mass index (BMI) at any given age [35]. The entire single exon of the melanocortin-4 receptor (MC4-R) was evaluated by using five primer pairs. Direct sequencing identified a proband in which a heterozygous frame-shift mutation resulted in a nonfunctional truncated receptor. The proband's family was screened, and additional relatives with the mutation were identified. All of these relatives had similar levels of adiposity. Age of individuals is indicated to side of symbol, and BMI is below the symbol.

OBESITY, ADRENAL INSUFFICIENCY, AND RED HAIR PIGMENTATION ASSOCIATED WITH *POMC* MUTATIONS IN MAN: PATIENT 1

Obesity of very early onset, red hair, ACTH deficiency ACTH deficiency led to clinical presentation
Two mutations in exon 3:
Paternal allele:
G→T at nt 7013 leads to premature stop codon 79 (complete absence of ACTH, α-MSH, β-endorphin
Maternal allele:
1–base pair deletion nt 7133 leads to a frame-shift–disruptiing binding motif of ACTH and αMSH.

FIGURE 15-26. Mutations in the *POMC* gene lead to a syndrome of adrenal insufficiency, red hair pigmentation, and obesity. Preproopiomelanocortin is the precursor for many peptides, including adrenocorticotropin hormone (ACTH), melanocyte-stimulating hormone (MSH), and beta-endorphin. In the patient described here, two different POMC mutations led to interference with appropriate synthesis of ACTH and MSH. The adrenal insufficiency results from the absence of ACTH. Red hair results from the absence of MSH regulation of pigmentation in the hair follicle, which would be mediated by the melanocortin-1 receptor. Obesity results from the absence of centrally acting MSH, which would regulate eating through the melanocortin-4 receptor [36].

OBESITY, ADRENAL INSUFFICIENCY AND RED HAIR PIGMENTATION ASSOCIATED WITH POMC MUTATIONS IN MAN: PATIENT 2:

Obesity of very early onset, red hair, ACTH deficiency ACTH deficiency led to clinical presentation
Homozygous C→A transversion at nt 3804 leads to out-of-frame start codon
Abolishment of translation of wild-type protein

FIGURE 15-27. A syndrome of obesity, adrenal insufficiency, and red hair pigmentation was seen in another patient described by Krude *et al.* [36]. This patient was homozygous for a mutation that abolished preproopiomelanocortin translation. ACTH—adrenocorticotropin hormone.

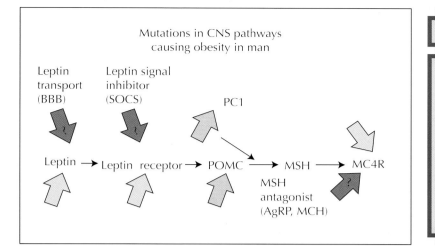

Mutations in CNS pathways
causing obesity in man

FIGURE 15-28. Summary of mutations in central nervous system pathways that may be associated with obesity in humans. Blue arrows point to mutations that have been identified. Gray arrows with question marks point to sites where mutations may occur but that have not yet been confirmed. AgRP—agouti-releasing peptide; BBB—blood–brain barrier; MC4-R—melanocortin-4 receptor; MCH—melanin concentrating hormone; MSH—melanocyte-stimulating hormone; PC1—prohormone convertase-1; POMC—preproopiomelanocortin; SOCS—suppressors of cytokine signaling.

PROHORMONE CONVERTASE 1 GENE AND OBESITY

1. Extreme childhood obesity
2. Abnormal glucose homeostasis, hypogonadotropic, hypogonadism, hypocortisolism, elevated plasma proinsulin level, low insulin level, elevated POMC level
3. Compound heterozygote in PC1

   Gly→Arg 483 prevents processing of prepro PC1 and retention in endoplasmic reticulum

   A→C + 4 intron 5-splice site, skipping of exon 5, loss of 26 residues, frameshift, and premature stop codon
4. Similarity in genetic abnormality and phenotype to fat/fat mouse

FIGURE 15-29. At least one severely obese patient with a prohormone convertase-1 (PC1) mutation has been described. The patient was a compound heterozygote for the *PC1* gene [37]. This patient's clinical syndrome was very similar to that seen in the fa/fa rat. POMC—preproopiomelanocortin.

PPAR-GAMMA2

358 unrelated German persons

121 were obese, (BMI >29)

Examined for mutations at or near serine phosphorylation site at amino acid 114. This site negatively regulates transcriptional activity of the protein.

Mutation identified—proline→glutamine at position 115.

  4 of 121 obese persons had this mutation

  0 of 237 non–obese persons had this mutation.

Overexpression of the mutant gene in fibroblasts led to synthesis of a phosphorylation defective protein and accelerated differentiation of cells into adipocytes.

FIGURE 15-30. Peroxisome proliferator-activated receptor (PPAR)-gamma is an important regulator of adipocyte differentiation. In a large study of German patients, four obese patients with a missense mutation in PPAR-gamma were identified [38]. This mutation resulted in the conversion of proline at position 115 to a glutamine. Overexpression of the mutant gene in mouse fibroblasts revealed that the mutant protein is defective in phosphorylating a serine in position 114. Fibroblasts expressing the mutant gene showed accelerated differentiation into adipocytes. BMI—body mass index.

Treatment of Obesity

NIH ASSESSMENT CONFERENCE: METHODS OF VOLUNTARY WEIGHT LOSS CONTROL, AND BETHESDA, MARYLAND, 1992

40% of women and 24% of men attempt weight loss at any time

Most people can lose 10% of initial weight

One third to one half regained weight within 1 year, and most regained weight within 5 years

For many overweight persons, achieving and maintaining a healthy weight is a lifelong challenge.

FIGURE 15-31. The treatment of obesity poses major challenges. A large proportion of the U.S. population is trying to lose weight at any given time. Although most persons lose a modest amount of weight, weight loss is not usually maintained.

RATIONALE FOR LONG TERM USE OF OBESITY MEDICATIONS

Obesity is a chronic disease with morbid consequences.

If medications are effective at weight loss, affect morbid consequences, and are safe, they should be used.

Precise cut-off point for use of therapy must be determined through clinical trials, as is the case with therapies for other conditions (eg, hypertension, diabetes, hyperlipidemia).

FIGURE 15-32. Obesity is a chronic illness associated with complications. Some chronic illnesses, such as hypertension, may respond to dietary maneuvers (eg, reduction in salt intake). However, patients may be unable to make the necessary changes or the response may be inadequate. Safe medications that help obese individuals achieve sustained weight loss would substantially affect the morbidity and mortality associated with obesity.

RECENT AND FUTURE APPROACHES TO WEIGHT LOSS

Sibutramine (meridia) - novel serotonin and norepinephrine reuptake

Orlistat (Xenical)—inhibitor of intestinal fat absorption

Old standbys—phentermine, diethylpropion, mazindol

β-3 adrenergic agonists

Leptin or leptin analogues/mimics

Centrally acting agents based on new discoveries

Antagonists of melanin-concentrating hormone, orexin, neuropeptide Y, galanin

Agonists of melanocortin-4 receptor, corticotropin-releasing hormone receptors

Inhibitors of leptin resistance

FIGURE 15-33. Many medications are potentially available for the treatment of obesity. The odds of successful pharmacologic therapy are increased when drug therapy is combined with a behavior modification program. Commercial programs may be as effective as hospital-based programs. Sibutremine [39] leads to effective weight loss in a subset of motivated patients; its effectiveness appears to be similar to that of phentermine used as a sole agent. The Food and Drug Administration has just approved orlistat .One-year trials of orlistat with doses of 120 mg three times daily revealed that in the treatment group, weight loss at 1 year was approximately 50% greater than that in the control group (10.3 kg compared with 6.1 kg) [40]. Although the drug was effective in large clinical trials, its effectiveness in patients seen in a standard office practice has not yet been evaluated. Novel therapies, such as beta-three adrenergic agonists or leptin mimetics, or agents based on neuropeptide regulation are the subject of intense investigation.

OBESITY PHARMACOTHERAPY: TIME LINE

Amphetamines used in 1950s and 1960s

No new drugs approved between 1973 and 1996

Major controversy about attitude of FDA toward

Weintraub study published, 1992:

Double blind, controlled trial of the efficacy of fen-phen

Redux approved in 1996: fen-phen and Redux take off

1997

July 8—Mayo reports 24 cases of valvular disease

September 15—Voluntary withdrawal of fenfluramine and dexfenfluramine

November 14—Interim guidelines from CDC, FDA, and NIH:

History and physical examination, with or without, echocardiography

1998—Further follow-up

FIGURE 15-34. Few drugs directed at the treatment of obesity have been introduced in the past several decades. This partly reflects resistance to treating obesity as a chronic illness. A long-term trial of phentermine and fenfluramine was the subject of a series of reports in 1992 [41], which demonstrated effectiveness and initiated a renewed interest in these agents. Dexfenfluramine [42] was introduced in 1996. Although the association of treatment with fenfluramine and phentermine (fen-phen) and pulmonary hypertension was known, new studies showed that therapy with fenfluramine and dexfenfluramine led to the development of valvular heart disease [43]. This led to withdrawal of both agents from the market. CDC—Centers for Disease Control and Prevention; FDA—Food and Drug Administration; NIH—National Institutes of Health.

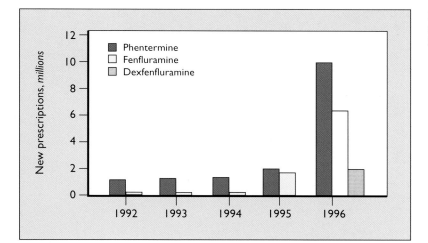

FIGURE 15-35. From 1992 to 1996, the number of prescriptions of anorexiant drugs increased substantially. This increase demonstrates the potential demand for safe and effective drugs.

FOLLOW-UP STUDIES ON FEN-PHEN AND VALVULAR DISEASE

Khan *et al.* 233 patients and 233 matched controls

  All regimens were associated with increased prevalence

  12-26–fold increase, mainly in trace and mild atrial insufficiency

  Clinical significance, natural history unknown

Hick *et al.* Population-based follow-up and case-control study in United Kingdom on recipients

  6532 Redux recipients, 2371 fenfluramine recipients, 862 phentermine recipients

  Redux or fenfluramine <3 months—7/10,000 exposed

  Redux or fenfluramine > 4 months—35/10,000 (mainly atrial insufficiency)

  Asymptomatic cases not ascertained

Weissman *et al.*

  Modification of double-blind, placebo-controlled trial

  1072 patients, Echocardiograms added

  2–3 months of Redux-therapy associated with small increase in mild or trace atrial insufficiency (17% compared with 12%)

  Mild or greater atrial insufficiency

  Atrial insufficiency and moderate or greater myocardial infarction not significant

FIGURE 15-36. The report by Kahn *et al.* [43] showed that 23% of patients treated with fenfluramine or dexfenfluramine developed valvular disease (53 of 223). Subsequent studies confirmed the occurrence of valvular disease, but at a lower incidence [44].

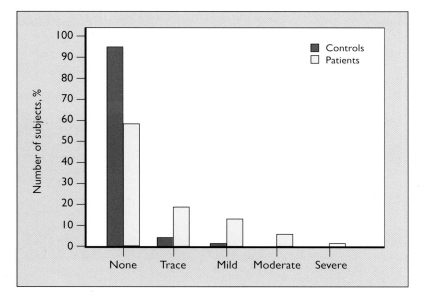

FIGURE 15-37. Reported incidence of valvular heart disease in the study by Kahn *et al.* Risk for valvular disease increased with duration of treatment.

SUMMARY

1. The molecular mechanisms regulating body weight and obesity are beginning to be understood.

2. Specific mechanisms have been defined in a few cases.

3. Most human obesity is likely to be caused by dysregulation of several or many factors. As our understanding of the mechanisms involved in the regulation of body weight increases, identification of factors responsible for obesity will be possible.

4. Although some treatments are available, none are ideal; success of long-term therapy is mixed at best.

FIGURE 15-38. Understanding of the molecular mechanisms of obesity in the general population will improve as our understanding of the regulators of eating behavior improves. Although current treatments are limited, the potential for new specific treatments based on the identification of specific molecular targets has increased.

Relative Risk for Obesity

RELATIVE RISK FOR OBESITY ASSOCIATED WITH BODY MASS INDEX AND FAT DISTRIBUTION IN MEN

BMI	Waist Hip Ratio		
	<0.85	0.85–1.0	>1.0
20 to <25	Very low	Low	Medium
25 to <30	Low	Medium	High
30 to <35	Medium	High	Very high
35 to <40	High	Very high	Very high
>40	Very high	Very high	Very high

FIGURE 15-39. Relative risk for obesity varies with fat distribution. For any particular body mass index (BMI), the lower the waist-to-hip ratio: *ie,* the smaller the intra-abdominal deposits, the lower the risk.

Acknowledgement

I would like to thank Dr. Jeffrey Flier for the use of his figures on therapeutic agents used in obesity (Figs. 15-33 through 15-37).

References

1. Flegal KM, Carrp MD, Kuczmarski RJ, et al.: Overweight and obesity in the United States: prevalence and trends, 1960-1994. *Int J Obesity* 1998, 22:39–37.

2. Vanitallie TB: Body weight, morbidity and longevity. In: *Obesity.* Edited by Bjorntorp P, Brodoff BN. Philadelphia: JB Lippincott; 1992.

3. Smith SR: Regional fat distribution. In: Nutrition, Genetics and Obesity. Edited by Bray GA, Ryan DH. Baton Rouge, LA: Louisiana State University Press; 1999:433–458.

4. Goodpaster B, Thaete F, Somoneau J, et al.: Subcutaneous abdominal fat and thigh muscle composition predict insulin sensitivity independently of visceral fat. *Diabetes* 1997, 46:1579–1585.

5. Ravussin E, Lillioja S, Anderson TE, et al.: Determinants of 24-h energy expenditure in man. *J Clin Invest* 1986, 778:1568–1578.

6. Prentice AM, Black AE, Coward WA, et al. High levels of energy expenditure in obese women. *Br Med J* 1986, 292:983–987.

7. Flatt JP: Importance of nutrient balance in body weight regulation. *Diabetes Metab Rev* 1988, 4:571–581.

8. Flatt JP, Gupte S. In: *Nutrition, Genetics and Obesity.* Edited by Bray GA, Ryan DH. Baton Rouge, LA: Louisiana State University Press; 1999:73–88.

9. Anand BK, Brobeck JR: Hypothalamic control of food intake in rates and cats. *Yale J Biol Med* 1951, 24:123.

10. Hetherignton A, Ranson SW: Hypothalamic lesions and adiposity in the rat. *Anat Rec* 1940, 78:149.

11. Qu D, Ludwig DS, Gammeltoft S, et al.: A role for melanin concentrating hormone in the central regulation of feeding behavior. *Nature* 1996, 380:243–246.

12. Sakurai T, Amemiya A, Ishii M, et al. Orexins and orexin receptors: a family of hypothalamic neuropeptides and G protein-coupled receptors that regulate feeding behavior. *Cell* 1998, 92:1 page following 696.

13. Turton MD, Oshea D, Bloom SR: Central effects of neuropeptide Y with emphasis on its role in obesity and diabetes. In: *Neuropeptide Y and Drug Development.* Edited by Grundemar L, Bloom SR. San Diego: Academic Press; 1997:15–39.

14. Stanley BG, Kyrkouli SE, Lampert S, et al.: Neuropeptide Y chronically injected into the hypothalamus: a powerful neurochemical inducer of hyperphagia and obesity. Peptides 1986, 7:1189–1192.

15. Billington CJ, Briggs JE, Grace M, et al.: Effects of intracerebroventricular injection of neuropeptide Y on energy metabolism. Am J Physiol 1991, 260(2 Pt 2):R321–R327.

16. Zhang Y, Proenca R, Maffei M, et al.: Positional cloning of the mouse obese gene and its human homologue. Nature 1994, 372:425–432.

17. Halaas JL, Gajiwala KS, Maffei M, et al.: Weight reducing effects of the plasma protein encoded by the obese gene. Science 1995, 269:543–546.

18. Ahima RS, Prabakaran D, Mantzoros C, et al.: Role of leptin in the neuroendocrine response to fasting. Nature 1996, 383:250–252.

19. Shimada M, Tritos NA, Lowell BB, et al.: Mice lacking melanin concentrating hormone are hypophagic and lean. Nature 1998, 396:670–674.

20. Ericson JC, Clegg KE, Palmiter RD: Sensitivity to leptin and susceptibility to seizures in mice lacking neuropeptide Y. Nature 1996, 381:415–418.

21. Erickson JC, Hollopeter G, Palmiter RD: Attenuation of the obesity syndrome of ob/ob mice by the loss of neuropeptide Y. Science 1996, 274:1704–1707.

22. Tartaglia LA, Dembski M, Weng X, et al.: Identification and expression cloning of a leptin receptor, OB-R. Cell 1995, 83:1263–1271.

23. Elias CF, Saper CB, Maratos-Flier E, et al.: Chemically defined projection linking the mediobasal hypothalamus and the lateral hypothalamic area. J Comp Neurol 1998, 402:442–459.

24. Mountjoy KG, Robbinsa LS, Mortrud MT, et al.: The cloning of a family of genes that encode the melanocortin receptors. Science 1992, 257:1248–1251.

25. Montague CT, Farooqi IS, Whitehead JP, et al.: Congenital leptin deficiency is associated with severe early-onset obesity in humans. Nature 1997, 387:903–908.

26. Clement K, Vaisse C, Lahlou N, et al.: A mutation in the human leptin receptor gene causes obesity and pituitary dysfunction. Nature 1998, 392:398–401.

27. Tsujii S, Bray GA: Acetylation alters the feeding response to MSH and beta-endorphin. Brain Res Bull 1989, 23:165–169.

28. Yen TT, Gill AM, Frigeri LG, et al.: Obesity, diabetes and neoplasia in the yellow Avy/- mice: ectopic expression of the agouti gene. FASEB J 1994, 8:481–488.

29. Blanchard SG, Harris CO, Ittoop OR, et al. Agouti antagonism of melanocortin binding and action in the B16F10 murine melanoma cell line. Biochemistry 1995, 34:10406–10411.

30. Lu D, Willard D, Patel IR, et al.: Agouti protein is an antagonist of the melanocyte-stimulating hormone receptor. Nature 1994, 371:799–802.

31. Huszar D, Lynch CA, Fairchild-Huntress V, et al.: Targeted disruption of the melanocortin-4 receptor results in obesity in mice. Cell 1997, 88:131–141.

32. Shutter JR, Graham M, Kinsey AC, et al.: Hypothalamic expression of ART, a novel gene related to agouti, is up-regulated in obese and diabetic mutant mice. Genes Dev 1997, 11:593–602.

33. Ollmann MM, Wilson BD, Yang YK, et al.: Antagonism of central melanocortin receptors in vitro and in vivo by agouti-related protein. Science 1997, 281:135–138.

34. Yeo GS, Farooqi IS, Aminian S, et al.: A frameshift mutation in MC4R associated with dominantly inherited human obesity. Nat Genet 1998, 20:111–112.

35. Vaisse C, Clement K, Guy-Grand B, et al.: A frameshift mutation in human MC4R is associated with a dominant form of obesity. Nat Genet 1998, 20:113–114.

36. Krude H, Biebermann H, Luck W, et al.: Severe early-onset obesity, adrenal insufficiency and red hair pigmentation caused by POMC mutations in humans. Nat Genet 1998, 9:155–157.

37. Jackson RS, Creemers JW, Ohagi S, et al.: Obesity and impaired prohormone processing associated with mutations in the human prohormone convertase 1 gene. Nat Genet 1997, 16:303–306.

38. Ristow M, Muller-Wieland D, Pfeiffer A, et al.: Obesity associated with a mutation in a genetic regulator of adipocyte differentiation. N Engl J Med 1998, 339:953–959.

39. Bray GA, Blackburn GL, Ferguson JM, et al.: Sibutramine produces dose-related weight loss. Obes Res 1999, 7:189–198.

40. Hauptman J, Guerciolini R, Nichols G: Orlistat: a novel treatment for obesity. In: Nutrition, Genetics and Obesity. Edited by Bray GA, Ryan DH. Baton Rouge, LA: Louisiana State University Press; 1998.

41. Weintraub M: Long-term weight control: the National Heart, Lung, and Blood Institute funded multimodal intervention study. Clin Pharmacol Ther 1992, 51:581–585.

42. Guy-Grand B: INDEX (international dexfenfluramine study) as a model for long-term pharmacotherapy of obesity in the 1990s. Int J Obes Relat Metab Disord 1992, 16 Suppl 3:S5–S14.

43. Khan MA, Herzog CA, St Peter JV, et al.: The prevalence of cardiac valvular insufficiency assessed by transthoracic echocardiography in obese patients treated with appetite-suppressant drugs. N Engl J Med 1998, 339:713–718.

44. Weissman NJ, Tighe JF Jr, Gottdiener JS, et al.: An assessment of heart-valve abnormalities in obese patients taking dexfenfluramine, sustained-release dexfenfluramine, or placebo. Sustained-Release Dexfenfluramine Study Group. N Engl J Med 1998, 339:725–732.

Index

A

Acidosis. *See also* Diabetic ketoacidosis (DKA)
    laboratory evaluation of, 34
Ackee fruit, hypoglycemia and, 112
Acromegaly, 180-181
    acute and delayed effects of supraphysiologic growth hormone on carbohydrate metabolism and, 180
    growth hormone-induced hepatic and peripheral insulin resistance and, 181
    octreotide effects on glucose homeostasis in, 181
    response to oral glucose testing in, 180
Adrenal insufficiency, obesity and red hair pigmentation and, 198
Advanced glycation endproducts (AGEs), 126-128
    albumin permeability of glomerular basement membrane and, 127
    diabetic nephropathy and, 156
    inhibition of, amelioration of abnormalities by, 128
    macromolecular endocytosis due to, 127
    mechanisms of damage caused by, 127, 128
    potential pathways leading to formation of, 126
    putative receptors for, 127
Age, resting blood flow and, 169
Agouti protein, obesity and, 196-197
AKT kinase, as downstream effector of insulin action, 20
Albumin
    glomerular basement membrane permeability to, advanced glycation endproducts and, 127
    microalbuminuria detection and, 152
Albumin excretion rate (AER), urinary, in diabetic nephropathy, 87
Alcoholic ketosis, laboratory evaluation of, 34
Aldose reductase
    diabetic nephropathy and, 156
    hypoglycemic damage and, 123-124
        function in nondiabetic and diabetic cells and, 123
        nerve conduction velocity and, 124
        under oxidative stress, 123
Amino acids, insulin secretion and, 9
Amputation, in small-fiber neuropathy, 171
Amyloid deposits, insulin secretion in type 2 diabetes and, 11
Aneurysms, sustained microaneurysms in type 1 diabetes and, 65
Angle closure glaucoma, clinical presentation of, 136
Anorexiant drugs, 200-201
    available drugs, 200
    fen-phen, 201
    new, lack of, 200
    usage of, 201

Antiatherogenic gene expression, insulin resistance in vascular cells and, 130
Antihypertensive agents, for diabetic nephropathy, 158
Antilipolysis, insulin regulation of, 25
Apoptosis, insulin action and, 16
Arginine, insulin secretion in type 2 diabetes and, 9
Arrhythmia, sinus, loss of, in autonomic neuropathy, 172
Autonomic nervous system
    of heart, 173
    insulin secretion and, 9
Autonomic neuropathy, 172-173
    autonomic nervous system of heart and, 173
    cardiac, RR intervals and, 172
    model of effects on heart rate, 172
    segmental loss of sympathetic fibers in heart and, 173

B

Bergman minimal model, 72
ß-cells, 1
    electron micrograph of, 4
    endogenous hyperglucagonemia effects on, 183
    fatty acid influence on, 8
    glucose-induced electrical activity of, in mice, 7
    glucotoxicity and, insulin secretion in type 2 diabetes and, 12
    insulin secretion by, mechanisms of, 7
    lipotoxicity and, insulin secretion in type 2 diabetes and, 12
    lymphokine model for destruction of, in type 1 diabetes, 55
    nutrient sensing and insulin secretion by, in type 2 diabetes, 76
    population of, mechanisms responsible for maintenance of, 4
    rapid destruction of, in pathogenesis of type 1 diabetes, 54
    stages of decomposition of, insulin secretion in type 2 diabetes and, 12
ß tropic virus-viral superantigen model, of viral role in type 1 diabetes, 56
Bicarbonate, for diabetic ketoacidosis, 39
Biostator, 114
Blindness, in diabetic retinopathy, 141-143
    causes of, 141
    neovascularization of iris and, 143
    ophthalmic complications associated with, 141-143
Blood flow, resting, age and, 169
Blood glucose
    disposal of
        oxidation and nonoxidative, dose-response curve for action of insulin on, 99
        peripheral, 98

gluconeogenesis contribution to fasting plasma glucose concentration and, 97
high. *See* Hyperglycemia; Hyperglycemic entries
insulin levels and levels of, 73
low. *See* Hypoglycemia
peripheral utilization of, in Cushing syndrome, 182
plasma glucose responses to glucagon and, in patients with insulinoma and normal patients and, 114
plasma levels of, intravenous, subcutaneous, and intramuscular low-dose insulin regimens and, in diabetic ketoacidosis, 38
turnover in fasting stage, insulin resistance and, 96
in type 1 diabetes, with nonphysiologic insulin replacement, 61
utilization of, pheochromocytoma and, 184
variables involved in control of, 72
Blood pressure
    insulin and, 106
    insulin resistance and, 104
Blood volume, insulin and, 106
Brain, glucose supply to, maintenance of, 35

C

Calcium-channel blockers, for diabetic nephropathy, 158
Calories, consumed and expended, balance between, 192
Carbohydrate metabolism, acute and delayed effects of supraphysiologic growth hormone on, in acromegaly, 180
Cardiac output, insulin and, 106
Cardiovascular disease, 90-92. *See also* Heart, autonomic neuropathy and; Vascular disorders
    fen-phen and, 201
    management of, multifactorial approach to, 92
    mortality due to, in type 2 diabetes, 91
    pathogenesis and clinical features of, 90
Cardiovascular dysmetabolic syndrome, 83
Carpal tunnel syndrome, 165
Cataracts, clinical presentation of, 136
Cell death, insulin action and, 16
C-fiber dysfunction, in small fiber neuropathy, 169-171
    age and resting blood flow and, 169
    clinical presentation of, 170
    management of, 171
    nerve fibers in skin and, 170
    vasodilation and, 169
Charcot neuroarthropathy, hot foot of, 171, 172
Coma, hyperosmolar and hypoglycemic, laboratory evaluation of, 34
Continuous subcutaneous insulin infusion therapy (CSII), 59

Lymphokine model for ß-cell destruction, in type 1 diabetes, 55

M

Macular edema, 135
  clinical manifestations of, 136, 140
  treatment of, 145
Male sexual dysfunction, 90
Maturity-onset diabetes of the young, typical pedigree of family with, 75
Mechanoreceptor function, nerve fibers in skin and, 170
Median entrapment, 165
Melanin concentrating hormone, obesity and, 196
Melanocortin-4 receptor, obesity and, 197, 198
Mental status, serum osmolality related to, in diabetic ketoacidosis, 37
Messenger RNA, insulin regulation of, 25
Metformin, for type 2 diabetes, site of action of, 81
Methanol intoxication, laboratory evaluation of, 34
Microalbuminuria, detection of, 152
Microaneurysms, sustained, in type 1 diabetes, 65
Microvascular insufficiency, diabetic neuropathy and, 164
Molecular mimicry model, of viral role in type 1 diabetes, 56
Mononeuritis, 165
Motor neuropathy, proximal, 165
Multiple daily injection therapy (MDI), 59
Muscle wasting, in large fiber neuropathy, 167-168

N

Necrolytic migratory erythema, 183
Neovascularization
  of iris
    clinical presentation of, 136
    in proliferative diabetic retinopathy, 143
  retinal, growth factors and, 148-149
Nephropathy. *See* Diabetic nephropathy
Nerve conduction velocity, aldose reductase and hypoglycemic damage and, 124
Neuroarthropathy, 171-172
  hot foot of, 171, 172
  prediction of foot ulcers versus, 171
Neuropathy. *See* Diabetic neuropathy
Neuropeptide Y (NPY)
  leptin suppression of, 193
  production of, 194
Neurovascular dysfunction, in neuropathy, 168
Non-insulin-dependent diabetes.
    See Type 2 diabetes
Nonproliferative diabetic retinopathy (NPDR).
    See Diabetic retinopathy, nonprolific
Nutrient sensing, by ß-cells, in type 2 diabetes, 76

O

Obesity, 191-203
  genetic predisposition to type 2 diabetes and, interaction with, 76

insulin resistance and, 104
  in type 2 diabetes, 80
molecular mechanisms of, 192-194, 202
  energy homeostasis and, 193
  hypothalamic regulation of eating behavior and, 193
  neuropeptide Y and, 194
  requirements for stable weight and, 192
monogenic mechanisms of, 194-199
  agouti protein and, 196-197
  central nervous system pathway mutations associated with, 199
  eating and pigmentation and, 196-198
  in humans, 194, 195
  leptin deficiency and, 196
  melanocortin-4 receptor and, 197, 198
  obesity, adrenal insufficiency, and red hair pigmentation and, 198
  peptides regulating eating and, 195
  peroxisome proliferator-activated receptor-gamma and adipocyte differentiation and, 199
  POMC gene mutations and, 198
  in rodents, 194, 195
  peroxisome proliferator-activated receptor-gamma and, 199
prevalence of, 191
regional fat deposits and, 192
relative risk for, 202
risk for other diseases and, 192
treatment of, 199-202
  fen-phen and, 201
  long-term use of medications for, 200
  medications available for, 200
  utilization of medications for, 201
Octreotide, effects on glucose homeostasis, in acromegaly, 181
Ocular complications. *See* Diabetic retinopathy; Eye complications
Oral glucose testing
  in acromegaly, 180
  hypoglycemia and, 115
Oxidative stress
  aldose reductase and hypoglycemic damage under, 123
  diabetic nephropathy and, 155

P

Pancreas
  differentiation of, 2
  embryologic origin of, 2
  in type 1 diabetes, 49
Pancreatic transplantation
  for diabetic nephropathy, 159
  for type 1 diabetes, 68-69
    islet transplantation compared with, 69
    results with, 68-69
Pancreatoprivic diabetes, 186
Papillopathy, clinical presentation of, 136
PC-1, modulation of insulin action by, 27
Peptides, regulating eating behavior, 195

Perception, sensory, nerve fibers in skin and, 170
Peroxisome proliferator-activated receptor (PPAR)-gamma, obesity and, 199
Pheochromocytoma, 184
  glucose intolerance and, 184
  glucose production and utilization and, 184
Phosphate, for diabetic ketoacidosis, 39
Phosphatidylinositol 3-kinase (PI 3-K), 77
  binding to insulin receptor substrate, 19
  insulin receptor substrate/phosphatidylinositol 3-kinase pathway and, 17
Phosphorylation
  insulin action and, 16
  insulin receptor substrate sites of, 18
Photocoagulation, laser
  for macular edema, 145
  for proliferative diabetic retinopathy, 144
  side effects and complications of, 146-147
  therapeutic efficacy of, 146
Pigmentation, eating behavior related to, 196-198
  agouti protein and, 196-197
  melanocortin-4 receptor and, 197, 198
  POMCgene mutations and, 198
Plantar entrapment, 165
Plasma expanders, for diabetic ketoacidosis, 42
POMC gene mutations, obesity and, 198
Prenatal development, insulin resistance and, 104
Prohormone convertase-1 gene mutation, obesity and, 199
Proinsulin
  limits of plasma levels of, hypoglycemia and, 113
  processing of, 5
Proliferative diabetic retinopathy (PDR).
    See Diabetic retinopathy, proliferative
Protein kinase C (PKC)
  diabetic nephropathy and, 156
  as downstream effector of insulin action, 20
  hypoglycemic damage and, 124-125
Protein tyrosine phosphatases, modulation of insulin action by, 26
Proteinuria, screening and treatment recommendations for, 160
p70 S6 kinase, insulin regulation of, 21
Pylol pathway, redox changes induced by, potential relationship with other mechanisms underlying diabetic complications, 129

R

Rad, modulation of insulin action by, 27
Ras/mitogen-activated protein kinase (MAPK) pathway, 17
Ras signaling pathway, insulin activation of, 21
Reactive oxygen species (ROS)
  increase in, by hyperglycemia, 122
  potential relationship with other mechanisms underlying diabetic complications, 129
  protein kinase C activation by, 124
Renal disease. *See* Diabetic nephropathy
Retinal detachment, clinical presentation of, 136

Color Plates

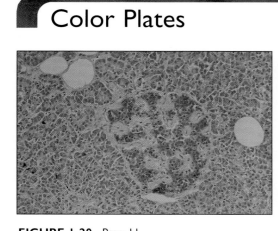
FIGURE 1-20. Page 11

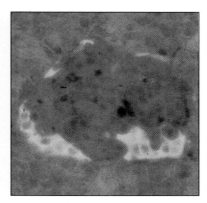
FIGURE 3-2A. Page 30

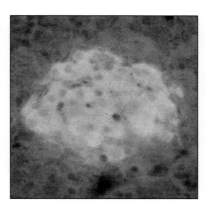
FIGURE 3-2B. Page 30

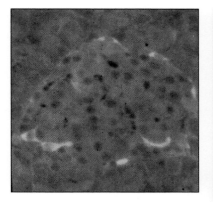
FIGURE 3-2C. Page 30

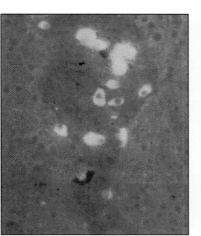
FIGURE 3-2D. Page 30

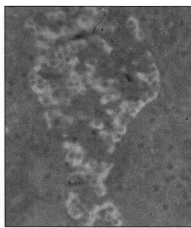
FIGURE 3-2E. Page 30

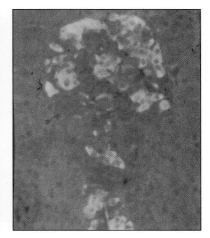
FIGURE 3-2F. Page 30

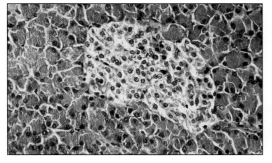
FIGURE 3-4A. Page 32

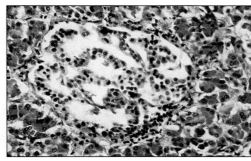
FIGURE 3-4B. Page 32

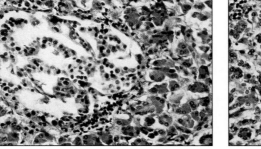
FIGURE 3-4C. Page 32

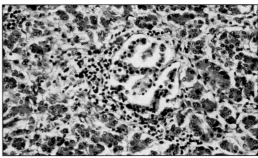

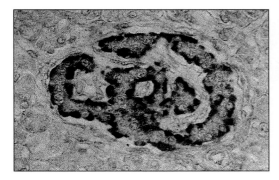
FIGURE 4-11C. Page 49

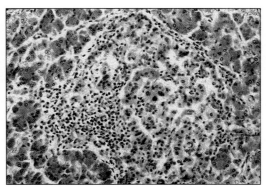
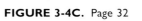
FIGURE 4-11D. Page 50

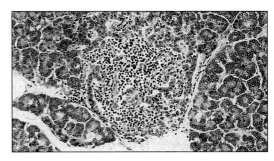
FIGURE 4-12. Page 50

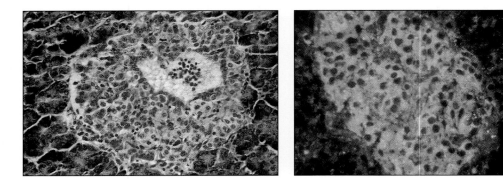

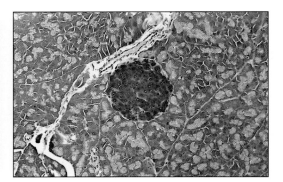

FIGURE 4-13. Page 50

FIGURE 4-14. Page 50

FIGURE 4-20A. Page 52

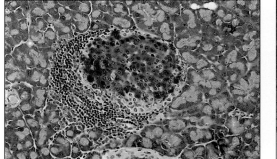

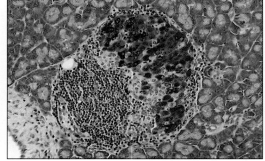

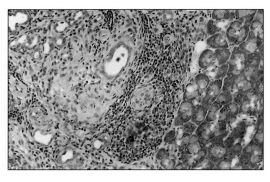

FIGURE 4-20B. Page 52

FIGURE 4-20C. Page 53

FIGURE 4-20D. Page 53

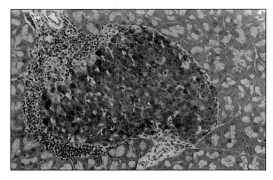

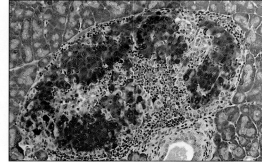

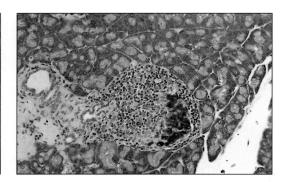

FIGURE 4-20E. Page 53

FIGURE 4-20F. Page 53

FIGURE 4-20G. Page 53

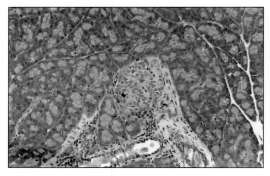

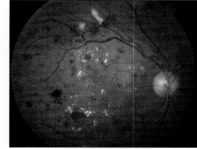

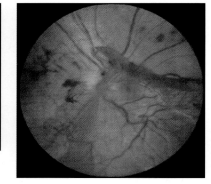

FIGURE 4-20H. Page 53

FIGURE 7-5. Page 86

FIGURE 7-6. Page 87

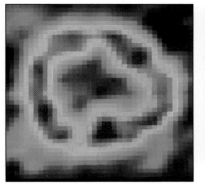

FIGURE 8-9A. Page 98

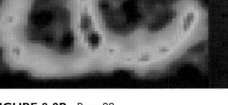

FIGURE 8-9B. Page 98

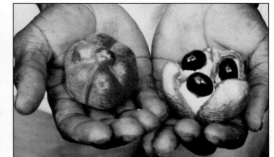

FIGURE 9-6. Page 112

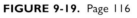

FIGURE 9-15. Page 115

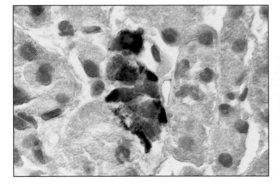

FIGURE 9-19. Page 116

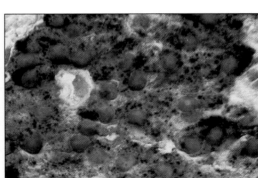

FIGURE 9-20. Page 117

FIGURE 9-21. Page 117

FIGURE 9-22A. Page 117

FIGURE 9-22B. Page 117

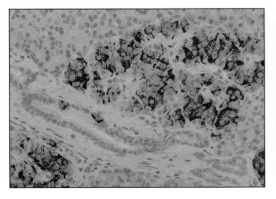

FIGURE 9-23. Page 118

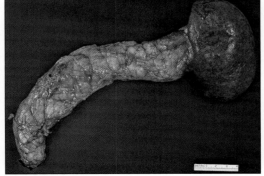

FIGURE 9-24. Page 118

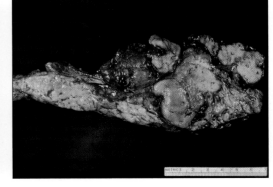

FIGURE 9-25. Page 118

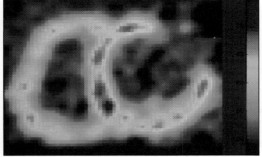
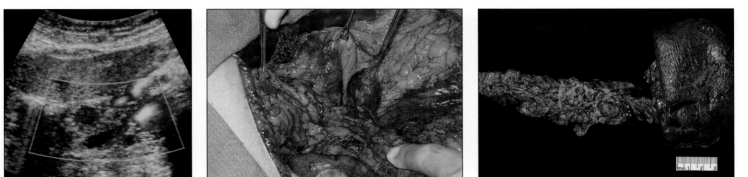

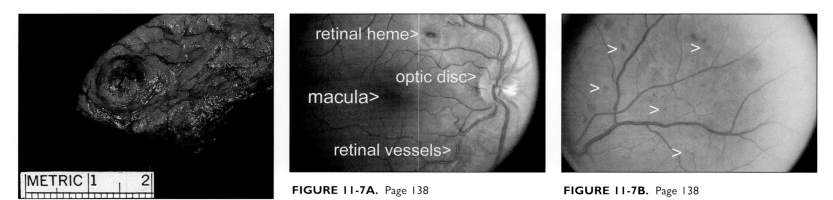

FIGURE 9-26. Page 118

FIGURE 11-7A. Page 138

FIGURE 11-7B. Page 138

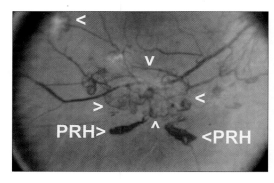

FIGURE 11-7C. Page 139

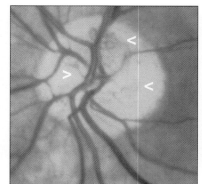

FIGURE 11-7D. Page 139

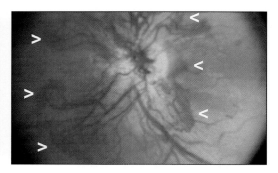

FIGURE 11-9A. Page 140

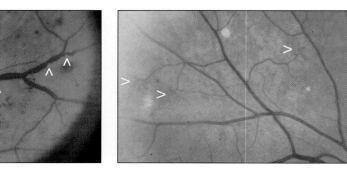

FIGURE 11-9B. Page 140

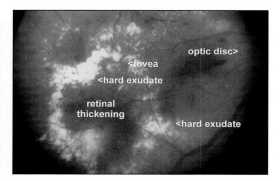

FIGURE 11-9C. Page 140

FIGURE 11-10B. Page 140

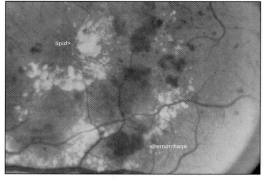

FIGURE 11-12B. Page 141

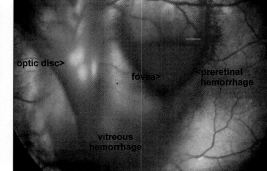

FIGURE 11-12C. Page 142

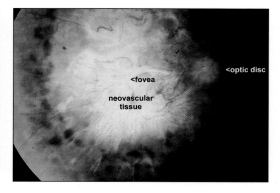

FIGURE 11-12D. Page 142

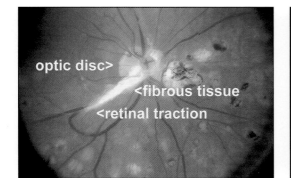

FIGURE 11-13A. Page 142

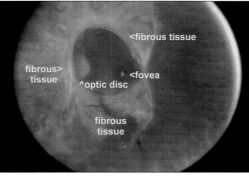

FIGURE 11-13B. Page 142

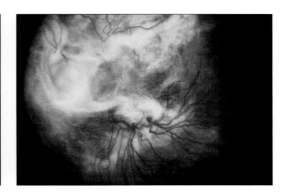

FIGURE 11-13C. Page 143

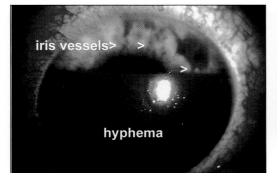

FIGURE 11-14A. Page 143

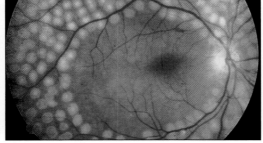

FIGURE 11-15A. Page 144

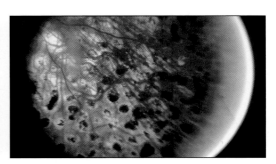

FIGURE 11-15B. Page 144

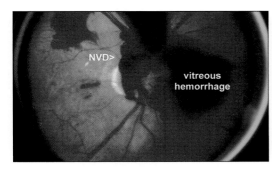

FIGURE 11-15C. Page 144

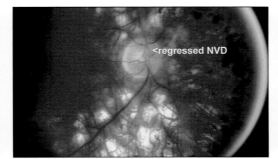

FIGURE 11-15D. Page 144

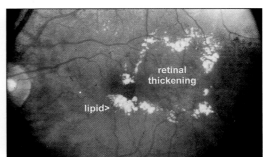

FIGURE 11-16A. Page 145

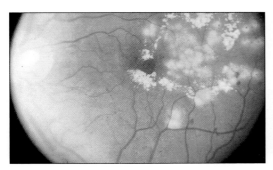

FIGURE 11-16C. Page 145

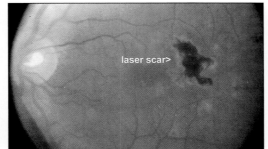

FIGURE 11-16D. Page 145

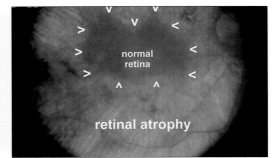

FIGURE 11-18A. Page 146

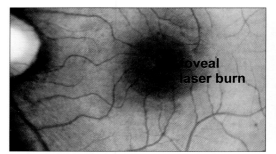

FIGURE 11-18C. Page 147

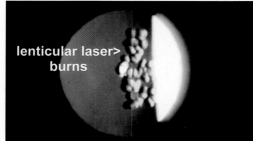

FIGURE 11-18D. Page 147

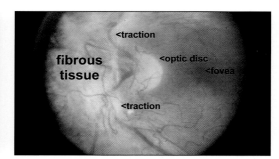

FIGURE 11-19B. Page 147

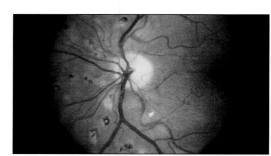

FIGURE 11-19C. Page 147

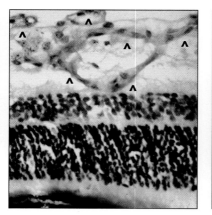

FIGURE 11-22A. Page 149

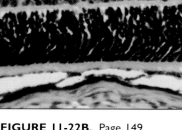

FIGURE 11-22B. Page 149

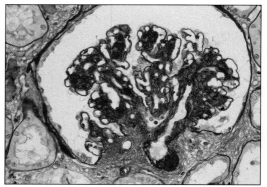

FIGURE 12-6A. Page 153

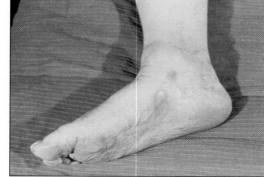

FIGURE 13-19. Page 171

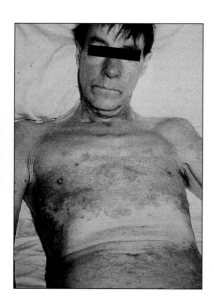

FIGURE 14-10A. Page 183

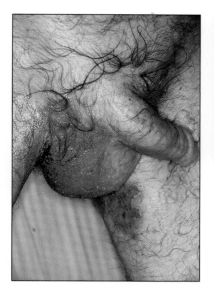

FIGURE 14-10B. Page 183

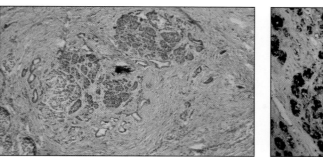

FIGURE 14-16. Page 186

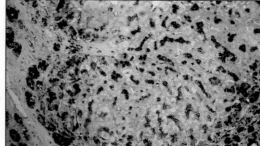

FIGURE 14-17A. Page 186

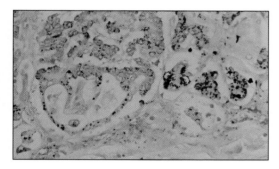

FIGURE 14-17B. Page 186